Contents

Contributors to Fourth Edition

Dr R Mark Beattie
BSc MBBS FRCPCH MRCP
Consultant Paediatric Gastroenterologist, Paediatric Medical Unit, Southampton General Hospital, Southampton

Dr Sarah A L Williams
MA MB ChB MRCPCH
SpR Paediatric Gastroenterology, Paediatric Gastroenterology Department, Southampton General Hospital, Southampton

Dr Joanne Borbone
MB ChB MRCPCH
SpR Paediatrics, Southampton General Hospital, Southampton

Dr Reynella Anne Morenas
MBBS BSc MRCPCH
SpR Paediatrics, Royal Hampshire County Hospital, Hampshire

Dr Helen C Fielder
MBBS MRCPCH
Consultant Neonatologist, Princess Anne Hospital, Southampton

The publishers and Authors would also like to thank the following contributors to the previous editions for their contribution:

Dr Nick Brown
Consultant Paediatrician, Salisbury District Hospital, Wiltshire

Dr Tracey Farnon
Consultant Paediatrician, Salisbury District Hospital, Wiltshire

Dr A B Acharya
Senior Registrar, Peterborough District Hospital, Peterborough

Dr D L I Ellis
Senior House Officer, Peterborough District Hospital, Peterborough

Dr L J Phillips
Senior House Officer, Peterborough District Hospital, Peterborough

Dr A T Tidswell
Senior House Officer, Peterborough District Hospital, Peterborough

MRCPCH 1 Questions with Individual Subject Summaries

Fourth Edition

R Mark Beattie
BSc MBBS FRCPCH MRCP

Sarah A L Williams
MA MB ChB MRCPCH

Joanne Borbone
MB ChB MRCPCH

© 2011 PASTEST LTD
Egerton Court
Parkgate Estate
Knutsford
Cheshire
WA16 8DX
Telephone: 01565 752000

First published 1997
Second edition 2000
Third edition 2006, Reprinted 2010
Fourth edition 2011

ISBN: 1905635745
9781905635740

A catalogue record for this book is available from the British Library.

Text prepared in the UK by Carnegie Book Production, Lancaster
Printed and bound in the UK by CPI Antony Rowe, Chippenham, Wiltshire

Introduction

We hope that this text will prove invaluable in your preparation for MRCPCH Part 1 or Diploma in Child Health. We have personally found earlier editions of this book essential in the preparations for both of these qualifications.

The format of the questions in this edition has been totally revised in accordance with the structure of the new style examination, with a higher percentage of EMQs (extended matching questions) and BOFs (best of fives) whilst updating the multiple choice questions to reflect the distribution of question types you will encounter in both Paper 1A and 1B. All the material has been updated and over 20% of the questions are entirely new to this edition. All the subject summaries are succinct but comprehensive overviews of the areas essential to cover in preparation for the exam as well as clinically relevant for all doctors working in paediatrics today.

We would like to acknowledge the many authors who have enthusiastically contributed to this book over its number of editions and pay special thanks to the significant contribution made in this edition by Reynella Morenas and Helen Fielder as well as Lily Martin at PasTest for her patience and expertise in helping pull this new edition together.

We hope that you will find this text just as invaluable in your preparation as we did in the past and wish you ever success in both your examinations and future careers.

Mark Beattie

Sarah Williams

Joanne Borbone

October 2011

CHAPTER 1

Cardiology

Multiple True–False Questions

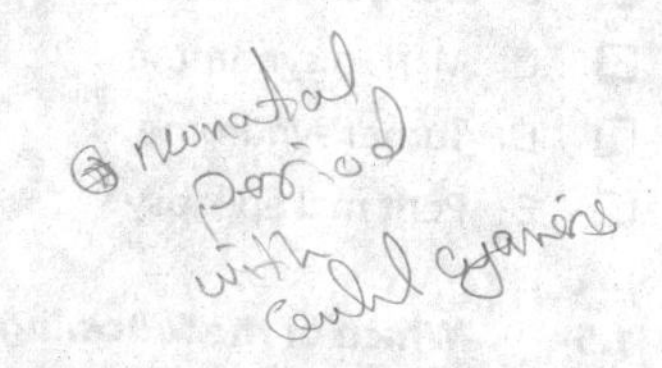

1.1 Which of the following conditions can present in the neonatal period with central cyanosis?

- ❑ A Eisenmenger syndrome
- ❑ B Pulmonary atresia
- ❑ C Hypoplastic left heart
- ❑ D Transposition of the great arteries
- ❑ E Critical aortic stenosis

1.2 With regard to the paediatric ECG

- ❑ A Neonates have right axis deviation
- ❑ B Congenital complete heart block is associated with maternal systemic lupus erythematosus
- ❑ C Right bundle-branch block is seen in coarctation of the aorta
- ❑ D Romano–Ward syndrome produces prolongation of the PR interval
- ❑ E A resting heart rate in newborns of 180 is a tachycardia

1.3 Which of the following chest radiograph findings would support the paired diagnosis?

- ❑ A Atrioseptal defect and coeur en sabot (heart in a boot)
- ❑ B Patent ductus arteriosus (PDA) and rib notching
- ❑ C Truncus arteriosus and absent thymus
- ❑ D Total anomalous pulmonary venous drainage and cottage loaf appearance
- ❑ E Scimitar syndrome and dextrocardia

1.4 Which of the following conditions are associated with an increased incidence of heart disease?

- ❑ A Kawasaki disease
- ❑ B Congenital rubella
- ❑ C Marfan syndrome
- ❑ D Turner syndrome
- ❑ E Petit mal epilepsy

1.5 Which of the following statements are true?

- ❑ A The most common congenital cardiac lesion is an ASVD
- ❑ B Tetralogy of Fallot is associated with plethoric lung fields
- ❑ C The Blalock–Taussig shunt gives rise to a continuous murmur
- ❑ D Nitrous oxide can be used to treat persistent pulmonary hypertension
- ❑ E Ebstein anomaly is an anomaly of the tricuspid valve

1.6 Concerning the fetal circulation

- ❑ A The umbilical vein carries deoxygenated blood to the placenta from the fetus
- ❑ B Fetal superior vena caval blood preferentially flows across the foramen ovale into the left atrium
- ❑ C Forty per cent of right ventricular outflow enters the lungs via the pulmonary arteries
- ❑ D The descending aorta is connected to the pulmonary artery via the ductus venosus
- ❑ E Gas exchange occurs in the fetal lungs

1.7 Which of the following statements are true?

- ❑ A Patients with cyanotic congenital heart disease grow normally
- ❑ B Immunisation is contraindicated in children with congenital heart disease
- ❑ C The combined oral contraceptive pill is contraindicated in patients with cyanotic congenital heart disease
- ❑ D Two per cent of patients with congenital heart disease have a chromosomal abnormality
- ❑ E Thirty per cent of infants with chromosomal defects have heart defects

1.8 Which of the following cardiac defects and teratogens are correctly paired?

- ☐ A Alcohol and transposition of the great arteries
- ☐ B Sodium valproate and tetralogy of Fallot
- ☐ C Furosemide and PDA
- ☐ D Phenytoin and coarctation of the aorta
- ☐ E Lithium and Ebstein anomaly

1.9 Which of the following are causes of circulatory failure in the first week of life?

- ☐ A Arrhythmias
- ☐ B Hypoplastic left heart
- ☐ C Birth asphyxia
- ☐ D Severe anaemia
- ☐ E Fluid overload

Best of Five Questions

1.10 With regard to advanced life support and resuscitation in children with cardiac arrest, which of the following statements is most factually correct?

- ☐ A **Basic life support with high concentration oxygen should be continued throughout any resuscitation with the minimum of interruptions**
- ☐ B **Ventricular fibrillation is the most common cardiac arrest rhythm in children**
- ☐ C **It is important that a child's airway is secured during an arrest situation, so it is acceptable for basic life support to be interrupted for as long as it takes to intubate the child**
- ☐ D **The resuscitation dose of adrenaline is 0.1 µg/kg and should be administered at 4-minute intervals in asystolic arrests with the third dose being given as a higher dose of 1 mg/kg if no response is seen**
- ☐ E **In a paediatric arrest associated with PEA a 2 J/kg synchronised DC shock should be given every 2 minutes while reversible causes are being sought and treated**

1.11 A 14-year-old girl is referred to the paediatric outpatient clinic with a 4-month history of palpitations.

She is normally fit and well and has not experienced any recent illness or weight loss. She is in her final year at an all girls' private school but is generally achieving good grades in all her classes. She describes her symptoms as a racing heart rate that comes on gradually and will slowly decrease back to normal after several hours. She has not had associated chest pain or collapses and her symptoms usually present during school hours. She has had no episodes associated with exercise or during her time at home. She has a sensation of difficulty breathing during the attacks and has described 'pins and needles' in her hands during her episodes. She has no significant past medical history of cardiac disease but does have mild asthma. She has no family history of heart disease, sudden death or deafness. She had an entirely normal examination including a normal pulse rate (70 beats/min regular); blood pressure and 12-lead ECG in clinic were within normal limits.

Which of the following outcomes from this consultation is the most appropriate?

- ❑ A Referral to paediatric cardiologist for further investigation of cardiac arrhythmia
- ❑ B FBC, U&Es, TFTs and 24-hour urinary catecholamine collection with follow-up in general paediatric clinic to exclude medical causes for her palpitations
- ❑ C Reassurance that her palpitations do not have a significant cause, advice about relaxation and stress control during exam season, and discharge to follow-up from clinic
- ❑ D Referral to child and adolescent psychiatry for treatment of anxiety disorder
- ❑ E Initiation of propranolol treatment for panic attacks

1.12 An 18-month-old girl is admitted to the paediatric assessment unit with a 3-week history of worsening shortness of breath and difficulty feeding accompanied by weight loss.

She had had symptoms of a cold and mild gastroenteritis a week before the onset of symptoms from which she had initially appeared to recover. She had become increasingly lethargic, seemed unsettled and had increased work of breathing when laid flat, relieved by being in an upright position or sleeping in a propped-up position in her buggy. She had previously been a well, thriving child with no significant past medical history. On examination she had a low-grade fever of 37.8°C and a heart rate of 190 beats/min while settled. She had increased work of breathing with bibasilar crepitations. She had a respiratory rate of 50 beats/min with mild intercostal recession and normal oxygen saturations of 98% in air. On auscultation of her heart no murmurs were heard but she was thought to have a gallop rhythm. On examination of her abdomen a 4 cm palpable liver was found.

From the following list choose the most likely explanation for her current symptoms.

- ❑ A Supraventricular tachycardia
- ❑ B Pneumonia with hyperinflation of her thorax
- ❑ C Viral myocarditis
- ❑ D Large VSD with cardiac failure
- ❑ E Cystic fibrosis

1.13 Which of the following statements about ECG changes associated with electrolyte abnormalities is most factually correct?

- ❑ A ECG changes associated with hyperkalaemia are progressive with the severity of hyperkalaemia leading to the absence of p waves, broadening of QRS complexes, and VF or VT
- ❑ B Hyperkalaemia is associated with increased height of U waves
- ❑ C ECG changes seen in hypocalcaemia mimic those seen in hypokalaemia
- ❑ D Hypernatraemia is associated with reduced QT interval on ECG
- ❑ E Hypocalcaemia is associated with a shortened QTc and in severe cases sudden death

1.14 With regard to aortic stenosis, which of the following statements is most factually correct?

- ❑ A Aortic stenosis is the most common cardiac lesion associated with Down syndrome
- ❑ B Right ventricular hypertrophy is a common finding in a child with aortic stenosis
- ❑ C An ejection click on auscultation suggests that the stenosis is supravalvular
- ❑ D The most common treatment for aortic stenosis in childhood is aortic valve replacement
- ❑ E There is an association with sudden death in patients with aortic stenosis

1.15 Which of the following statements about Williams syndrome is most factually correct?

- ❑ A The most common cardiac lesion associated with Williams syndrome is an atrioseptal defect
- ❑ B Williams syndrome is caused by a microdeletion on chromosome 11, which encodes for the elastin gene
- ❑ C Diagnosis of Williams syndrome can be confirmed by fluorescence *in situ* hybridization (FISH) studies
- ❑ D Williams syndrome is associated with normal development and IQ
- ❑ E Hypercalcaemia is required to make the diagnosis of Williams syndrome in a neonate

1.16 Which of the following statements about cardiovascular disease associated with Down syndrome is most factually correct?

- ❑ A The most common cardiac lesion associated with Down syndrome is an atrial septal defect
- ❑ B Echocardiography is indicated in all cases of Down syndrome for identification of congenital cardiac disease even if a murmur is not present
- ❑ C Up to 20% of all cases of Down syndrome have associated heart defects
- ❑ D Cardiac disease in Down syndrome becomes symptomatic earlier than isolated congenital heart disease due to the high prevalence of pulmonary arterial hypertension
- ❑ E The cardiac defects associated with Down syndrome are the sole cause of pulmonary vascular disease in this population

1.17 Which of the following statements concerning transposition of the great arteries is most factually correct?

- ☐ A Transposition of the great arteries is associated with decreased pulmonary blood flow and pulmonary oligaemia on chest radiograph
- ☐ B Transposition of the great arteries is the most common cause of cyanotic congenital heart disease in the neonatal period
- ☐ C Transposition of the great arteries is associated with a metabolic alkalosis at presentation
- ☐ D The vast majority of cases of transposition of the great arteries are diagnosed on routine antenatal ultrasonography
- ☐ E Transposition of the great arteries occurs together with a recognized paediatric syndrome in 80% of cases

1.18 Which of the following statements regarding tetralogy of Fallot is most factually correct?

- ☐ A The murmur heard in a patient with tetralogy of Fallot becomes louder during cyanotic spells
- ☐ B Cyanotic spells associated with tetralogy of Fallot usually begin around 4–6 months of age
- ☐ C An atrial septal defect is one of the four major components of tetralogy of Fallot
- ☐ D Finger clubbing usually develops within the first few months of life
- ☐ E Most patients with tetralogy of Fallot have a left-to-right shunt across the VSD

1.19 Which of the following statements concerning atrial septal defects is most factually correct?

- ☐ A Ostium primum defects are more common than ostium secundum defects
- ☐ B Atrial fibrillation is a common associated complication in the first decade of life
- ☐ C In a secundum defect the ECG shows right bundle-branch block and left axis deviation
- ☐ D In children with ASDs the pulmonary vascular resistance increases in early childhood, leading to pulmonary hypertension typically in the first decade of life
- ☐ E A pulmonary to systemic flow ratio of more than 2:1 is an indication for surgical or more commonly percutaneous transcatheter device closure

1.20 Which of the following statements about ventricular septal defects (VSDs) is most factually correct?

- ❑ A VSDs are most commonly located in the muscular part of the ventricular septum
- ❑ B VSDs will cause an audible flow murmur across the defect, usually audible from birth
- ❑ C Infective endocarditis is a complication seen in approximately 10% of all children with VSDs
- ❑ D VSDs are associated with higher oxygen content in the blood of the right ventricle than the right atrium
- ❑ E VSDs are associated with right ventricular volume overload

1.21 Which of the following interventions would produce the best clinical outcome for a child at risk of developing Eisenmenger syndrome?

- ❑ A Surgical correction of a VSD when cardiac catheter demonstrates significant pulmonary hypertension
- ❑ B Nocturnal oxygen supplementation
- ❑ C Sildenafil to help control pulmonary hypertension
- ❑ D Correction of the VSD before the development of pulmonary hypertension
- ❑ E Total heart and lung transplantation

1.22 Which of the following statements about patent ductus arteriosus is most factually correct?

- ❑ A The incidence of persistent ductus arteriosus is increased in males compared with females
- ❑ B Cardiac catheter coil placement is the treatment of choice for symptomatic infants with persistent ductus arteriosus post term
- ❑ C PDA can be treated with prostaglandins
- ❑ D PDA usually closes spontaneously in term infants
- ❑ E The incidence of PDA is increased in preterm infants and those with perinatal hypoxia and/or distress

1.23 Which of the following statements concerning coarctation of the aorta is most factually correct?

- ☐ A It is rare to diagnose duct-dependent coarctation on antenatal ultrasonography
- ☐ B Coarctation of the aorta is associated with rib notching on chest radiograph in infancy
- ☐ C Coarctation is commonly associated with a tricuspid aortic valve
- ☐ D Coarctation of the aorta is more common in females
- ☐ E Adult-type coarctation of the aorta is associated with blood pressure discrepancy between the upper and lower limbs

1.24 Which of the following statements about childhood hypertension is most factually correct?

- ☐ A A systolic pressure greater than the 75th centile for age and sex is defined as hypertension
- ☐ B Primary hypertension is more common than secondary hypertension in children
- ☐ C In infants the most common cause of hypertension is renal parenchymal disease
- ☐ D Children with hypertension are usually symptomatic
- ☐ E More than 25% of children with secondary hypertension will have symptoms of headache at presentation

1.25 Which of the following statements concerning infective endocarditis is most factually correct?

- ☐ A Infective endocarditis is associated with a 13–20% mortality rate
- ☐ B Antibiotic prophylaxis is indicated to cover dental procedures in children with congenital heart disease
- ☐ C Splinter haemorrhages in the nailbeds are an almost universal finding
- ☐ D The diagnosis of infective endocarditis is excluded if echocardiography is normal
- ☐ E The right side of the heart is most commonly affected

1.26 Which of the following statements about cardiomyopathy is the most factually correct?

- ❑ A Hypertrophic obstructive cardiomyopathy is most commonly inherited as an X-linked disorder
- ❑ B Dilated cardiomyopathy is associated with doxorubicin toxicity in children
- ❑ C Restrictive cardiomyopathy is the commonest cardiomyopathy in childhood
- ❑ D Endocardial fibroelastosis is a form of hypertrophic cardiomyopathy
- ❑ E There is an increased incidence of dilated cardiomyopathy in infants of mothers with diabetes

1.27 Which of the following statements about rheumatic fever is most factually correct?

- ❑ A Rheumatic fever is caused by an infection with group A α-haemolytic *Streptococcus* species
- ❑ B The most common cardiac manifestation of rheumatic fever is an isolated endocarditis, occurring in over 50% of cases
- ❑ C The most commonly occurring major criterion for diagnosing rheumatic fever is polyarthritis
- ❑ D PR prolongation on the ECG is one of the major diagnostic criteria
- ❑ E Prophylactic antibiotics should be stopped after 3 months

1.28 A 5-year-old girl is referred to a paediatric outpatient clinic for assessment of a murmur heard incidentally when she was reviewed by her GP with a 48-hour history of fever and cough.

In clinic she is heard to have a 2/6 systolic murmur, heard loudest in the left sternal edge. The murmur is loudest on lying flat but is audible in the sitting position. She has no symptoms of breathlessness or exercise intolerance. She is active – dances and swims after school with her older siblings. There is no family history of cardiac disease and she has never been admitted to hospital.

What is the most appropriate follow up for this young girl with regard to her murmur?

- ❑ A Immediate referral for paediatric cardiology review
- ❑ B ECG and chest radiograph
- ❑ C Exercise stress test
- ❑ D Outpatient referral to paediatric cardiology
- ❑ E Reassurance that the murmur is innocent and discharge from follow-up

1.29 A 3-month-old child presents to the emergency department with a 20-minute history of severe shock – pale but responsive with a peripheral capillary refill time of 4 seconds and a central capillary refill time of 3 seconds.

She is found to have a tachycardia of 290 beats/min with a narrow complex on the ECG. Vascular access is difficult to obtain. High-flow oxygen has been administered by the ambulance.

What is the most appropriate next management step?

- ❑ A Asynchronous DC shock of 2 J/kg
- ❑ B Intramuscular ceftriaxone
- ❑ C Place an intraosseous needle and administer adenosine 100 μg/kg
- ❑ D Synchronous shock of 1 J/kg
- ❑ E Amiodarone given via an intraosseous needle

1.30 Which of the following statements about Wolff–Parkinson–White syndrome is most accurate?

- ❑ A Wolff–Parkinson–White syndrome is most commonly found in patients with congenital heart disease, most commonly with corrected transposition of the great arteries
- ❑ B The ECG of a patient with Wolff–Parkinson–White syndrome, when the patient is in normal rhythm, is indistinguishable from normal
- ❑ C Digoxin is useful in the long-term treatment of patients with Wolff–Parkinson–White syndrome
- ❑ D Radiofrequency ablation of the accessory pathway is potentially curable
- ❑ E Wolff–Parkinson–White syndrome has an equal sex distribution

1.31 Which of the following statements about the paediatric ECG is most accurate?

- ❑ A The PR interval is prolonged in hyperkalaemia
- ❑ B The normal PR interval in infancy is 0.2–0.3 s
- ❑ C It is normal to have upright T wave in lead V1 until approximately 3 months of age
- ❑ D A prolonged QTc is considered to be > 0.35 s
- ❑ E The normal range for the axis of a neonatal QRS complex is 160–210°

1.32 Which of the following statements about prolonged QT syndrome is most factually correct?

- ❑ A There is a significant risk of sudden death associated with prolonged QT syndrome but 90% of cases of sudden death will have had symptoms before the fatal event
- ❑ B Erythromycin should be avoided in patients with prolonged QT syndrome
- ❑ C Sixty per cent of cases of prolonged QT syndrome will present between 30 and 50 years of age
- ❑ D Romano–Ward syndrome is an autosomally dominant, inherited syndrome associated with prolonged QT and congenital deafness
- ❑ E A normal ECG excludes the diagnosis of prolonged QT syndrome in a patient with a positive family history

1.33 Which symptom from the following list is the MOST important when considering a diagnosis of Kawasaki disease?

- ❑ A Gallbladder hydrops
- ❑ B High-grade fever for >5 days
- ❑ C Thrombocytosis
- ❑ D Petechial rash
- ❑ E Bilateral exudative conjunctivitis

1.34 Which is a sign of subacute bacterial endocarditis (SBE)?

- ❑ A Splinter haemorrhages
- ❑ B Extensor surface nodules
- ❑ C Eosinophilia
- ❑ D Cervical nodes
- ❑ E Renal artery bruit

1.35 A 3-month-old baby boy is admitted to hospital breathless with poor feeding. On arrival the main findings are: pale with pulse of 240/min, liver enlarged at 3 cm below costal margin and saturation in air of 88%. Which is the MOST appropriate first action?

- ❑ A Intravenous adenosine
- ❑ B Intravenous β blocker
- ❑ C Application of ice pack over face
- ❑ D Oxygen
- ❑ E Intranasal adenosine

1.36 A 4-day-old baby girl is admitted from home with increasing cyanosis. On examination, she is deeply cyanosed (saturation in air 78%), and has mild subcostal recession. She is alert and not distressed. What is the MOST likely diagnosis?

- ❑ A Large ventricular septal defect
- ❑ B Tricuspid atresia
- ❑ C Diaphragmatic hernia
- ❑ D Persistent fetal circulation
- ❑ E Transposition of the great arteries

1.37 A 4-month-old is referred to the outpatient clinic with stridor since birth and faltering growth. The baby is thin with a soft ejection systolic and diastolic murmur. What is the investigation MOST likely to yield a unifying diagnosis in this clinical setting?

- ❑ A Sweat test
- ❑ B Barium swallow
- ❑ C Direct laryngoscopy
- ❑ D ECG
- ❑ E Arteriography

1.38 A 2-year-old, fully immunised boy is referred with suspected measles. He has a week-long history of fever and malaise and has developed a generalised morbilliform rash.

On arrival he is miserable, febrile (temperature 40.1°C), cervical lymphadenopathy, conjunctivitis, desquamation over palms. Bloods apart from a high plasma viscosity are normal.

What is the MOST appropriate first-line management?

- ❑ A Full infection screen including lumbar puncture and urine and broad-spectrum antibiotic cover
- ❑ B Vitamin A
- ❑ C High-dose aspirin and parenteral immunoglobulin
- ❑ D Parenteral steroids
- ❑ E High-dose aspirin alone

Extended Matching Questions

1.39–1.41 Theme: Neonatal cyanosis

- ❑ A Congenital pneumonia
- ❑ B Methaemoglobinaemia
- ❑ C Acrocyanosis
- ❑ D Persistent pulmonary hypertension of the newborn
- ❑ E Diaphragmatic hernia
- ❑ F Transposition of the great arteries
- ❑ G Obstructed total anomalous pulmonary venous connection (TAPVC)
- ❑ H Truncus arteriosus
- ❑ I Pulmonary atresia
- ❑ J Pneumothorax

For each of the following clinical scenarios pick the most likely diagnosis from the list above. Each option may be used once, more than once or not at all.

1.39

A 41-week gestation baby boy was born weighing 3.96 kg after a labour lasting 36 hours. Rupture of the membranes occurred 30 hours before delivery; his mother did not receive antibiotics intrapartum and remained apyrexial throughout labour. The baby was noted to have central and peripheral cyanosis at birth. After 5 minutes he was noted to have a good respiratory effort and received facial oxygen which improved his cyanosis. At an hour after delivery he would not latch on to feed and was noted to be grunting with a recurrence of his cyanosis, tachycardia at 180 beats/min, with increased respiratory rate of 80 beats/min and intercostal and subcostal recession and nasal flaring. He was hypothermic with a temperature of 35.0°C. His saturation at the time was 88% in air but improved to 98% in 100% oxygen.

1.40

A 39-week gestation male infant was born by spontaneous vaginal delivery after a labour lasting 36 hours. His mother had had full normal antenatal care with no concerns on any of her antenatal scans. Rupture of membranes occurred 6 hours before delivery. The baby was born in good condition and was noted to have mild acrocyanosis but was initially feeding well. At 12 hours of age he was noted to be blue around his eyes and mouth by his parents. At this time he had good respiratory effort with a respiratory rate of 60 beats/min and no increased work of breathing. He had equal air entry bilaterally but saturations were noted to be 66% in air. His cardiovascular examination was unremarkable with a heart rate of 160 beats/min but no murmurs audible and palpable brachial and femoral pulses. On delivery of 100% oxygen via a neonatal non-rebreathe bag no improvement in his saturations was seen.

1.41

A term baby girl is born by spontaneous vaginal delivery after an uncomplicated labour of 6 hours duration. She is found to have some cyanosis (sats 88%) at delivery with mild tachypnoea and respiratory distress, which partially corrects with facial oxygen. Over the next couple hours of life she becomes increasingly cyanosed with increased respiratory rate of 80bpm and marked intercostal and subcostal recession and grunting. On auscultation of her heart a gallop rhythm is heard and she appears to have 2 cm of hepatomegaly by 5 hours of age. Oxygen saturations at 5 hours of age are 66% in air but partially correct to 80% in air with 100% facial oxygen.

1.42–1.44 Theme: Illness with cardiac manifestations

- ❑ A Cardiomyopathy
- ❑ B Endocarditis
- ❑ C Rheumatic fever
- ❑ D Pericarditis
- ❑ E Malaria
- ❑ F Nephrotic syndrome
- ❑ G Juvenile chronic arthritis
- ❑ H Intrauterine infection
- ❑ I SLE
- ❑ J None of the above

Choose the best options from the list above for the three situations described below. Each option may be used once, more than once or not at all.

1.42

A 14-year-old boy, treated for a rhabdomyosarcoma at age 3 years with complete recovery, presents with shortness of breath over some months. On examination he appears tired and tachypnoeic. There is triple rhythm and raised jugular venous pressure. Chest radiograph shows cardiomegaly.

1.43

A 4-week-old baby presents with a gradual onset of tachypnoea, tachycardia and enlargement of the liver. Heart failure is suspected. Chest radiograph, ECG and echo show some ventricular dilatation but a structurally normal heart. Other basic investigations including full blood count (FBC), biochemistry and culture of blood, urine and cerebrospinal fluid (CSF) are all within normal limits for age.

1.44

An 8-year-old boy is referred with a painful swollen right knee having recovered from a swollen painful left elbow 24 hours previously. He was febrile on admission with a temperature of 38.8°C with an unusual pink ring-like rash affecting his trunk. He was the fifth child of a currently single mother who had no significant past medical or family history of note. He was well grown but had had a sore throat 2 weeks before admission, from which he had completely recovered before the onset of his current symptoms. He was heard to have a new mid-diastolic murmur on examination, and was found to have first-degree heart block on ECG on admission.

1.45–1.47 Theme: Cardiac investigations

- ❑ A 24-hour ECG
- ❑ B Echocardiography
- ❑ C Cardiac catheter
- ❑ D Thoracic computed tomography (CT) scan
- ❑ E Thoracic magnetic resonance (MR) scan
- ❑ F Chest radiograph
- ❑ G Arterial compliance studies
- ❑ H ECG
- ❑ I Stress test
- ❑ J None of the above

Choose the best investigation from the list above for the three situations described below. Each option may be used once, more than once or not at all.

1.45

A 2-year-old boy, who is sent to outpatients with a murmur, is well and pink with normal pulses. There is a soft systolic murmur at the right supraclavicular area, louder on sitting.

1.46

A 14-year-old girl with recurrent 'panic attacks' has a fast heart rate of 'at least 120 at rest'. On examination she is well with a normal cardiac examination.

1.47

A 5-year-old boy, who had an aortic stenosis repaired at age 18 months, presents with increasing shortness of breath. There is a systolic murmur on examination best heard over the 'aortic' area.

1.48–1.50 Theme: Syncope

- ❑ A Reassurance that the event is a simple faint and discharge to follow-up
- ❑ B ECG and immediate referral of patient to paediatric cardiologist with presumed long QT syndrome
- ❑ C 12-lead ECG with cardiac referral if abnormality is reported
- ❑ D 12-lead ECG and outpatient EEG with review and appropriate referral if abnormal
- ❑ E Start treatment with β blockers to decrease frequency of events
- ❑ F Referral to child and adolescent health service for assessment with regard to psychogenic events
- ❑ G EGC and referral to cardiologist for investigation of possible myocarditis
- ❑ H 12-lead ECG and investigation with external digital loop cardiac monitor if ECG normal
- ❑ I 12-lead ECG and investigation with exercise if ECG normal
- ❑ J 12-lead ECG and if normal advice to restrict exercise, and increase salt and fluid intake in the future to avoid further events

From the list above, choose the BEST option for the ongoing investigation and management of each of the patients in the following three clinical scenarios. Each option may be used once, more than once or not at all.

1.48

A 14-year-old girl is referred with a history of recurrent collapses at school over the preceding 3 months. All episodes have occurred during the school day over the summer months. The process of standing at the end of a class to move from one lesson to another can precipitate a feeling of dizziness followed by a drop to the floor. She has not sustained any significant injuries in the falls but one such episode was witnessed by a first aider at school, and she was seen to go pale and sink to the floor after standing up and was witnessed to have several jerks in her arms while on the floor. She fully recovered within minutes back to her normal self. There is no significant family history of cardiac disease, sudden death, epilepsy or deafness.

1.49

A 14-year-old boy is referred after a loss of consciousness during a swimming lesson at school. He had been diving into the pool and was witnessed to lose consciousness on entering the water but did not hit his head before the dive or once he had entered the pool. He was retrieved from the pool by the lifeguard on duty and had a strong cardiac output when assessed on the side of the pool before the start of any resuscitation. He has no recollection of chest pain or dizziness associated with the event, and can clearly remember diving into the pool but nothing else until recovering on the side of the pool. He had never experienced any similar events previously and he is normally fit and active. He has a good exercise tolerance usually, and has been swimming many times before.

1.50

A 2-year-old girl is seen in the accident and emergency department after a collapse following a head injury in the garden. The child ran into a wooden garden table while playing with her older sister and cousin. She was reported by her cousin (13 years) to cry out in pain and then almost instantly fall limply to the floor. She was described as being deathly pale for about a minute and her eyes were seen to deviate upwards and her posture became stiff with her arms extended and her hands clawed for several seconds before relaxing. She came round after a few seconds and was confused initially but then became more lucid. She then fell asleep in the ambulance but had normal pulse, rhythm strip and saturations in the ambulance on the trip to hospital. There is no family history of sudden death or epilepsy or significant cardiac abnormalities. Her mother was said to have severe temper tantrums as a preschool child and these would occasionally lead to faints.

1.51–1.53 Theme: Chest pain

- ❑ A Aortic stenosis
- ❑ B Pneumonia
- ❑ C Acute asthma
- ❑ D Precordial catch syndrome
- ❑ E Costochondritis
- ❑ F Anxiety
- ❑ G Gastro-oesophageal reflux disease
- ❑ H Hypertrophic cardiomyopathy
- ❑ I Kawasaki disease
- ❑ J Anomalous coronary artery

Choose the best diagnosis from the list above for each of the following case descriptions. Each option can be used once, more than once or not at all.

1.51

A 16-year-old girl, RC, is referred to paediatric outpatients with a 12-month history of recurrent severe chest pain. The pain is localised to the left side of the chest and does not radiate. Attacks can occur up to every couple of days but she can go weeks between attacks. The pain is so severe during an attack that she can have trouble breathing for its duration. The pains are self-resolving and last up to a couple of minutes in each instance. RC is a well-grown active girl with no significant findings on a thorough physical examination including normal blood pressure. She has no family history of significant cardiac problems.

1.52

A 14-year-old boy was brought to the accident and emergency department after collapsing during a regional rugby final. When he arrived in the department he had regained consciousness and described a crushing central chest pain developing after a period of sprinting, followed by sweatiness, light-headedness and collapse. He has never had any similar symptoms before and is a regular member of the under-16 first XV. On examination he is found to have an ejection click and ejection systolic murmur heard maximally at the upper right sternal edge, with radiation into the carotid arteries bilaterally. There were no other significant findings during his initial examination. ECG revealed left ventricular hypertrophy.

1.53

A 12-year-old girl presents to her GP with a 2-week history of left-sided anterior chest pain exacerbated by exercise and deep breathing. She has never had similar symptoms in the past and has no history of cough, fever, trauma or preceding illness. On examination she has a normal cardiovascular, respiratory and GI examination and normal ECG. On examination of her anterior chest wall there is no obvious swelling or bruising seen but she has point tenderness over the 2nd costochondral junction, similar in nature to her presenting complaint.

1.54–1.56 Theme: Murmurs heard beyond the neonatal period

- ❑ A Atrial septal defect
- ❑ B Ventricular septal defect
- ❑ C Patent foramen ovale
- ❑ D Patent ductus arteriosus
- ❑ E Tricuspid regurgitation
- ❑ F Still's murmur
- ❑ G Venous hum
- ❑ H Coarctation of the aorta
- ❑ I Aortic valve stenosis
- ❑ J Innocent pulmonary flow murmur

For each of the following clinical scenarios choose the most appropriate diagnosis from the list above. Each option may be used once, more than once or not at all.

1.54

A 6-year-old boy is seen in outpatients after a murmur was heard by his GP during a febrile illness. The boy is well grown and has a good exercise tolerance, and competes in his school's football team regularly. When he is seen in outpatients he is clinically well and has fully recovered from his febrile illness. He has no family history of cardiac problems and no relevant past medical history. On examination in clinic he is found to have a soft systolic murmur (2/6) heard in the upper left sternal edge and a heave palpable at the left sternal border. He has a normal S1 and fixed splitting of his second heart sound. There was no change in the examination findings on standing. The rest of his cardiovascular and systemic examination was unremarkable. ECG revealed right bundle-branch block and mild right ventricular hypertrophy.

1.55

A 6-year-old girl was seen in outpatients after a murmur was detected by her GP during a febrile illness. She is well grown and has a good exercise tolerance, participating in regular ballet and gymnastic classes outside school. When she is reviewed in outpatients she is well and has fully recovered from her viral illness. She has no family history of heart disease or early sudden death and has no relevant past medical history. On examination she has a soft (2/6) midsystolic musical murmur in the lower left sternal edge, with no increased activity palpable in her precordium. She had a normal S1 with obvious splitting of S2 which varied with respiration. On standing the intensity of the murmur decreased. The rest of her cardiovascular and systemic examination was unremarkable. ECG revealed partial right bundle-branch block but no other abnormalities.

1.56

A 13-year-old girl is referred to paediatric outpatients for assessment when a murmur is heard during examination for a chest infection. When she is seen in outpatients her chest infection has entirely resolved and she is well. She has no symptoms of fatigue or exercise intolerance, and has not had an excess of childhood chest infections. She has no family history of cardiac abnormalities or sudden death at an early age. On examination in clinic she has an ejection systolic murmur heard loudest at the upper left sternal edge in a subscapular area, and is also heard radiating through to her back in the subscapular area. On auscultation of her heart sounds an ejection click is heard in the aortic area (upper right sternal edge). Her blood pressure is measured as 150 systolic in both arms with a systolic of 110 in both legs. On simultaneous palpation of her pulses there is an obvious delay in her femoral pulse compared with her brachial pulse. Her ECG and chest radiograph were entirely normal.

1.57–1.59 Theme: Differential diagnosis of heart failure

- [ ] A Severe anaemia
- [ ] B Large AV malformation
- [ ] C Myocarditis
- [ ] D Supraventricular tachycardia-induced cardiac failure
- [ ] E Duchenne muscular dystrophy
- [ ] F VSD
- [ ] G Bronchiolitis
- [ ] H Dilated cardiomyopathy
- [ ] I Aortic stenosis
- [ ] J Friedreich ataxia

For each of the following clinical scenarios choose the most appropriate diagnosis from the list above. Each option may be used once, more than once or not at all.

1.57

An 11-month-old baby presents to the paediatric assessment unit with a 4-week history of increasing dyspnoea with feeding. She was born at term and had thrived on the 75th centile since birth. Four weeks before her admission she had suffered from a viral illness with a fever of 38°C lasting 4 days, with associated coryzal symptoms and mild gastroenteritis from which she recovered; from that time, however, she did not appear to regain her premorbid appetite, struggling to take her morning and evening 6-oz bottles of formula. She was noted by her parents to be increasingly sweaty while feeding and was much more reluctant to crawl than before her illness. On examination she was tachycardic and apyrexial, with a pulse rate of 180 beats/min and no obvious clinical murmurs on auscultation. She had tachypnoea with a respiratory rate of 60 beats/min and saturations of 99% in air. She had mild intercostal recession and on auscultation had bilateral wheeze. She had palpable but universally weak peripheral pulses and cool peripheries. On examination of her abdomen she had 4 cm hepatomegaly. Her weight now plots on the 25th centile for age.

1.58

A 16–year-old boy presents after an episode of collapse during a games lesson at school. He had been a very active and sporty child, participating in the school football team until the last 12 months. He had gained a significant amount of weight and developed chest discomfort on exertion, with shortness of breath over the last 12 months. His parents had thought that his weight gain had left him less fit than previously. He had a family history of a first cousin who was born with hypoplastic left heart, but there was no other history of heart disease and no history of unexplained sudden death at an early age. On arrival in hospital he was conscious, and oriented in time, place and person. He said that he had experienced chest pain on running just before his collapse. On examination he was mildly tachycardic with a rate of 100 beats/min. He was heard to have an ejection systolic murmur in his upper right sternal edge, radiating to his carotid artery. There was an associated ejection click and a thrill palpable in the suprasternal notch. He had mild tachypnoea at rest and bilateral wheeze on auscultation of his chest. ECG showed left ventricular hypertrophy.

1.59

A 3-month-old baby presents to a paediatric assessment unit referred due to faltering growth. He was born at term after a normal antenatal course and no problems were reported on antenatal screening or on his 4-week postnatal check. His birth weight was on the 50th centile and he was entirely bottle fed from birth. He grew along the 50th centile for the first 2 months of life but started to drop off this centile over the last month. His parents described him as increasingly sweaty with feeds and becoming fatigued halfway through his bottles, having previously tolerated them well. On examination he was tachycardic with a pulse rate of 180 beats/min at rest. He was tachypnoeic with a respiratory rate of 80 beats/min. He has a pansystolic murmur loudest over the lower left sternal boarder with palpable 3 cm hepatomegaly.

CHAPTER 2

Community Paediatrics and Child Psychiatry

Multiple True–False Questions

2.1 Concerning the social development of children

- ☐ A By 18 months a child should be able to have interactive play and be turn taking
- ☐ B It is normal for a child to show shyness towards a stranger at 9 months
- ☐ C Symbolic play should not be expected at 3 years
- ☐ D A child should be waving bye-bye by 1 year of age
- ☐ E A child should be smiling spontaneously by 1 week of age

2.2 Concerning attention deficit hyperactivity disorder

- ☐ A It is successfully controlled by dietary restriction
- ☐ B It can lead to poor academic achievement
- ☐ C It can be exacerbated by anticonvulsant treatment
- ☐ D It is more common in boys
- ☐ E The use of drug therapy can cause sleep disturbance

2.3 Psychiatric referral is indicated for

- ☐ A A 15-year-old girl who has taken an overdose of paracetamol
- ☐ B A 14-year-old boy off school with recurrent morning headaches
- ☐ C Grief reaction in a 6-year-old boy lasting for a year
- ☐ D A 9-year-old who is afraid of the dark
- ☐ E Encopresis in a 7-year-old boy where constipation has been excluded

2.4 Concerning child sexual abuse

- ☐ A It occurs in up to 10% of children
- ☐ B Child sexual abusers often have a history of being abused as a child
- ☐ C Girls are 20 times more likely to be abused than boys
- ☐ D It is associated with an increased incidence of anal fissures
- ☐ E Reflex anal dilatation is pathognomonic

2.5 Concerning physical abuse in children

- ☐ A Fathers are more likely to be abusers than mothers
- ☐ B It is more common in first-born children
- ☐ C Children with learning difficulties are at increased risk
- ☐ D The head and neck are the most common sites of injury
- ☐ E The majority of non-accidental fractures occur in children of school age

2.6 Concerning childhood schizophrenia

- ☐ A It is rare
- ☐ B Long-term remission occurs in 90%
- ☐ C Delusions are a feature
- ☐ D Family history is often positive
- ☐ E It is associated with a lifetime increased risk of suicide

2.7 Causes of developmental regression include

- ☐ A Down syndrome
- ☐ B Cerebral palsy
- ☐ C Gaucher disease
- ☐ D Subacute sclerosing panencephalitis
- ☐ E Human immunodeficiency virus (HIV) infection

2.8 A child of 12 months would be expected to

- ☐ A Pick up a sugar cube between the finger and thumb
- ☐ B Be dry during the day
- ☐ C Feed with a biscuit
- ☐ D Use at least two different words with meaning
- ☐ E Wave bye-bye

Best of Five Questions

2.9 The following statements refer to oppositional defiant disorder. Select the MOST appropriate.

- ❑ A It can be least evident with adult and peers that the child knows well
- ❑ B It often includes behaviour that violates the law
- ❑ C It is classically seen in teenagers
- ❑ D Toddler tantrums are a form of this
- ❑ E Comorbidity with other disruptive behaviours is uncommon

2.10 The following statements refer to enuresis. Select the MOST appropriate.

- ❑ A Primary enuresis is more likely than secondary enuresis to have an underlying organic cause
- ❑ B Enuresis is defined as continued wetting beyond the age of 3 years
- ❑ C Nocturnal enuresis can by treated with antidiuretic hormone
- ❑ D Restricting fluid throughout the day should be encouraged in primary enuresis
- ❑ E It is more common in girls than in boys

2.11 The following statements refer to parental responsibility. Select the MOST appropriate.

- ❑ A Parents lose parental responsibility when their children are voluntarily taken into local authority care
- ❑ B Only the mother holds parental responsibility if parents are unmarried
- ❑ C A father loses parental responsibility if he divorces the mother of his child
- ❑ D A stepfather has automatic parental responsibility for his wife's children
- ❑ E Parental responsibility is automatically given to the mother

2.12 A 4-year-old girl is referred to children's outpatients with a 2-month history of passing irregular hard stool.

It has been causing her such distress that her mother is presently not sending her to school. On examination she has a soft abdomen but a small anal fissure.

What is the BEST advice to give the parents?

- ☐ A To keep her off school until the constipation is completely treated; she doesn't have to legally go to school until she is 5 years of age
- ☐ B She will need to be admitted to hospital to have an enema to get on top of it and get her back to school
- ☐ C Her anal fissure is a worrying sign of possible abuse and will need further investigation
- ☐ D Her constipation is likely to need treatment for several months to get her stool soft and regular and allow her anal fissure to heal
- ☐ E Advise mum to increase her fluid and fibre intake

2.13 A 15-year-old girl presents with severe weight loss over the last 6 months.

Her mum reports that she has been exercising excessively and has not menstruated for several months. A number of investigations including TFTs (thyroid function tests) and coeliac screen have not showed any abnormality. She has a resting heart rate of 40/min and a marked postural drop in her blood pressure. She is cool peripherally.

What is the BEST advice to give parents?

- ☐ A A diagnosis of anorexia nervosa is possible and she will need to be admitted to hospital for management of her acute state
- ☐ B A diagnosis of anorexia nervosa is possible and you will refer her on to a psychiatric outpatients
- ☐ C A diagnosis of anorexia nervosa is not likely but she appears dehydrated and therefore her mother should encourage her to take fluids
- ☐ D Advise her mother to stop her daughter exercising so much
- ☐ E To keep a food diary over the next few weeks and come back to see you later that month

2.14 The following statements refer to scoliosis. Select the MOST appropriate.

- [ ] A Initiation of treatment is required once the curvature is greater than 35°
- [ ] B Scoliosis repair is not advisable in patients with Duchene muscular dystrophy due to the reduced life expectancy
- [ ] C Neuromuscular scoliosis accounts for >75% of cases
- [ ] D Idiopathic scoliosis is more common in girls
- [ ] E Scoliosis is a lateral and rotational curvature of the thoracic and lumbar spine, measuring >20°

2.15 A 7-year-old boy has a diagnosis of attention deficit hyperactivity disorder.

Over the last 2 years his parents have had parental training to manage his condition and he has had psychological, behavioural and educational intervention. Despite this he continues to have problems both at home and at school with his hyperactivity, and of late his teachers feel that it is having an adverse effect on his attainment at school.

Select the MOST appropriate next step.

- [ ] A Stop the psychological intervention and start medication
- [ ] B To advise eliminating artificial colouring and additives from the diet
- [ ] C Discuss with parents the use of medication as part of a comprehensive treatment plan
- [ ] D Reassure parents that he is likely to grow out of his condition, given time
- [ ] E Treat his mother for depression

2.16 The following statements refer to school refusal. Select the MOST appropriate statement.

- [ ] A Parents are not aware of their child's absence from school
- [ ] B Family stress may be a precipitating factor
- [ ] C Associated physical symptoms are uncommon
- [ ] D These are often low achieving pupils
- [ ] E The absence from school is often intermittent

2.17 A 15-year-old boy is referred to a general paediatric outpatients clinic.

His mother has become increasingly concerned about his low mood. He no longer goes out with his friends and has become increasingly isolated and anxious about school. She is particularly concerned with his sleep because he is sleeping poorly and having problems getting to sleep and waking early in the morning. The 15 year old is difficult to engage in clinic but denies any drug or alcohol consumption.

What is the MOST likely diagnosis?

- ❑ A Normal teenage behaviour
- ❑ B Childhood depression
- ❑ C Schizophrenia
- ❑ D Drug missuse
- ❑ E Bipolar disorder

2.18 The following statements refer to childhood squint. Select the MOST appropriate.

- ❑ A They occur in <1% of pre-school children
- ❑ B They can only lead to amblyopia of the affected eye if the squint is paralytic
- ❑ C There is an absolute indication for testing of visual acuity
- ❑ D Paralytic squint is more common than non-paralytic squint
- ❑ E Non-paralytic squint rarely requires corrective surgery

2.19 The following statements refer to hearing assessments and screening. Select the MOST appropriate.

- ❑ A A distraction test is an appropriate hearing assessment for a 3-month-old child
- ❑ B Neonatal hearing screening in the UK involves automated otoacoustic emission (AOAE)
- ❑ C A normal neonatal hearing screen excludes hearing impairment as a cause of speech and language delay
- ❑ D Early detection and treatment of hearing impairment have no effect on developmental and educational outcome
- ❑ E After bacterial meningitis, a formal hearing assesment should be preformed approximately 1 year after the illness

2.20 The following statements refer to hearing impairment. Select the MOST appropriate statement.

- ❑ A Glue ear is an uncommon cause of hearing impairment in children
- ❑ B Alport syndrome is associated with conductive hearing loss
- ❑ C Hearing aids are not appropriate for children aged <6 months
- ❑ D Children presenting aged >2 years with hearing impairment will not have a genetic cause for their impairment
- ❑ E Hearing loss of <20 dB is unlikely to affect development

2.21 The following statements refer to sudden infant death syndrome. Select the MOST appropriate.

- ❑ A The majority of SIDS occurs in babies over the age of 6 months
- ❑ B Prematurity is a risk factor
- ❑ C The risk is increased with increasing maternal age
- ❑ D It is more common in girls
- ❑ E It is associated with the use of pacifiers or dummies

2.22 The following statements refer to speech delay in childhood. Select the MOST appropriate statement.

- ❑ A Speech delay is more common in girls
- ❑ B Speech delay is common in autism
- ❑ C Speech delay is associated with tongue-tie
- ❑ D Speech delay is more common in first-born children
- ❑ E Speech delay is uncommon in pre-school children

2.23 A 9-month-old child is referred to a paediatric outpatient clinic by a health visitor because her mother has concern about the child's development.

On examination the child can be pulled to sit with no head lag and will sit unaided; he is not yet pulling himself to stand, although will stand if held. The child will grasp objects in both hands and bang them together, although does not yet appear to have a pincer grip. His mother reports that he does babble and say Dada but has concern that does not yet use this specifically for his father. He appears a sociable child and plays peek-a-boo with you, although his mother reports that he is not yet waving or drinking from a cup.

Select the MOST appropriate statement.

- ☐ A The child has global developmental delay
- ☐ B The child has normal development
- ☐ C The child has delayed gross motor development
- ☐ D The child has delayed fine motor deveolpment
- ☐ E The child has delayed speech and language

2.24 The following statements refer to what would be expected of a 3-year-old child. Select the MOST appropriate.

- ☐ A Copy a square
- ☐ B Write his or her own name
- ☐ C Ride a bicycle
- ☐ D Go up stairs one foot per step
- ☐ E Recognise numbers up to 20

2.25 The following statements refer to children who toe walk. Select the MOST appropriate.

- ☐ A It is uncommon in children under the age of 2 years
- ☐ B An underlying neurological cause is most likely in these children
- ☐ C Treatment is usually required
- ☐ D Botulinum toxin is not useful in these children
- ☐ E It may be caused by congenital shortening of the Achilles tendon

2.26 You receive a referral letter for your general paediatric clinic from a GP to see a 12-year-old girl who attends the local fee-paying grammar school.

She complains of excessive tiredness for the last 4 months and her school attendance has fallen to less than 20% of expected. She experiences frequent waking overnight and daytime drowsiness. There is no history of weight loss or any systemic symptoms of note. Examination is unremarkable. The GP has already requested the following blood tests, all of which are normal: full blood count (FBC) and film, erythrocyte sedimentation rate (ESR), C-reactive protein (CRP), urea and electrolytes (U&Es), liver function tests (LFTs) and TFTs, creatine kinase (CK), glucose and Epstein–Barr virus serology. Urinalysis is also normal. The GP thinks that the diagnosis is one of chronic fatigue syndrome.

Which course of action would be MOST appropriate?

- ❑ A Pass the referral to the Child and Adolescent Mental Health Services (CAMHS) so that they can institute family therapy and explore the possibility of an underlying depressive illness
- ❑ B See in clinic before requesting ongoing follow-up by the physiotherapists to commence a graded exercise programme, to try to restore a more normal level of day-to-day activity for the child
- ❑ C After thorough history and examination in clinic, reassure the family and patient that there is no evidence of serious underlying pathology. Explain variable timescale and prognosis. Develop a management plan with patient and family agreement that addresses issues of concern, and arrange regular reviews of progress
- ❑ D Assess in clinic and arrange further investigations to rule out underlying pathology. At review, reassure patient and family that no organic cause has been found and problems will resolve with time
- ❑ E After review in clinic, prescribe low-dose antidepressants to try to normalise sleep pattern in an attempt to improve school attendance

2.27 Choose the MOST appropriate statement regarding separation anxiety from the list below.

- ❑ A It is developmentally normal until the age of approximately 8 years
- ❑ B It is more common in girls than boys
- ❑ C Presence of separation anxiety disorder in teenagers is most likely to present as school refusal and somatic symptoms
- ❑ D Separation anxiety disorder has a poor prognosis even with early intervention and treatment
- ❑ E To be diagnosed as a disorder (according to *Diagnostic and Statistical Manual of Mental Disorders* [DSM]-IV criteria), symptoms must have been present for a minimum of 3 months

2.28 Select the MOST appropriate statement from the following with regard to somatoform disorders in childhood.

- ❑ A They are often appropriately managed solely by the mental health services
- ❑ B They rarely have any long-term consequences for the child or family
- ❑ C They overlap with factitious disorders and malingering
- ❑ D They occur more frequently in children whose parents have a physical illness
- ❑ E Medical investigations are rarely helpful

2.29 The following statements refer to sleep disorders in childhood. Select the MOST appropriate statement.

- ❑ A Melatonin is a drug licensed for treating sleep disturbance in children
- ❑ B Sleep laboratory studies are helpful in defining the nature of most sleep disorders in childhood
- ❑ C Sleepwalking is rare in prepubertal children
- ❑ D Insomnia is the most frequent sleep disorder seen in postpubertal children with depression
- ❑ E Night terrors are short-lived episodes occurring during the first few hours of sleep, which terminate spontaneously and of which the child has poor recollection the following day

2.30 A school nurse discusses a 6-year-old boy with you, who teachers have noticed appears to be clumsier than his peers in the classroom and on the playground. He struggles in particular with his handwriting and he is not achieving at the same level as his classmates. What would be the MOST appropriate course of action to recommend?

- ❑ A Request educational psychology opinion to look for the presence of underlying learning difficulties
- ❑ B Make direct contact with teachers to establish level of concern before arranging a multidisciplinary assessment of child's abilities with the consent of the parents
- ❑ C Referral to paediatric neurologist to rule out a possible underlying neurological disorder
- ❑ D Assess in clinic to obtain a full history and perform examination in order to make an application for a Statement of Special Educational Needs
- ❑ E Ask for an occupational therapy assessment and treatment programme to be drawn up to follow in the classroom for improving the child's fine motor skills

2.31 In prospective cohort studies, the BIGGEST drawback is:

- ❑ A Bias
- ❑ B Confounding
- ❑ C Need for frequent measures
- ❑ D Tolerability of intervention
- ❑ E Loss to follow-up

2.32 In randomised controlled trials, the MAIN aim of randomisation is to:

- ❑ A Reduce bias
- ❑ B Reduce cost
- ❑ C Increase compliance
- ❑ D Reduce confounding
- ❑ E Increase generalisability

Extended Matching Questions

2.33–2.35 Theme: Psychiatric disorders

- ❑ A ADHD
- ❑ B Gilles de la Tourette syndrome
- ❑ C Oppositional defiant disorder
- ❑ D Conduct disorder
- ❑ E Autism
- ❑ F Depression
- ❑ G Obsessive–compulsive disorder
- ❑ H Generalised anxiety disorder

For each of the following clinical scenarios choose the MOST likely diagnosis from the list above. Each option may be used once, more than once or not at all.

2.33

A 4-year-old boy with speech and language delay who is having difficulty settling into school. He has not yet formed any friendships with his peers. His teacher remarks that he seems to enjoy playing with the bricks but will only line them up in patterns.

2.34

A 14-year-old boy who has had a number of facial tics including eye blinking and some uncontrollable vocalisation for the last 18 months. He is now reluctant to go out with his friends due to being overly self-conscious.

2.35

A 16-year-old boy with 2-year history of disobedient defiant behaviour at both home and school. He has run away from home, been in trouble with the police for breaking and entering properties, and has been recently excluded from school for fighting.

2.36–2.38 Theme: Allied professionals

- ❑ A Speech and language therapist
- ❑ B Occupational therapist
- ❑ C Physiotherapist
- ❑ D Health visitor
- ❑ E Dietician
- ❑ F Psychologist
- ❑ G Psychiatrist
- ❑ H School nurse

Choose the best option from the list above for each of the three statements given below. Each option may be used once, more than once or not at all.

2.36

Provides assessment of fine motor control and advice on appliances to aid daily living.

2.37

Provides health promotion for the prevention of illness from birth and additional services to vulnerable families, and is part of the primary healthcare team

2.38

Provides assessment of safety of swallow and all aspects of communication, both verbal and non-verbal.

2.39–2.41 Theme: Trial design

- ❑ A Ecological
- ❑ B Case–control
- ❑ C Prospective cohort
- ❑ D Nested case–control
- ❑ E Randomised controlled trial
- ❑ F Cross-sectional
- ❑ G Retrospective cohort
- ❑ H Case report

Choose the best option from the list above for each of the three situations described below. Each option may be used once, more than once or not at all.

2.39

Generating hypothesis for the importance of regional differences in alcohol consumption and oral cancers.

2.40

Studying the relationship between rare trace element deficiencies preconceptually and abdominal wall defects.

2.41

Ascertaining association between head circumference at birth and IQ at the age of 40 years.

2.42–2.44 Theme: Statistical methods

- ☐ A *t* test
- ☐ B Mann–Whitney rank sum test
- ☐ C Pearson correlation coefficient
- ☐ D Survival analysis
- ☐ E Odds ratio
- ☐ F Relative risk
- ☐ G Chi-squared (χ^2)
- ☐ H Multiple regression

Choose the best method from the list above for each of the three situations described below. Each option may be used once, more than once or not at all.

2.42

Comparing growth parameters between two groups.

2.43

Comparing time to readmission after discharge with asthma on two different treatments.

2.44

Examining relationship between body mass index (BMI) and peak flow rates.

2.45–2.47 Theme: Accidental injury

- ❑ A Burns and scalds
- ❑ B House fire
- ❑ C Choking
- ❑ D Poisoning
- ❑ E Drowning
- ❑ F Falls
- ❑ G Baby walkers
- ❑ H Road traffic accidents
- ❑ I Cycling

Choose the best option from the list above for each of the three statements given below. Each option may be used once, more than once or not at all.

2.45

The cause of the largest number of accidental deaths of children in the home each year.

2.46

The cause behind the largest number of non-fatal accidental injuries in children under the age of 15 years.

2.47

The cause of the majority of childhood accidental deaths per annum.

2.48–2.50 Theme: Developmental problems

- ❑ A Genetic studies for fragile X syndrome
- ❑ B Chromosomal analysis for Down syndrome
- ❑ C Blood lead level
- ❑ D Genetic studies for Rett syndrome
- ❑ E Genetic studies for Williams syndrome
- ❑ F Genetic studies for Wolf–Hirschhorn syndrome
- ❑ G Plasma very-long-chain fatty acid levels
- ❑ H Neuroimaging

Choose the most appropriate diagnostic test from the list above for each of the three case scenarios described below. Each option may be used once, more than once or not at all.

2.48

A 6-week-old baby girl is referred by the GP after attending for routine developmental assessment. The GP is concerned about the presence of dysmorphic features and poor growth. The baby has frontal bossing and a high frontal hairline in association with a broad, beaked nose and hypertelorism. The growth chart reveals that the weight is only just maintained on the 2nd centile and the head circumference has dipped beneath the 0.4th centile.

2.49

A 3-year-old boy is referred by the health visitor due to concerns about behaviour and development. The health visitor has been unable to review the child for over 6 months as the family have been in temporary accommodation out of area while waiting to be rehoused. The health visitor is concerned that his development appears to have regressed and, in particular, he is still managing to use single words only when communicating. His mother complains that he seems to be much more short-tempered than previously and he has developed problematic constipation.

2.50

You are referred a 2-year-old girl by her GP. Parents report an abrupt deterioration in her language skills over the previous 6 weeks so that she is now communicating by grunts and gestures, whereas she had previously been able to put two words together with meaning. She has developed a tendency to bring her hands repeatedly to her mouth but is no longer able to feed herself or hold a beaker. They also describe episodes where she is hyperventilating and stares with no response to her parents' voice.

CHAPTER 3

Dermatology

Multiple True–False Question

3.1 With regard to scabies

- ☐ A It is caused by infestation with the mite *Sarcoptes scabiei*
- ☐ B Failure to respond to treatment is usually due to incorrect diagnosis
- ☐ C In children under the age of 2 years, the head and neck area should be omitted when applying scabicide treatment
- ☐ D Lindane is the treatment of choice
- ☐ E Itching may persist for up to 6 weeks after successful treatment

Best of Five Questions

3.2 A 3-year-old boy presents with a several week history of multiple, discrete, circular, pearly white, papular lesions on his lower trunk and upper thigh. On closer inspection they all have a small central depression. They are causing him no discomfort.

What is the MOST likely diagnosis?

- ☐ A Molluscum contagiosum
- ☐ B Papular urticaria
- ☐ C Scabies
- ☐ D Keratosis pilari
- ☐ E Eczema

3.3 A pregnant woman with atopic eczema and asthma, who has a 4-year-old child with moderately severe eczema, requests advice about reducing the risk of eczema in her unborn child. Select the MOST appropriate advice from the following.

- ☐ A There is good clinical and epidemiological evidence to support the delayed introduction of potential food allergens in weaning foods (eg milk protein and eggs)
- ☐ B In high-risk families, there is evidence to support prolonged exclusive breastfeeding (ie beyond 6 months) as a preventive measure
- ☐ C If breastfeeding is not possible, soya-based formulae should be used in preference to cows' milk preparations
- ☐ D Removing certain known food allergens from the mother's diet during pregnancy does not reduce the risk or prevent the onset of atopic eczema
- ☐ E Taking measures to minimise exposure to house-dust mite have been shown to reduce the risk of the development of eczema after birth

3.4 A 6-week-old baby attending for developmental assessment is noted to have a well-circumscribed lesion on the bridge of his nose measuring 5 mm diameter and with a bluish hue.

The GP refers the child to the ward. The mass feels firm to the touch. Her parents say it was not present at birth and have noticed that it temporarily increases in size when the baby cries. Appearances are consistent with a capillary haemangioma.

What is the MOST appropriate advice to give to these parents?

- ☐ A Inform parents that no further follow-up is required as the majority spontaneously involute by school age
- ☐ B Referral to a plastic surgeon is required for consideration of removal of the lesion
- ☐ C Commence a course of oral steroids to limit the growth of the lesion
- ☐ D Reassure parents that it is likely to heal without scarring with time
- ☐ E Arrange follow-up for the child in the outpatient clinic to monitor the growth of the lesion over the coming weeks

Extended Matching Questions

3.5–3.7 Theme: Infections

- ❑ A *Staphylococcus aureus*
- ❑ B *Mycoplasma pneumoniae*
- ❑ C Epstein–Barr virus
- ❑ D Coxsackie virus
- ❑ E *Candida albicans*
- ❑ F Group A streptococcus
- ❑ G Herpes simplex virus
- ❑ H Adenovirus

Choose the most likely causative infective agent from the list above for each of the three case scenarios described below. Each option may be used once, more than once or not at all.

3.5

A 4-month-old baby boy has a 72-hour history of low-grade fever and bilateral purulent conjunctivitis. Large flaccid bullae are present in the groins and axillae, with some areas of sloughing on the neck, revealing a moist, erythematous base.

3.6

A 2-year-old girl is admitted with a high fever and refusal of any oral intake for 24 hours. Florid vesicles with an erythematous base are noted on the lips, gums and palate. Cervical lymphadenopathy is present. Inflammation and vesicle formation are also noted around the nailbed of one thumb.

3.7

A 6-year-old boy is seen with a blanching, urticarial-looking rash present for 48 hours. It started on the palms of both hands, spreading proximally, and now involves the trunk and face. It is confluent in places. His mother describes lesions as starting off as discrete, raised areas that blister centrally before developing central pallor. There is no mucosal involvement. The child is otherwise well with normal systemic examination.

CHAPTER 4

Endocrinology and Syndromes

Multiple True–False Questions

4.1 Down syndrome is associated with an increased incidence of

- ❑ A Alzheimer disease
- ❑ B Coeliac disease
- ❑ C Acute leukaemia
- ❑ D Hirschsprung disease
- ❑ E Oesophageal atresia

4.2 Complications of type 1 diabetes include

- ❑ A Tall stature
- ❑ B Hypoglycaemia
- ❑ C Lipoatrophy
- ❑ D Proximal myopathy
- ❑ E Cataract

4.3 Causes of a delayed bone age are

- ❑ A Obesity
- ❑ B Growth hormone deficiency
- ❑ C Central precocious puberty
- ❑ D Social deprivation
- ❑ E Chronic asthma

4.4 Features of Noonan syndrome include

- ❑ A Webbing of the neck
- ❑ B Pulmonary valve stenosis
- ❑ C Learning disability in 80%
- ❑ D Delayed puberty
- ❑ E Normal final adult height

4.5 Causes of gynaecomastia include

- ❑ A Normal child
- ❑ B Klinefelter syndrome
- ❑ C Noonan syndrome
- ❑ D Growth hormone deficiency
- ❑ E Cimetidine

4.6 The following are known to stimulate growth hormone secretion

- ❑ A Glucagon
- ❑ B Arginine
- ❑ C Aldosterone
- ❑ D Thyroxine
- ❑ E Insulin

4.7 Concerning central (true) precocious puberty

- ❑ A It is more common in boys than in girls
- ❑ B Computed tomography (CT) head scanning is indicated in all boys
- ❑ C It is usually idiopathic in girls
- ❑ D Testicular volume would be expected to be increased in boys
- ❑ E It is gonadotrophin independent

4.8 In achondroplasia

- ❑ A Bowing of the legs is common
- ❑ B Length of the vertebral spine is decreased
- ❑ C Diagnostic radiological features are present at birth
- ❑ D Inheritance is autosomal recessive
- ❑ E Macrocephaly occurs

Best of Five Questions

4.9 The following statements refer to Addison disease. Select the MOST appropriate.

- ❑ A It is more common in boys
- ❑ B Fatigue is a common presenting feature
- ❑ C Serum renin is characteristically low
- ❑ D The short Synacthen test is normal
- ❑ E It can present with hyperglycaemia if in crises

4.10 The following are features of classic homocystinuria. Select the MOST appropriate.

- ❑ A Autosomal dominant inheritance
- ❑ B Hyperextendable joints
- ❑ C Abnormal from birth
- ❑ D Predisposition to vascular thrombosis
- ❑ E Aortic root dilatation

4.11 Select the MOST appropriate statement regarding congenital hypothyroidism

- ❑ A It is usually due to dyshormonogenesis
- ❑ B It is usually symptomatic in the neonatal period
- ❑ C The incidence is 1 in 4000
- ❑ D A high thyroid-stimulating hormone (TSH) and normal T_4 on treatment suggest poor compliance
- ❑ E Screening is at the 6-week check

4.12 Concerning Klinefelter syndrome select the MOST appropriate statement.

- ❑ A The karyotype is 47 XYY
- ❑ B There is increased risk of leukaemia
- ❑ C Infertility is rare
- ❑ D Gynaecomastia is an uncommon finding in adolescents
- ❑ E The testes are large

4.13 For Turner syndrome select the MOST appropriate statement.

- ☐ A Fetal loss in the first trimester is common
- ☐ B Hypogonadotrophic hypogonadism is a feature
- ☐ C The incidence increases with advancing maternal age
- ☐ D Spontaneous puberty is never seen
- ☐ E Infants are usually large for dates

4.14 With regard to type 1 diabetes mellitus, select the MOST appropriate statement.

- ☐ A It has a peak incidence at 9–10 years of age
- ☐ B It is more common in children who possess the HLA-B3 antigen
- ☐ C It is associated with islet cell antibodies in 30% at diagnosis
- ☐ D It has a peak incidence during the summer months in the UK
- ☐ E It is associated with an increased risk of diabetes in siblings of the affected case

4.15 The following statements refer to aldosterone. Select the MOST appropriate statement.

- ☐ A Secretion is stimulated by a fall in serum sodium
- ☐ B It is secreted in response to a rise in blood pressure
- ☐ C Deficiency is a cause of hypokalaemia
- ☐ D It acts on the ascending limb of the loop of Henle
- ☐ E Levels are normal in pseudohypoaldosteronism

4.16 The following refer to features of Graves disease. Select the MOST appropriate.

- ☐ A Male predominance
- ☐ B Constipation
- ☐ C Peak incidence in early childhood
- ☐ D Association with HLA-DR3
- ☐ E Inappropriate weight gain

4.17 A 13-year-old boy attends outpatient clinic because he is concerned that many of his friends are now taller than him and he does not seem to have grown as they have.

He is worried. On examination he has some sparse dark coarse hair over the junction of the pubes and reports that he has noticed some enlargement of his penis and growth of his testis. He has a testicular volume of 8 ml.

Select the MOST likely diagnosis.

- ❑ A Delayed puberty
- ❑ B Normal puberty
- ❑ C Precocious puberty
- ❑ D Premature adrenache
- ❑ E Premature thelarche

4.18 Concerning 21-hydroxylase deficiency, select the MOST appropriate statement from the following.

- ❑ A Its inheritance is autosomal dominant
- ❑ B Hypertension is common
- ❑ C A reduced serum 17OH-progesterone is characteristic
- ❑ D Plasma potassium is low in salt losers
- ❑ E It can present as premature isosexual development in boys

4.19 Regarding fragile X syndrome, choose the MOST appropriate statement.

- ❑ A It occurs as a consequence of allelic expansion
- ❑ B It is a cause of micro-orchidism in boys
- ❑ C It is asymptomatic in carrier girls
- ❑ D It causes more severe learning difficulties in girls than boys
- ❑ E It is associated with small ears

4.20 The following statements refer to growth hormone deficiency. Choose the MOST appropriate statement.

- ❑ A It is the cause of short stature in Cushing syndrome
- ❑ B Treatment with growth hormone can improve final height
- ❑ C It does not require investigation of other hypothalamic–pituitary function
- ❑ D It can lead to boys having large genitalia
- ❑ E It is usually evident at birth

4.21 The following statements refer to galactosaemia. Choose the MOST appropriate statement.

- ❑ A It has an incidence of 1 in 1000 live births
- ❑ B Clinical manifestations can occur before a baby has been fed
- ❑ C It can lead to delayed puberty
- ❑ D Hepatic failure is rare
- ❑ E It is treated with a dairy-free diet

4.22 Select the MOST appropriate statements regarding the use of insulin pumps.

- ❑ A They reduce the need for blood sugar monitoring
- ❑ B Less education is required because with a continuous pump the regimen is stable
- ❑ C Diabetic ketoacidosis will take longer to develop in those patients using them because they generally have improved control
- ❑ D They can be useful in infants where small alterations in insulin is difficult with standard insulin pens
- ❑ E They reduce lifestyle flexibility due to the pump having to be continuously attached

4.23 In nutritional rickets, which of the following is MOST likely to occur?

- ❑ A It leads to increased mineralisation of the growing bone
- ❑ B Hyperphosphataemia is a cause
- ❑ C Exclusive breastfeeding may be protective
- ❑ D Craniosynostosis is a clinical feature
- ❑ E Vitamin D deficiency is the most common cause

4.24 Which of the following is MOST likely to cause hypercalcaemia?

- ❑ A Vitamin D deficiency
- ❑ B Hyperparathyroidism
- ❑ C Phenytoin
- ❑ D Di George syndrome
- ❑ E Hypothyroidism

4.25 Following a neonatal delivery, a midwife is unable to decide on the gender of the baby due to ambiguous genitalia. Select the MOST appropriate course of action.

❑ A Suggest to the midwife that it is likely that the baby is the gender it most looks like so she should inform the parents of this most likely gender, because it will cause them unnecessary distress to make them wait

❑ B After examination of the baby inform the parents of the most likely gender, because it will cause them unnecessary distress to make them wait

❑ C Inform the parents that the chromosomes will need to be done and after this result they will be informed what gender the child should be reared as

❑ D Inform the parents that a number of investigations will need to be performed and that they will need to wait before a sex is assigned

❑ E Inform the parents that a definitive diagnosis will be reached

4.26 The following statements refer to osteogenesis imperfecta. Choose the MOST appropriate statement.

❑ A Blue sclerae are diagnostic

❑ B Type II is likely to be mild

❑ C Bisphosphonate infusion is potentially curative

❑ D Compression vertebral body fractures can be seen

❑ E Alkaline phosphatase levels will be raised

4.27 With regard to an infant who has been diagnosed with phenylketonuria after neonatal screening, select the MOST appropriate statement from the following.

❑ A The infant will be severely affected at birth

❑ B The urine is odourless

❑ C It is caused by an inability to produce phenylalanine

❑ D Seizures can occur

❑ E Untreated individuals have a normal IQ

4.28 Which is the MOST appropriate statement about type 2 diabetes in childhood?

❑ A It does not pose a significant problem in western society

❑ B It is usually associated with weight loss at presentation

❑ C It is seen in association with acanthosis nigricans

❑ D It is rarely associated with the microvascular complications as seen in type 1 diabetes

❑ E It is always treatable with dietary measures and oral hypoglycaemic agents

4.29 Select the MOST appropriate statement regarding hypoglycaemia in neonates.

- ❑ A Intramuscular glucagon is the treatment of choice
- ❑ B Increased glycogen stores in large-for-date babies, such as infants of diabetic mothers, are protective
- ❑ C The best time to take blood and urine samples is after the correction of a hypoglycaemic episode
- ❑ D Long-term consequences include lowered IQ and decreased head size
- ❑ E A bolus of 2.5 ml/kg of 50% dextrose should be used to correct the abnormality

4.30 With regard to McCune–Albright syndrome, which is the MOST appropriate statement?

- ❑ A Precocious puberty caused by this condition is more commonly seen in girls than boys
- ❑ B Fibrous dysplasia commonly results in pathological fracture
- ❑ C Café-au-lait pigmentation is typically present at birth
- ❑ D Precocious puberty is primarily due to central gonadotrophin-dependent causes
- ❑ E A family history of café-au-lait pigmentation supports the diagnosis

4.31 Select the MOST appropriate statement about sexual determination and differentiation.

- ❑ A Gender identity should be determined by the phenotypic appearance
- ❑ B Gonadal differentiation *in utero* occurs in the second trimester
- ❑ C Androgen insensitivity syndrome leads to an undermasculinised male
- ❑ D Labial adhesions are a cause of ambiguous genitalia
- ❑ E If palpable gonads are present, the infant can be assigned the male sex

4.32 Select the MOST appropriate statement listed below about obesity in childhood.

- ❑ A The various strategies that are used to tackle obesity (ie dietary modification and increased physical activity) have a strong evidence base supporting their use
- ❑ B It is defined as a body mass index (weight in kilograms/[height in metres]^2) >30
- ❑ C Weight loss is the most frequently recommended course of action to prevent long-term health complications
- ❑ D It is a greater problem in girls than boys in the UK population
- ❑ E It is a risk factor for subclinical coronary artery sclerosis and atherosclerosis in childhood

Extended Matching Questions

4.33–4.35 Theme: Syndromes

- ❑ A Prader–Willi syndrome
- ❑ B Cri-du-chat syndrome
- ❑ C Noonan syndrome
- ❑ D Fragile X syndrome
- ❑ E Cornelia de Lange syndrome
- ❑ F Down syndrome
- ❑ G Treacher Collins syndrome
- ❑ H Angelman syndrome
- ❑ I Silver–Russell syndrome

Choose the BEST diagnoses from the list above for each of the cases described below. Each option may be used once, more than once or not at all.

4.33

A child who at birth was noted to be small for gestational age and floppy. Over the first 6 months of life the child had failure to thrive. Now 5 years of age the child has had rapid weight gain and is obese with mild learning difficulties. The child is noted to have almond-shaped eyes and small hands and feet. On genetic testing the child is noted to have an abnormality in chromosome 15.

4.34

A child who at birth was noted to be small for gestational age. Postnatally the child failed to thrive and now at 5 years of age has short stature, microcephaly, hearing impairment and moderate learning difficulties. The child is noted to have arched eyebrows with synophrys. The child has a small upturned nose, low-set ears and small widely spaced teeth.

4.35

A child who at birth was noted to be small for gestational age with an abnormal cry. Postnatally the child failed to thrive. At 5 years of age the child has microcephaly and severe learning difficulties. The child is noted to have wide set eyes, micrognathia and abnormally folded external ears.

4.36–4.38 Theme: Diabetes mellitus

The following are complications/associations of diabetes mellitus and its treatment:

- ❑ A Hypoglycaemia
- ❑ B Cerebral oedema
- ❑ C Diabetic ketoacidosis
- ❑ D Eating disorder
- ❑ E Peripheral neuropathy
- ❑ F Microalbuminuria
- ❑ G Coeliac disease
- ❑ H Autoimmune thyroiditis

Choose the MOST likely diagnosis from the list above for each of the cases described below. Each option may be used once, more than once or not at all.

4.36

A 3-year-old child with type 1 diabetes is admitted to a paediatric assessment unit with a 5-day history of diarrhoea and vomiting. He has had diabetes for 12 months and this is the first time that his parents have had to deal with an intercurrent illness. Initially they had been managing at home using a standard regimen for when he has an illness (sick day rules) but have found it increasingly difficult to manage him over the last 12 hours. On admission he was peripherally cool and has a blood sugar of 28 and a pH of 7.11. Over the next 4 hours he is given intravenous fluids and insulin. Two hours later the nurses are concerned that he is very sleepy; they report that before this he was awake but complaining of a headache. His blood sugar is 5. He has a heart rate of 60/min and a blood pressure of 120/60.

4.37

A 17-year-old boy who has had type 1 diabetes for the last 13 years. His average HbA1c is 12%. On routine screening in clinic he is well with a blood sugar of 13. His early morning urinary albumin/creatinine ratio is 4 g/mmol.

4.38

A 12-year-old girl who has had diabetes for the last 4 years attends for her routine outpatient clinic. Her HbA1c is 6.9%, her blood sugar 6, and she uses an insulin pump. You note that over a 60-month period she has lost 4 kg in weight. Clinically she has no goitre and her tissue transglutaminase is positive.

4.39–4.41 Theme: Causes of hypoglycaemia

- ☐ A Hypothyroidism
- ☐ B Glycogen storage disease
- ☐ C Beckwith–Wiedemann syndrome
- ☐ D Sepsis
- ☐ E Medium-chain acyl-CoA dehydrogenase deficiency (MCAD)
- ☐ F Congenital hypopituitarism
- ☐ G Fructose-1,6-bisphosphatase deficiency
- ☐ H Insulinoma
- ☐ I Alcohol ingestion

Choose the best diagnoses from the list above for each of the case scenarios described below. Each option may be used once, more than once or not at all.

4.39

A 15-year-old boy presents having woken in the morning feeling light-headed. His parents report that he seemed disoriented. On arrival in the emergency department he had a blood sugar of 1.8, raised C-reactive peptide and raised insulin level.

4.40

A 3-month-old child presents sleepy and lethargic; her blood sugar is 1.6. Other bloods taken at the time of her hypoglycaemia show a lactic acidosis, hyperuricaemia and hyperlipidaemia. Urine dipstick shows ketones. On examination she has hepatomegaly and is noted to be on the 0.4th centile. Her mother expresses that she has had concern about her child's growth and she has had episodes of being sleepy and sweaty in the past.

4.41

A 6-month-old child presents having been unwell for 12 hours with a coryzal illness. His mother reports that he has been off his food and vomited twice; he has taken little in orally in the preceding hours. On arrival he is floppy and quiet with a blood sugar of 1.3. On further testing he has no ketones in his urine, raised liver enzymes and elevated urinary organic acids

4.42–4.44 Theme: Fluid balance

- ❑ A Syndrome of inappropriate ADH
- ❑ B Primary polydipsia
- ❑ C Nephrotic syndrome
- ❑ D Excessive sodium intake
- ❑ E Gastroenteritis
- ❑ F Central diabetes insipidus
- ❑ G Nephrogenic diabetes insipidus
- ❑ H Diuretic induced

Choose the BEST diagnoses from the list above for each of the set of results and clinical findings described. Each option may be used once, more than once or not at all.

4.42

A 3-year-old boy who is peripherally cool, with generalised oedema. Results show plasma sodium 132 mmol/l, urinary sodium 4 mmol/l and raised protein in his urine.

4.43

A 5-year-old boy post head injury has an increased urine output. Results show plasma sodium of 152 mmol/l; he appears intravascular depleted. He has a low urinary osmolality but high plasma osmolality.

4.44

A 12-year-old boy with pneumonia has a plasma sodium of 128 mmol/l and urinary sodium of 30 mmol/l; he does not appear intravascularly compromised. He has a low urine output and high urinary osmolality. His urea and creatinine are within normal limits for his age and size.

4.45–4.47 Theme: Growth and development

- ❑ A Russell–Silver syndrome
- ❑ B Turner syndrome
- ❑ C Constitutional delay of growth and puberty
- ❑ D Kallmann syndrome
- ❑ E Familial short stature
- ❑ F Growth hormone deficiency
- ❑ G Williams syndrome
- ❑ H Noonan syndrome
- ❑ I Hypopituitarism

Choose the best diagnoses from the list above for each of the case scenarios described below. Each option may be used once, more than once or not at all.

4.45

A 13-year-old girl is seen in clinic for an opinion with regard to her short stature and pubertal development. Her growth chart reveals that she was of low birthweight (2.2 kg). Her height had been maintained on the 2nd centile for age until age 11 years, when it fell below the 0.4th centile. She is currently 130 cm tall. She has stage 2 pubic hair, but no breast bud development. Her mother is 173 cm tall and her father 181 cm tall. The target centile range, given the parents' heights, is calculated as between the 25th and 98th centiles. The result of a bone age radiograph requested by the GP has already been reported and has the appearance is equivalent to 12 years and 8 months of age. She has elevated levels of FSH and LH.

4.46

A 10-week-old baby girl is referred by the health visitor with feeding problems and faltering growth. The baby was of low birthweight (2.4 kg at term) and is struggling to take the suggested volumes of high-energy formula to maintain adequate weight gain along the 0.4th centile, although the head circumference is increasing steadily along the 25th centile. The health visitor feels that the baby appears slightly dysmorphic with a high forehead and micrognathia, giving a triangular appearance to the facies. The baby is noted to be slightly floppy on handling. Her parents report that she has been smiling for the last 2 weeks. A murmur was heard on the postnatal check but an echocardiogram revealed no abnormality and the murmur has since resolved. Serum electrolytes including calcium levels and a 24-hour blood glucose profile are within normal limits.

4.47

A 15-year-old boy is seen in clinic due to short stature. Growth charts, which are available from birth, show that his birthweight and length were on the 50th centile. Over the first year of life his height and weight fell to the 9th centile where his growth was maintained until the last 18 months, when his height has fallen to just beneath the 2nd centile. Examination reveals testicular volume of <10 ml with the presence of sparse pubic and axillary hair. There are no dysmorphic features and systemic examination is otherwise unremarkable. Random growth hormone levels requested by the GP are just beneath the lower end of the normal range for his age. Thyroid function is normal, along with full blood count, biochemical profile and erythrocyte sedimentation rate (ESR). Bone age is delayed 3 years. His mother recalls that her menarche occurred at the age of 16 years.

4.48–4.50 Theme: Hypocalcaemia

- ☐ A Hypoparathyroidism
- ☐ B Di George syndrome
- ☐ C Vitamin D deficiency
- ☐ D Pseudohypoparathyroidism
- ☐ E Chronic renal failure
- ☐ F Pseudopseudohypoparathyroidism
- ☐ G Fanconi syndrome

Choose the best diagnosis from the list above for each of the three scenarios described below. Each option may be used once, more than once or not at all.

4.48

A 4-week-old baby is referred by the GP with a history of twitching movements. The baby has also only just regained his birthweight and is described by mum as difficult to feed. A murmur is heard and he is noted to have low-set ears on examination.

4.49

A 15-month-old girl is referred by the health visitor with concerns about delayed development. The child is on the 91st centile for weight and the 2nd centile for height. The fourth and fifth digits of both hands appear shorter than the other fingers and both radii are slightly bowed. Parents do not report any abnormal movements. Baseline biochemistry including FBC, renal function, calcium, phosphate, alkaline phosphatase and thyroid function is all within normal limits. Chromosomal analysis is also normal.

4.50

A 3-year-old eastern European refugee girl attends the accident and emergency department (A&E) after a fall. A radiograph is taken of her tibia and fibula due to localised tenderness over this area. The bones appear osteopenic but no other bony abnormality is seen. She is referred for a paediatric opinion because she appears thin and malnourished. In view of the radiological appearances, the A&E doctors have requested a bone profile, which reveals a low corrected serum calcium and elevated serum phosphate. Parathyroid hormone levels returned subsequently are elevated.

CHAPTER 5

Gastroenterology and Nutrition

Multiple True–False Questions

5.1 ***Helicobacter pylori***

- ☐ A It is a Gram-positive bacterium
- ☐ B It causes chronic antral gastritis
- ☐ C It causes a nosocomial infection
- ☐ D It is best diagnosed on culture
- ☐ E It is a common cause of recurrent abdominal pain

5.2 **Characteristic features of Crohn disease include**

- ☐ A Aphthous mouth ulcers
- ☐ B Ankylosing spondylitis
- ☐ C Sclerosing cholangitis
- ☐ D Raised inflammatory indices
- ☐ E Growth retardation

5.3 **Recognised consequences of abetalipoproteinaemia include**

- ☐ A Failure to thrive
- ☐ B Autosomal dominant inheritance
- ☐ C Ataxia secondary to vitamin D deficiency
- ☐ D Child is normal at birth
- ☐ E Retinitis pigmentosa

5.4 Characteristic features of acrodermatitis enteropathica include

- ☐ A Malabsorption of copper
- ☐ B Autosomal dominant inheritance
- ☐ C Recurrent infections
- ☐ D Alopecia
- ☐ E Rapid response to treatment with zinc sulphate

5.5 Vitamin A

- ☐ A Deficiency is the most common cause of visual loss worldwide
- ☐ B It is fat soluble
- ☐ C It has an important role to play in resistance to infection
- ☐ D It is present in milk
- ☐ E It is beneficial in the management of severe measles

5.6 Immunoglobulin A

- ☐ A Makes up 50% of serum immunoglobulins
- ☐ B Predominates on respiratory and gastrointestinal surfaces in its secretory form
- ☐ C Selective deficiency is rare with a prevalence of less than 1 in 10 000
- ☐ D Deficiency is associated with an increased risk of infection
- ☐ E Deficiency is associated with an increased risk of atopic disease

5.7 The following statements are true

- ☐ A Starch is a glucose polymer
- ☐ B Lactose is a disaccharide made up of galactose and glucose
- ☐ C Carbohydrate digestion is dependent on pancreatic secretion
- ☐ D Sucrase hydrolyses sucrose into glucose and fructose
- ☐ E Glucose, galactose and fructose are all absorbed by an active transport mechanism

5.8 Causes of partial villous atrophy on small bowel biopsy include

- ☐ A Coeliac disease
- ☐ B Giardiasis
- ☐ C Cows' milk sensitive enteropathy
- ☐ D Inflammatory bowel disease
- ☐ E Autoimmune enteropathy

5.9 Gilbert syndrome

- ❑ A It causes unconjugated hyperbilirubinaemia
- ❑ B It causes bilirubinuria
- ❑ C It can progress to cirrhosis
- ❑ D It has a prevalence of 6%
- ❑ E It episodes of jaundice are precipitated by acute infections

Best of Five Questions

5.10 Which of the following statements about complementary feeding (weaning) is most factually correct?

- ❑ A Exclusive breastfeeding of infants until 6 months is associated with a decreased incidence of infection
- ❑ B There is clear evidence that the introduction of certain foods between 4 and 6 months is associated with an increased prevalence of food allergy
- ❑ C There are newly emerging concerns that exclusive breastfeeding until 6 months is associated with iron deficiency anaemia
- ❑ D Exclusive breastfeeding for at least 6 months is associated with a decreased incidence of coeliac disease in later life compared with the introduction of gluten between 4 and 6 months
- ❑ E The reported percentage of mothers in the UK who exclusively breastfeed their babies for 6 months is around 15%

5.11 Which of the following statements with regard to acute abdominal pain in children is most factually correct?

- ❑ A The rate of perforation of the appendix at diagnosis falls from 80% to 30% between the first and second decades of life
- ❑ B Acute appendicitis is the most common surgical cause of an acute abdomen in the under-5 age group
- ❑ C Acute appendicitis is most common in the second decade of life
- ❑ D Abdominal ultrasonography is rarely helpful in diagnosis but can help to identify alternative pathology, including ovarian problems in girls
- ❑ E The classic presentation of central colicky abdominal pain localising to the lower right quadrant occurs in about 70% of patients

5.12 Which of the following statements with regard to iron deficiency anaemia in children is most factually correct?

- ❑ A The bioavailability of iron in breast milk is low
- ❑ B Iron-rich foods include egg yolk, red meat, fortified breakfast cereals, and dried fruit, green vegetables, beans and pulses
- ❑ C Malabsorption is the major cause for iron deficiency in children in the UK
- ❑ D The most likely cause for non-response to oral iron treatment is an undiagnosed pathological aetiology, eg coeliac disease, blood loss or chronic inflammation
- ❑ E Follow-on milks should be encouraged in all children to prevent iron deficiency anaemia

5.13 A 20-month-old Asian boy of non-consanguineous parents presents with a history of swelling of the wrists. He complains of pain in his limbs and since mobilising his parents have become concerned about his 'bandy legs'. He was breastfed from birth and had solids introduced into his diet at 6 months of age. He had a green-stick fracture of his radius at the age of 12 months secondary to a fall at nursery. Which of the following diagnoses is most likely in this case?

- ❑ A Juvenile idiopathic arthritis
- ❑ B X-linked hypophosphataemic rickets
- ❑ C Non-accidental injury
- ❑ D Vitamin D-deficient rickets
- ❑ E Acute lymphoblastic leukaemia

5.14 A 2-year-old boy presents to the GP with a 3-month history of recurrent episodes of small amounts of bright red blood per rectum.

He is well grown and does not have any associated symptoms of abdominal pain, diarrhoea or constipation. There is no family history of GI bleeding and he does not appear clinically anaemic. He has no other cutaneous signs on examination and has normal cardiovascular, respiratory and abdominal examinations in clinic.

What is the most likely diagnosis from the list below?

- ❑ A Constipation with anal fissure
- ❑ B Peutz–Jegher syndrome
- ❑ C Juvenile polyp
- ❑ D Familial adenomatous polyposis coli
- ❑ E Juvenile polyposis

5.15 Which of the following statements about breastfeeding is MOST accurate?

- ☐ A Breastfeeding offers clear benefits in the prevention of lower respiratory tract infections
- ☐ B A diagnosis of PKU is an absolute contraindication to breastfeeding
- ☐ C Maternal HIV, hepatitis C and hepatitis B are contraindications to breastfeeding in developed countries
- ☐ D Breastfeeding reduces the rate of gastrointestinal infections of infants while it continues
- ☐ E Breastfeeding increases IQ equally in both low-birthweight and normal-birthweight infants

5.16 Which of the following statements is the most factually correct with regard to the administration of vitamin K to babies in the neonatal period?

- ☐ A Vitamin K deficiency bleeding is a potentially fatal disorder that is virtually preventable with one dose of vitamin K given intramuscularly at birth
- ☐ B The vast majority of vitamin K deficiency-associated bleeding occurs within the first week of life
- ☐ C If an oral regimen is undertaken, a single dose of oral vitamin K is recommended in all formula-fed babies
- ☐ D Significant bleeding in the neonatal period normally occurs in children with significant risk factors for vitamin K deficiency bleeding
- ☐ E There is good evidence to support an increased risk of childhood leukaemia in babies given vitamin K in the neonatal period

5.17 Which of the following statements with regard to testing for carbohydrate malabsorption is most factually correct?

- ☐ A Resolution of symptoms on removal of the suspected carbohydrate from the diet is conclusive evidence of the presence of lactose intolerance
- ☐ B Non-resolution of symptoms on removal of suspected carbohydrate from the diet excludes the diagnosis of carbohydrate intolerance
- ☐ C Reducing substances of 0.05% in the stool are indicative of carbohydrate intolerance
- ☐ D An early peak of hydrogen in a hydrogen breath test, followed by a secondary peak, may be indicative of small bowel bacterial overgrowth
- ☐ E Alkaline stool pH is indicative of carbohydrate intolerance

5.18 Which of the following statements is the most factually correct with regard to folate/folic acid?

- ☐ A Serum folate reflects the total body store of folate
- ☐ B Red cell folate is increased as part of the acute phase reaction
- ☐ C Methotrexate and trimethoprim are folate antagonists
- ☐ D Folic acid occurs in high levels in green vegetables
- ☐ E Supplementation with folic acid is recommended in all pregnancies with high risk of neural tube defects

5.19 Which of the following statements with regard to infant formula and breast milk is most factually correct?

- ☐ A The protein and carbohydrate components of colostrum are higher than those of mature breast milk
- ☐ B There is good evidence to show that casein-predominant formulas are more satisfying for hungrier babies
- ☐ C The fat content of breast milk varies throughout the day and throughout a feed
- ☐ D The iron content of first formula milks closely resembles that of breast milk
- ☐ E The renal solute load of a casein-based formula is similar to that of a whey-based formula

5.20 Which of the following statements concerning carbohydrate intolerance in childhood is most factually correct?

- ☐ A Carbohydrate intolerance is usually inherited in an autosomal dominant fashion
- ☐ B Symptoms of inherited carbohydrate intolerance are most common in the first 4 years of life
- ☐ C Symptoms of congenital carbohydrate intolerance always occur in the neonatal period
- ☐ D Symptoms of lactose intolerance often require total exclusion of all dairy products throughout life
- ☐ E Acquired post-enteritis lactose intolerance is usually transient

5.21 Which of the following statements about preterm and term formulae and breast milk is most factually correct?

- ❑ A Preterm formula has a lower sodium content than term formula
- ❑ B Preterm formula has the same protein content as term formula
- ❑ C Preterm babies fed with fortified breast milk show similar weight gain profiles to preterm babies fed on preterm formula milks
- ❑ D Preterm formula contains more fat, protein and electrolytes but the same amount of carbohydrate as term formula or unfortified breast milk
- ❑ E Babies fed on fortified breast milk have a decreased incidence of late-onset sepsis and necrotising enterocolitis when compared with babies fed on preterm formulae

5.22 Which of the following statements with regard to cows' milk, breast (human) milk and follow-on formulas is the most factually correct?

- ❑ A Cows' milk should not be introduced as part of the weaning diet in any way before the age of 1 year
- ❑ B Follow-on milk is essential to stop iron deficiency anaemia in the second year of life
- ❑ C Semi-skimmed cows' milk has the same vitamin content as full-fat cows' milk
- ❑ D Breast milk has the same energy content as unmodified cows' milk
- ❑ E Breast milk contains more protein and less carbohydrate than unmodified cows' milk

5.23 Which of the following statements with regard to nutritional supplements are the most factually correct?

- ❑ A Maxijul is a glucose polymer
- ❑ B Polycal contains MCT fats
- ❑ C Scandishakes is a cows' milk, protein-free, calorie supplement
- ❑ D Duocal contains carbohydrate, protein and fat
- ❑ E Calogen contains 250 kcal/100 g

5.24 Which of the following statements relating to Wilson disease is most factually correct?

- ❑ A Wilson disease is sporadically inherited
- ❑ B Wilson disease has a poor outcome even if diagnosed early and treated appropriately
- ❑ C A diet low in copper should be low in shellfish, liver and chocolate
- ❑ D The majority of patients with Wilson disease present with liver and renal impairment in early childhood
- ❑ E A presentation with psychiatric or neurological symptoms is rare

5.25 Which of the following statements with regard to neonatal hyperbilirubinaemia is most factually correct?

- ❑ A Babies who become jaundiced whilst breastfeeding are significantly at risk of dehydration and require supplementation with formula milk
- ❑ B Babies who have rhesus incompatibility and haemolysis will require exchange transfusion
- ❑ C Unconjugated hyperbilirubinaemia can present with dark urine, due to high levels of bilirubin in the urine
- ❑ D Neonates who develop jaundice within the first 24 h need urgent medical review to rule out underlying potentially severe aetiology for their jaundice
- ❑ E Clinical examination of neonates is an acceptable way to quantify the extent of neonatal jaundice and guide treatment

5.26 Which of the following statements with regard to coeliac disease is the most factually correct?

- ❑ A According to NICE guidelines type 1 diabetes mellitus is an indication for screening for coeliac disease
- ❑ B The majority of patients with coeliac disease present with irritability, pallor and malabsorption (diarrhoea and failure to thrive) in infancy after the introduction of gluten into the diet
- ❑ C Positive serology (IgA TTG, or IgG TTG if IgA deficient) is sufficient to make a diagnosis of coeliac disease
- ❑ D The effects of gluten on serology and small bowel mucosa are long lived so it is acceptable to advise patients with possible coeliac disease to exclude gluten whilst awaiting referral for definitive diagnosis and management
- ❑ E A family history of coeliac disease is present in 40% of people diagnosed with coeliac disease

5.27 Which of the statements about hepatitis B is the most factually correct?

- ❑ A Hepatitis B is a DNA virus
- ❑ B Transmission of hepatitis B is faeco-oral
- ❑ C Treatment of acute hepatitis B infection is by passive immunisation
- ❑ D Interferon-γ is a recognised treatment of the chronic carrier state
- ❑ E Anti-HBs antibodies suggest that a chronic carrier state has developed after acute infection

5.28 Which of the following statements concerning hepatitis A is the most factually correct?

- ❑ A Chronic liver disease commonly follows acute infection
- ❑ B Transmission is most commonly by exposure to contaminated blood at delivery
- ❑ C Passive immunisation produces lifelong immunity to infection
- ❑ D Hepatitis A is an RNA virus
- ❑ E Diagnosis of acute infection is by stool culture

5.29 Which of the following statements about hepatitis C is the most factually correct?

- ❑ A Maternal infection with hepatitis C is a contraindication to breastfeeding
- ❑ B Caesarean section is advised in all cases of hepatitis C in the developed world to reduce vertical transmission
- ❑ C Post-delivery immunisation is advised in all cases to decrease vertical transmission
- ❑ D Treatment with ribavirin as a monotherapy is currently recommended in the UK for children with moderate-to-severe liver disease
- ❑ E Transmission worldwide is most commonly by the vertical route

5.30 From the following list of infective agents and disease processes, which is most likely to cause the clinical picture of colitis with abdominal pain and bloody diarrhoea?

- ❑ A Rotavirus infection
- ❑ B *Giardia lamblia*
- ❑ C Peutz–Jegher syndrome
- ❑ D Non-typhoid *Salmonella* sp
- ❑ E Coeliac disease

5.31 Which of the following statements about *Giardia intestinalis* is the most factually correct?

- ❑ A *Giardia intestinalis* is a protozoal infection, the only host of which is humans
- ❑ B Infection with *Giardia intestinalis* can cause chronic diarrhoea, malabsorption, failure to thrive and intestinal histological changes similar to those seen in coeliac disease
- ❑ C *Giardia intestinalis* infection rate is highest in adolescents
- ❑ D *Giardia intestinalis* infection should be treated with erythromycin
- ❑ E Asymptomatic infection in developed countries should not be treated with antibiotics

5.32 Which of the following statements with regard to ulcerative colitis is most factually correct?

- ❑ A Half the patients presenting with ulcerative colitis present with classic colitic symptoms of abdominal pain and bloody diarrhoea
- ❑ B The pANCA blood tests are positive in 15% of cases of ulcerative colitis and 45% of cases of Crohn disease
- ❑ C FBC and inflammatory markers within the normal range almost always exclude a diagnosis of ulcerative colitis
- ❑ D Growth failure is a common presentation of ulcerative colitis and often precedes GI symptoms by months or even years
- ❑ E Ulcerative colitis is more common than Crohn disease in younger children and in Asian children

5.33 Which of the statements about recurrent abdominal pain in childhood is the most factually correct?

- ❑ A A family history of coeliac disease is common in these children
- ❑ B There is good evidence to suggest that the symptom of pain in these children is fictitious and made up for secondary gain
- ❑ C A family history of migraine is associated with a subset of children with recurrent abdominal pain
- ❑ D Introducing the biopsychosocial model of illness is best accepted at the later stages of management of these children when organic diagnoses have been excluded
- ❑ E A childhood history of recurrent abdominal pain is rarely associated with irritable bowel syndrome in adult life

5.34 Of the following causes of portal hypertension, which can be best described as being prehepatic?

- ❑ A Budd–Chiari syndrome
- ❑ B Constrictive pericarditis
- ❑ C Schistosomiasis
- ❑ D Portal vein thrombosis
- ❑ E Biliary atresia

5.35 Which of the following statements about rectal prolapse is the MOST correct?

- ❑ A It is associated with cystic fibrosis in most cases
- ❑ B It is usually painful
- ❑ C It requires reduction under general anaesthetic
- ❑ D It is most common in the pre-school-age group
- ❑ E It can always be resolved with a short course of laxatives and dietary advice

5.36 Which is the MOST appropriate statement about constipation?

- ❑ A It is usually associated with an underlying medical condition
- ❑ B It occurs occasionally in the pre-school-age group
- ❑ C It can be precipitated by a child's refusal to use school toilets
- ❑ D It should be investigated with rectal biopsy to exclude Hirschsprung disease
- ❑ E It can always be resolved with a short course of laxatives and dietary advice

5.37 Which is the MOST appropriate statement about pancreatitis in childhood?

- ❑ A It is commonly caused by gallstones in children
- ❑ B It can be caused by treatment with sodium valproate
- ❑ C It is a common cause of admission to hospital with abdominal pain in childhood
- ❑ D A mildly raised amylase level associated with abdominal pain is specifically diagnostic of pancreatitis
- ❑ E A normal ultrasound examination of the pancreas excludes the diagnosis

5.38 A 5-month-old baby with pH study-proven gastro-oesophageal reflux has not improved on treatment with Gaviscon. The centile chart now shows that the weight gain is beginning to falter. What would be the next MOST appropriate stage of treatment?

- ❑ A Addition of an acid suppressant, eg proton pump inhibitor
- ❑ B Referral for fundoplication
- ❑ C Trial of hydrolysed formula milk
- ❑ D Use of prokinetic agent such as domperidone
- ❑ E Reassurance that, with weaning, symptoms should improve

5.39 A 30-month-old girl is referred to clinic with a 6-month history of passing up to five watery stools per day.

Mother is particularly concerned as there are frequently recognisable food particles in the stools. The child's centile charts reveal that she is steadily gaining weight along the 50th centile for both height and weight. Dietary history reveals that she is a slightly fussy eater, tending to graze throughout the day rather than eating three full meals. She drinks up to 2.5 l of fruit squash per day via a bottle. Examination is unremarkable.

Which is the MOST appropriate course of action?

- ❑ A Collection of a stool sample for detection of reducing substances and implementation of a lactose-free diet
- ❑ B Arrange blood tests for full blood count, total IgA and anti-gliadin antibodies
- ❑ C Microbiological analysis of stool sample (culture and virology assessment) to exclude infective diarrhoea
- ❑ D Advice about dietary intake, especially with regard to the amount and type of fluids being offered with further follow-up to assess weight gain
- ❑ E Assay for faecal elastase to rule out pancreatic insufficiency

Extended Matching Questions

5.40–5.42 Theme: Constipation

- ❑ A Functional constipation
- ❑ B Hirschsprung disease
- ❑ C Tethered cord syndrome (neuro-orthopaedic syndrome)
- ❑ D Group A streptococcal perianal infection
- ❑ E Cows' milk intolerance
- ❑ F Hypothyroidism

- ❑ G Meconium ileus
- ❑ H Distal intestinal obstruction syndrome
- ❑ I Coeliac disease
- ❑ J Anal fissure

Choose the most likely diagnosis from the list above for each of the three clinical scenarios described below. Each option may be used once, more than once or not at all.

5.40

An 8-month-old baby boy with a known small muscular ventricular septal defect is seen in the general paediatric outpatient clinic with a history of recurrent episodes of abdominal distension in association with infrequent passage of stool, which have been present since birth. His weight has fallen from the 25th centile at birth to the 2nd centile at present. His mother describes frequent episodes of vomiting which have not improved with anti-reflux therapy. The cardiologists do not feel that his poor weight gain is related to his cardiac abnormality.

5.41

A 2-day-old term baby girl, born at home with birth weight 2.75 kg, is referred by the community midwife with a history of bilious vomiting and failure to open her bowels since birth. On palpation of her abdomen, which is moderately distended, there is a palpable mass in the right iliac fossa. Abdominal radiograph shows distended small intestinal loops, with a lower gastrointestinal contrast study revealing a microcolon with pellet-like meconium in the terminal ileum.

5.42

A 9-year-old girl presents to the paediatric outpatient clinic with a history of secondary incontinence and constipation. She has previously been fit and well. She had been dry by day and night at the age of 2 years and had not previously had any constipation. She had experienced a decrease in the frequency of her bowel motions and increased episodes of urinary incontinence over the previous 6 months. She had never been a particularly active child but her mother had noticed a particular reluctance to walk long distances over the previous year, and thought that her decreased activity may have contributed to her constipation. On examination she had some mild asymmetry of her gluteal muscles and absence of her ankle reflexes.

5.43–5.45 Theme: The causes of dysphagia in childhood

- ❑ A Guillain–Barré syndrome
- ❑ B Ingestion of caustic substance, causing oesophageal stricture
- ❑ C Oesophageal obstruction secondary to a swallowed foreign body
- ❑ D Globus hystericus
- ❑ E Pharyngeal abscess
- ❑ F Oesophageal web
- ❑ G Eosinophilic oesophagitis
- ❑ H Oesophageal candidiasis
- ❑ I Duchenne muscular dystrophy
- ❑ J Oesophageal stricture secondary to gastro-oesophageal reflux disease

Choose the most appropriate diagnosis from the list above for each of the three clinical scenarios. Each option may be used once, more than once or not at all.

5.43

A 9-year-old boy presents to the paediatric outpatient clinic with a 3-month history of progressive dysphagia for solid food. He has no problems swallowing liquids but has changed his diet over the 3 months of symptoms to avoid meat and similar solid food. He describes a feeling of food sticking in his upper oesophagus, and sometimes will regurgitate food once he has swallowed it. He is generally fit and well but has a past history of atopy with childhood eczema and mild asthma, not currently needing regular inhaled steroids to achieve good control.

5.44

A 3-year-old boy with learning difficulties presents with a sudden onset of dysphagia for solid food. He has not had significant gastroenterological symptoms in the past and does not have a history of atopy. He is systemically well at presentation with no indication of infection or trauma. He will regurgitate any solid food after attempted swallowing but swallows liquids without any problems.

5.45

A 3-year-old girl with severe cerebral palsy presents with weight loss and increasing vomiting and discomfort associated with feeds. She has been fed a normal diet by her mother since weaning, with no long-term concerns about her ability to safely chew and swallow her food. She previously enjoyed meal times but has suffered from irritability and vomiting in the past, and was diagnosed and treated for as gastro-oesophageal reflux as an infant. Over the last year her symptoms of irritability have been treated with various courses of muscle relaxants and antacids without much success. Having previously managed to maintain a weight on the 5th centile, she has recently lost weight and is now well below the 0.4th centile. She vomits/regurgitates food shortly after it is swallowed but has no problems swallowing liquids.

5.46–5.48 Theme: Vomiting in childhood

- ☐ A Urinary tract infection
- ☐ B Acute gastroenteritis
- ☐ C Acute appendicitis
- ☐ D Pyloric stenosis
- ☐ E Gastro-oesophageal reflux disease
- ☐ F Volvulus secondary to malrotation
- ☐ G Cows' milk protein sensitivity
- ☐ H Necrotising enterocolitis
- ☐ I Intussusception
- ☐ J Meningitis

For each of the following clinical scenarios choose the most appropriate diagnosis from the list above. Each of the options may be used once, more than once or not at all.

5.46

A 2-week-old baby boy presents acutely unwell with a 12-hour history of bile-stained vomiting, shock and metabolic acidosis. He was born at term with a normal antenatal history and had thrived on formula milk since delivery, regaining his birth weight by day 5 of life. He had been completely well up until 12 hours previously when he became very distressed and vomited recurrently, initially milk followed by bile-stained fluid. He had had normal bowel motions up to that day with two soft stools per day and no evidence of any blood associated with the stools. There was no significant history of bowel problems in the family and no contacts with infective gastroenteritis.

5.47

A 4-week-old baby boy is seen in the paediatric assessment unit due to a history of vomiting. He is the first-born child of non-consanguineous white parents. He was born at term and had initially gained weight well on formula milk from birth. He developed vomiting, which was infrequent initially at the end of his third week of life. Over the next 6 days his vomiting increased in frequency and amount. It was not bilious in nature and no blood was seen. He is currently forcefully vomiting after every feed but appears hungry after feeds; although initially alert he has become sleepier and mildly jaundiced. His frequency of bowel motions has decreased and on admission he had lost 400 g of weight in 4 days. On initial investigation his bloods show a metabolic alkalosis.

5.48

An 8-month-old girl presents with a 24-hour history of recurrent episodes of diarrhoea and vomiting. She has an elder brother of 3 years who attends preschool who was sent home with similar symptoms 24 hours before the onset of her symptoms. She has had eight episodes of vomiting over the preceding 24 hours through the day and night. There has been no associated bile or blood in the vomit. She has had eight episodes of watery diarrhoea over the preceding 24 hours but has no blood or mucus associated. She has a pulse rate of 140 beats/min at rest and is apyrexial. She has sunken eyes and decreased skin turgor and has not had a wet nappy in 12 hours. She is awake but lethargic.

5.49–5.51 Theme: Milk feed products

- A EO28
- B Modulen
- C Infatrini
- D Neocate
- E Nutramigen
- F InfaSoy
- G Enfamil AR
- H Neutiprem 2
- I Maxijul
- J Aptamil infant formula

Which of the above formula milks/supplements is most appropriate for a trial of treatment in each of the following clinical scenarios? Each may be used once, more than once or not at all.

5.49

A 2-month-old child presents to the GP with concerns about frequent watery stools, vomiting, colic and faltering growth. The child was initially breastfed for 3 weeks but, due to concerns about milk supply, he was changed to formula milk after 3 weeks. Subsequently his frequency of bowel movements increased and he became much more unsettled with drawing up of his legs and vomiting associated with feeds. He has mild infantile eczema and has a family history of asthma. His father was diagnosed with cows' milk protein intolerance as a baby and had soya milk throughout his first year.

5.50

A 9-month-old girl was seen by her GP after a prolonged illness associated with diarrhoea. She had developed diarrhoea and vomiting and mild pyrexia 24 hours after her older brother was sent home from school with diarrhoea and vomiting. Subsequently her mother and father developed diarrhoea and vomiting, but symptoms in her brother and parents entirely resolved within 7 days. She was now well in herself and had no symptoms of vomiting but had persisting diarrhoea – watery bowel motions during the day but not at night after her milk feeds four times a day. Her symptoms are now in their third week; she has lost weight but is now eating and drinking well.

5.51

A 3-week-old baby with a significant ventricular septal defect (VSD) has cardiac failure. He is struggling to gain weight despite continuous nasogastric feeds because he will vomit feeds above 100 ml/kg per day even if given continuously. He is currently on SMA White formula at 100 ml/kg per day continuous feed and his weight has remained static for 7 days of this regimen. He doesn't have any family history or personal history of atopy. He needs to maximise his nutrition and growth before definitive surgery for correction of his VSD.

5.52–5.54 Theme: Failure to thrive/faltering growth

- ❑ A Low birthweight
- ❑ B Diet-related iron deficiency anaemia
- ❑ C Neglect leading to malnutrition
- ❑ D Constitutionally small
- ❑ E Cows' milk protein allergy
- ❑ F Inadequate intake of calories
- ❑ G Turner syndrome
- ❑ H Coeliac disease
- ❑ I Restricted diet leading to malnutrition
- ❑ J Cerebral palsy

For each of the following clinical scenarios please choose carefully the most appropriate diagnosis from the list above. Each of the options may be used once, more than once or not at all.

5.52

An 8-week-old baby girl is seen in a paediatric assessment unit; she has been referred by the health visitor due to concerns about her weight gain. She was the first child born to non-consanguineous parents at a gestational age of 34 weeks after the spontaneous onset of preterm labour. She was born on the 9th centile for weight and had experienced a straightforward clinical course requiring only tube feeding for the first week of life as breastfeeding was established. She was discharged on day 8 of life, after 48 hours of demand breastfeeding and had continued to be exclusively breastfed since discharge. She was feeding every 2–3 hours during the day and feeds lasted up to 45 minutes. She did not have vomiting or diarrhoea but was not very settled in herself. Her mid-parental height centile plotted on the 50th centile and she had gained weight slowly after an initial drop and was now just below the 0.4th centile.

5.53

An 18-month-old child is referred to the outpatient clinic with a history of poor weight gain. He was born at term as the first child of vegetarian parents and was breastfed from birth. Mum was very careful to continue her vitamin supplementation from pregnancy into her period of breastfeeding, and had taken advice on the nutritional adequacy of her diet during pregnancy and breastfeeding. He was born on the 75th centile for height and length and crossed over to the 91st centile during his initial 6 months of exclusive breastfeeding. He had complementary feeding introduced at 6 months and progressed well on to three meals a day, including meat, and continued vitamin supplementation as per WHO advice. Around this time he appeared to become less settled and had experienced symptoms of loose stools and bloating of his abdomen. His weight gain slowed down and he fell from the 91st centile to the 25th centile for weight, but maintained a length on the 75th centile. He has no specific family history of gastrointestinal problems or allergy/atopy. On investigation he was found to have iron deficiency anaemia.

5.54

A 2-year-old girl, Poppy, presents to the paediatric outpatient department as a referral from her health visitor due to concerns about poor weight gain. She has failed to present on two previous occasions and on this occasion is accompanied by her mother and a social worker. She is the fifth (and youngest) child of this mother and has one sibling 13 months older than she is. Her mother is a single parent with little support from the father of this child, either financially or emotionally. Poppy was born on the 5th centile at 37 weeks' gestation, she was bottle-fed from birth and thrived on the 25th centile for weight. Her mid-parental centile plots just above the 50th centile. She has drifted down from the 25th centile to just below the 0.4th centile since weaning. The referral from the health visitor states that Poppy's mum is very caring but the household is chaotic, with no set meal times and variable amounts of food available in the house at different times. On examination Poppy is clean and tidy and has no evidence of injury, eczematous changes or stigmata of chronic disease. She has very little subcutaneous fat and appears pale with some angular stomatitis.

5.55–5.57 Theme: Neonatal jaundice

- ❑ A Biliary atresia
- ❑ B ABO incompatibility
- ❑ C Breast milk jaundice
- ❑ D Congenital hypothyroidism
- ❑ E Idiopathic neonatal hepatitis
- ❑ F Rhesus haemolytic disease
- ❑ G Congenital cytomegalovirus infection
- ❑ H Glucose 6-phosphate dehydrogenase deficiency
- ❑ I Neonatal haemochromatosis
- ❑ J *Escherichia coli* septicaemia

Choose the most likely diagnosis from the list above for each of the three scenarios described below. Each option may be used once, more than once or not at all.

5.55

A 5-day-old term baby boy of Mediterranean parents is referred with jaundice and poor feeding. Total serum bilirubin is 380 μmol/l, conjugated fraction <10%. His full blood count reveals haemoglobin of 10 g/dl, white cell count 12 × 10^9/l, platelets 400 and CRP <10. Maternal blood group is A rhesus positive and baby is O rhesus positive. On examination, the baby is found to have splenomegaly.

5.56

A 6-week-old breast- and formula-fed baby girl, born at term to Asian parents after a delivery complicated by prolonged rupture of membranes, is seen by her GP for routine developmental assessment. She is gaining weight along the 2nd centile, consistent with her birthweight. She is noted by the GP to be jaundiced and to have hepatosplenomegaly on examination, but otherwise handles normally and does not appear acutely unwell. Since the introduction of formula 2 weeks ago, the parents comment that her stools appear lighter in colour.

5.57

A baby girl is delivered at 35 weeks due to poor CTG (cardiotocography) in association with intrauterine growth retardation. The baby is in poor condition at birth, requiring intubation. Hepatosplenomegaly and petechiae are noted on initial examination. Broad-spectrum antibiotics are commenced after blood cultures have been taken. The baby becomes jaundiced within 24 hours of delivery and elevated liver enzymes are noted on liver function testing. A CT scan of the brain is performed subsequently, revealing bright areas in the periventricular region.

5.58–5.60 Theme: Rectal bleeding

- ❑ A Gardner syndrome
- ❑ B Constipation with anal fissure
- ❑ C Ulcerative colitis
- ❑ D Intussusception
- ❑ E Hirschsprung enterocolitis
- ❑ F Meckel diverticulum
- ❑ G Crohn disease
- ❑ H Henoch–Schönlein purpura
- ❑ I Allergic colitis
- ❑ J Rectal polyp

Choose the most likely diagnosis from the list above for each of the three scenarios described below. Each option may be used once, more than once or not at all.

5.58

A 5-year-old boy is brought to accident and emergency with abdominal pains of recent onset and parents report passage of fresh red blood per rectum. He has also complained of a sore left ankle over the same period of time. Systemic examination reveals a well-grown child on the 75th centile for height and weight. There is a palpable non-blanching rash on the shins. No masses are palpable per abdomen.

5.59

A 2-year-old girl presents acutely to A&E with a massive, bright-red bleed per rectum. She was previously fit and well growing along the 50th centile with a normal bowel habit and no history of atopy or abnormal bleeding. She is tachycardic on presentation and requires resuscitation and transfusion within the first hour of her admission. She has not experienced any recent change in bowel habit, abdominal pain or previous episodes of rectal bleeding in the past.

5.60

An 8-month-old baby boy presents with a 6-hour history of recurrent vomiting, pallor, repeated episodic drawing up of legs and screaming, and the passage of bloody jelly-like stools into his nappy. He has been formula fed from birth and is thriving on the 75th percentile for weight and length. On examination he is tachycardic with a reduced peripheral capillary refill of 3 seconds, and has a sausage-shaped mass palpable in his abdomen.

CHAPTER 6

Haematology, Oncology and Poisoning

Multiple True–False Questions

6.1 Sickle cell disease

- ❑ A It is associated with an increased risk of gallstones
- ❑ B It is associated with an increased risk of nocturnal enuresis
- ❑ C It can be diagnosed antenatally
- ❑ D It is an indication for prophylactic penicillin
- ❑ E It is associated with episodes of acute anaemia

6.2 Neonatal thrombocytopenia

- ❑ A It is an indication for cerebral ultrasound
- ❑ B It is an absolute indication for platelet transfusion after delivery
- ❑ C It may be caused by toxoplasmosis infection during pregnancy
- ❑ D It can occur in infants born to mothers with systemic lupus erythematosus
- ❑ E It may be associated with absent radii

6.3 Causes of neutropenia include

- ❑ A Hyperglycinaemia
- ❑ B Cytotoxic drug therapy
- ❑ C Chronic granulomatous disease
- ❑ D Kostmann syndrome
- ❑ E X-linked hypogammaglobulinaemia

6.4 Causes of bone pain and anaemia include

- ❑ A Vitamin C deficiency
- ❑ B Neuroblastoma
- ❑ C Langerhans cell histiocytosis
- ❑ D Acute lymphoblastic leukaemia
- ❑ e Sickle cell disease

6.5 Features of acute lymphoblastic leukaemia in childhood include

- ❑ A An incidence of 1 in 3500 in the first 10 years of life
- ❑ B Fever at presentation
- ❑ C Neutropenia
- ❑ D A better prognosis if the age is <2 years at presentation
- ❑ E Long-term survival in 80%

6.6 Aplastic anaemia can occur secondary to

- ❑ A Radiation
- ❑ B Chloramphenicol
- ❑ C Hepatitis A
- ❑ D Epstein–Barr virus
- ❑ E Parvovirus infection

6.7 Diseases with an increased risk of malignancy include

- ❑ A Ataxia telangiectasia
- ❑ B Bloom syndrome
- ❑ C Xeroderma pigmentosum
- ❑ D Down syndrome
- ❑ E Fanconi anaemia

6.8 Causes of a prolonged bleeding time include

- ❑ A Bernard–Soulier syndrome
- ❑ B Henoch–Schönlein syndrome
- ❑ C Haemophilia
- ❑ D Von Willebrand disease
- ❑ E Idiopathic thrombocytopenic purpura

Best of Five Questions

6.9 With regard to features of TAR syndrome, select the MOST appropriate.

- ❑ A X-linked inheritance
- ❑ B Normal platelet count
- ❑ C T-cell defect
- ❑ D Death from acute haemorrhage in late childhood
- ❑ E Digit deformities

6.10 With regard to tumour lysis syndrome, select the MOST appropriate statement.

- ❑ A It is more common in patients with a low tumour burden
- ❑ B Metabolic complications include hypokalaemia and hypercalcaemia
- ❑ C Treatment includes hyper hydration
- ❑ D Packed red blood cell transfusions are often indicated
- ❑ E Potassium should be added to all fluids

6.11 Concerning Hodgkin lymphoma, select the MOST appropriate statement

- ❑ A Lymphadenopathy is rare
- ❑ B Presentation tends to be in early childhood
- ❑ C More common in girls
- ❑ D Mediastinal masses can lead to airway obstruction
- ❑ E Bone marrow involvement occurs in >50% of patients

6.12 Chemotherapy side effects. Which of these statements is the MOST likely?

- ❑ A Asparginase leads to neurotoxicity
- ❑ B Vincristine leads to bladder toxicity
- ❑ C Cyclophosphamide leads to late effects on fertility
- ❑ D Bleomycin leads to encephalopathy
- ❑ E Asparginase leads to pulmonary toxicity

6.13 Glanzmann thrombasthenia. Select the MOST appropriate statement.

- ❑ A It is inherited as an autosomal dominant
- ❑ B Its gene locus is known
- ❑ C The platelet count is low
- ❑ D It requires long-term steroid treatment
- ❑ E Splenectomy may be beneficial

6.14 Concerning features of hereditary spherocytosis, select the MOST appropriate.

- ❑ A Splenomegaly
- ❑ B Conjugated hyperbilirubinaemia
- ❑ C Short stature
- ❑ D Haemolytic crises following fava bean ingestion
- ❑ E X-linked inheritance

6.15 Concerning vitamin B_{12}, select the MOST appropriate statement.

- ❑ A Deficiency can cause ataxia
- ❑ B Pernicious anaemia commonly occurs following terminal ileal resection
- ❑ C In deficiency the mean corpuscular volume is usually normal
- ❑ D Deficiency usually occurs in untreated coeliac disease
- ❑ E Extrinsic factor promotes absorption

6.16 Concerning rhesus haemolytic disease, select the MOST appropriate statement.

- ❑ A It cannot occur in first born children
- ❑ B It occurs as a consequence of the transplacental passage of IgM
- ❑ C The most common antibody type is anti-C
- ❑ D It can present as hydrops fetalis
- ❑ E It is an indication for elective caesarean section

6.17 In the case of anaemia of chronic disease, select the MOST appropriate statement.

- ❑ A The haemoglobin is usually <8 g/dl
- ❑ B The total iron binding capacity is raised
- ❑ C The anaemia is usually normocytic
- ❑ D The serum iron is usually increased
- ❑ E Iron supplements are contraindicated

6.18 Concerning blood transfusion, select the MOST appropriate statement.

- ❑ A Pyrexia is an absolute indication for stopping the transfusion
- ❑ B Back pain may be a symptom of severe transfusion reaction
- ❑ C Hypokalaemia is a well-recognised complication
- ❑ D White cell filters should be used for a patient's first transfusion
- ❑ E Hydrocortisone and antihistamines stop severe transfusion reactions in patients having regular transfusions

6.19 Thrombocytosis (platelet count >400 × 109/l) is MOST likely to be seen in which of the following.

- ☐ A The first week of Kawasaki disease
- ☐ B Aplastic anaemia
- ☐ C Post-splenectomy patients
- ☐ D Bernard–Soulier syndrome
- ☐ E Juvenile idiopathic arthritis

6.20 Concerning X-linked agammaglobulinaemia, select the MOST appropriate statement.

- ☐ A The gene locus is unknown
- ☐ B The thymus is hypoplastic or absent
- ☐ C T-cell function is abnormal
- ☐ D IgA, IgG and IgM are all reduced
- ☐ E Intravenous immunoglobulin therapy is not indicated

6.21 With regard to Di George syndrome, select the MOST appropriate statement.

- ☐ A Inheritance is autosomal recessive
- ☐ B The thymus is hyperplastic
- ☐ C It is associated with cardiac defects
- ☐ D The lymphocyte count is always reduced
- ☐ E Hypercalcaemia is common

6.22 Regarding osteosarcoma, select the MOST appropriate statement.

- ☐ A Usually presents in the first decade
- ☐ B Outcome <10% survival overall
- ☐ C Usually occurs in the metaphyseal region of growing bones
- ☐ D Lung metastasis at presentation occur in 80%
- ☐ E Fever at presentation is common

6.23 In accidental iron ingestion. What is MOST likely to occur?

- ☐ A Hypertension within 2 hours of ingestion
- ☐ B Hepatic necrosis within 30 minutes of ingestion
- ☐ C Haematemesis within 2 hours of ingestion
- ☐ D Pyloric stenosis 2 days after ingestion
- ☐ E Lactic acidosis within the first 2 hours

6.24 Carbon monoxide: select the MOST appropriate statement.

- ☐ A CO combines with haemoglobin to form carboxyhaemoglobin
- ☐ B CO shifts the oxygen dissociation curve to the right
- ☐ C CO toxicity occurs if the carboxyhaemoglobin level is 3–5%
- ☐ D Acute CO toxicity can cause neuropsychiatric problems
- ☐ E CO increases the oxygen-carrying capacity of the blood

6.25 In an overdose of tricyclic antidepressants, select the MOST likely.

- ☐ A Bradycardia precedes coma
- ☐ B Dialysis is effective at removing the drug
- ☐ C Cardiac arrhythmias are atrial and unlikely to cause significant clinical features
- ☐ D The pupils are constricted
- ☐ E Multiple doses of charcoal therapy can be used

6.26 Concerning aspirin overdose, select the MOST appropriate statement.

- ☐ A Gastric lavage and activated charcoal have no place in the management
- ☐ B Hyperkalaemia can occur
- ☐ C Hypoventilation is common
- ☐ D Normal biochemistry at 4 hours excludes significant overdose
- ☐ E Deafness is a recognised complication

6.27 Lead poisoning: what is MOST likely to occur?

- ☐ A Haematemesis
- ☐ B Encephalopathy
- ☐ C Thrombocytosis
- ☐ D Greying of the skin
- ☐ E Obesity

6.28 With regard to typical feature of sickle cell anaemia, select the MOST appropriate.

- ☐ A Massive splenomegaly at the age of 10 years
- ☐ B Short stature
- ☐ C Presentation in the first month of life
- ☐ D Increased susceptibility to group B streptococcal infections
- ☐ E Increased susceptibility to malaria

6.29 With regard to good prognostic signs in acute lymphoblastic leukaemia, select the MOST appropriate.

- ❑ A Less than 2 years at presentation
- ❑ B Male sex
- ❑ C High white cell count at diagnosis
- ❑ D Common cell type ALL
- ❑ E Mediastinal widening in chest radiograph

6.30 An otherwise well 2 year old presents with extreme pallor. Growth and development are normal. The child is pale but there is no lymphadenopathy or splenomegaly. Full blood count shows haemoglobin 4 g/dl (40 g/l), MCV 59. Other indices are normal. The MOST appropriate management is:

- ❑ A Start gluten-free diet
- ❑ B Small bowel technetium scan
- ❑ C Chelation therapy for lead
- ❑ D Bone marrow aspirate
- ❑ E Dietary review

6.31 In a child presenting with lymphadenopathy, which of the following is the BEST indicator of need for excision node biopsy?

- ❑ A Multiple anterior cervical nodes
- ❑ B Single supraclavicular node
- ❑ C Associated chronic fatigue
- ❑ D Post-auricular nodes
- ❑ E Known to have congenital heart disease

6.32 In chronic lead poisoning, what is MOST likely to occur?

- ❑ A Macrocytic anaemia
- ❑ B Osteomalacia
- ❑ C Pulmonary fibrosis
- ❑ D Cardiomyopathy
- ❑ E Delayed developmental milestones

Extended Matching Questions

6.33–6.35 Theme: Thrombocytopenia

- ❑ A Acute idiopathic thrombocytopenia purpura
- ❑ B Aplastic anaemia
- ❑ C Kassabach–Merrit syndrome
- ❑ D Wiskott–Aldrich syndrome
- ❑ E Acute lymphoblastic leukaemia
- ❑ F Folate deficiency
- ❑ G Langerhans cell histiocytosis
- ❑ H Disseminated intravascular coagulopathy

Choose the most likely diagnosis from the list above for each of the three descriptions below. Each option may be used once, more than once or not at all.

6.33

X-linked condition, associated with eczema and immunodeficiency. Platelet count is low and platelet size is also reduced.

6.34

Immune-mediated self-limiting condition. Haemoglobin and white cell count is normal, with platelet life span being shortened.

6.35

Low platelets, raised fibrin products, prolonged prothrombin time and partial thromboplastin time in a patient with widespread burns.

6.36–6.38 Theme: Anaemia

- ❑ A Iron deficiency anaemia
- ❑ B β Thalassaemia
- ❑ C Sickle cell disease
- ❑ D Glucose-6-phosphate dehydrogenase deficiency
- ❑ E Hereditary spherocytosis
- ❑ F Aplastic anaemia
- ❑ G Vitamin B_{12} deficiency
- ❑ H Diamond–Blackfan anaemia

Choose the most likely diagnosis from the list above for each of the three scenarios described below. Each option may be used once, more than once or not at all.

6.36

An 18-month-old child from the eastern Mediterranean presents with failure to thrive, hypochromic/microcytic anaemia and raised serum ferritin. Iron studies are normal.

6.37

An 18-month-old child with anaemia – hypochromic/microcytic. Other results show a low serum ferritin, low serum iron and increased total iron binding capacity.

6.38

An 18-month-old child presents acutely pale and jaundiced; his mother notes that she had given him broad beans for the first time and she recalls her grandfather had been unwell with these. Bloods show a low haemoglobin.

6.39–6.41 Theme: Common childhood cancers

- ❑ A Acute lymphoblastic leukaemia
- ❑ B Acute myeloid leukaemia
- ❑ C Non-Hodgkin lymphoma
- ❑ D Neuroblastoma
- ❑ E Medulloblastoma
- ❑ F Wilms tumour
- ❑ G Retinoblastoma
- ❑ H Osteosarcoma

Choose the most likely diagnosis from the list. Each option may be used once, more than once or not at all.

6.39

Embryonal tumour derived from neural crest tissue.

6.40

Embryonal tumour of the kidney.

6.41

Primitive neuroectodermal tumour occurring in the cerebellum.

6.42–6.44 Theme: Coagulopathy

- ❑ A Antiphospholipid antibody syndrome
- ❑ B Von Willebrand disease
- ❑ C Haemophilia A
- ❑ D Factor V Leiden
- ❑ E Protein C deficiency
- ❑ F Vitamin K deficiency
- ❑ G Antithrombin III deficiency

Choose the most likely diagnosis from the list above for each of the three descriptions below. Each option may be used once, more than once or not at all.

6.42

Autosomal dominant bleeding tendency, caused by an abnormality on chromosome 12. Equally common in boys and girls. Normal prothrombin time, prolonged bleeding time.

6.43

Hereditary prothrombotic disorder that caused activated protein C resistance.

6.44

X-linked bleeding disorder; can commonly lead to haemarthroses. Prolonged activated partial thromboplastin time but normal bleeding time.

6.45–6.47 Theme: Presenting symptoms of paediatric malignancies

- ❑ A Wilms tumour
- ❑ B Medulloblastoma
- ❑ C ALL
- ❑ D Osteosarcoma
- ❑ E Rhabdomyosarcoma
- ❑ F Hepatoblastoma
- ❑ G Hodgkin lymphoma
- ❑ H Histiocytosis X

Choose the most likely diagnosis from the list above for each of the three scenarios described below. Each option may be used once, more than once or not at all.

6.45

Acute limp.

6.46

Proptosis.

6.47

Pleomorphic rash.

6.48–6.50 Theme: Signs of poisoning

- ❑ A Mydriasis
- ❑ B Bradycardia
- ❑ C Haematemesis
- ❑ D Hyperacusis
- ❑ E Pruritus
- ❑ F Hyperventilation
- ❑ G Chorea
- ❑ H Abnormal odour

Choose the most likely sign from the list above for each of the three drug poisonings described below. Each option may be used once, more than once or not at all.

6.48

Iron.

6.49

Aspirin.

6.50

Tricyclic antidepressants.

CHAPTER 7

Infectious Diseases and Immunology

Multiple True–False Questions

7.1 Signs and symptoms of IgE-mediated food allergy include

- ❑ A Acute urticaria
- ❑ B Acute angio-oedema
- ❑ C Vomiting
- ❑ D Diarrhoea
- ❑ E Sneezing

7.2 Recognised causes of low immunoglobulins include

- ❑ A Nephrotic syndrome
- ❑ B Carbamazepine
- ❑ C Systemic lupus erythematosus
- ❑ D Primary intestinal lymphangiectasia
- ❑ E Congenital toxoplasmosis

7.3 The following are still notifiable diseases

- ❑ A Ophthalmia neonatorum
- ❑ B Leptospirosis
- ❑ C Relapsing fever
- ❑ D Dysentery
- ❑ E Mumps

7.4 With regard to anaphylaxis in children

- ☐ A Risk of death is increased in those with pre-existing asthma
- ☐ B Risk of death is increased by a delay in treatment with adrenaline
- ☐ C Subcutaneous adrenaline is indicated
- ☐ D Intramuscular adrenaline is indicated
- ☐ E Drug allergy is the most common cause

7.5 Concerning schistosomiasis

- ☐ A The intermediate host is a snail
- ☐ B Infected larvae are found in salt water
- ☐ C It causes an esinophilia
- ☐ D It can be diagnosed by stool culture
- ☐ E It can be diagnosed by urine culture

7.6 The following infections occur as a result of consuming unpasteurised milk or milk products

- ☐ A Brucellosis
- ☐ B Legionnaires disease
- ☐ C Listeria infection
- ☐ D Atypical mycobacterial infection
- ☐ E Campylobacter infection

7.7 Enteroviruses

- ☐ A They cause myocarditis
- ☐ B They cause hand, foot and mouth disease
- ☐ C They cause Guillain–Barré syndrome
- ☐ D They cause encephalitis
- ☐ E They are DNA viruses

7.8 Causes of recurrent bacterial meningitis include

- ☐ A Cranial dural defects
- ☐ B Spinal dural defects
- ☐ C Asplenia
- ☐ D Complement deficiencies
- ☐ E T-cell abnormalities

7.9 Features suggestive of a humoral immunodeficiency

- ❑ A Oesophageal candidiasis
- ❑ B Frequent urinary tract infection
- ❑ C Chronic diarrhoea with failure to thrive
- ❑ D Recurrent skin abscesses
- ❑ E Recurrent cold sores

7.10 Which of the following statements about cerebrospinal fluid (CSF) are correct:

- ❑ A A normal CSF glucose excludes bacterial meningitis
- ❑ B Red cells are a normal finding in the CSF of a child over the age of 6 years
- ❑ C CSF protein is higher in the neonate than in the older child
- ❑ D A spinal cord tumour can cause a lymphocytosis
- ❑ E The white cell count is always raised in bacterial meningitis

Best of Five Questions

7.11 A 2-year-old girl presents with a mild fever and an erythematous rash on her cheeks. The rash spreads to the trunk and persists for several days. What is the BEST advice?

- ❑ A This is a very mild childhood illness in healthy children
- ❑ B Avoid pregnant women, immunocompromised patients and those with haematological conditions
- ❑ C Exclude from nursery for 7 days after onset of rash
- ❑ D Blood testing is recommended to confirm diagnosis
- ❑ E None of the above

7.12 A 13-month-old boy has a high fever for 6 days, conjunctivitis, a macular rash and is miserable. He has induration at the site of his BCG scar. What is the MOST likely diagnosis?

- ❑ A Rubella
- ❑ B Measles
- ❑ C Kawasaki disease
- ❑ D Streptococcal infection
- ❑ E Toxic shock syndrome

7.13 A 6-year-old boy is involved in a road traffic accident and requires a splenectomy. What is the BEST advice to avoid future pneumococcal infections?

- ☐ A Recommend immunisation with 7-valent pneumococcal conjugate vaccine (PCV)
- ☐ B Recommend immunisation with 13-valent PCV
- ☐ C Recommend immunisation with 23-valent pneumococcal poysaccharide vaccine (PPV)
- ☐ D Treat suspected bacterial sepsis early and with intravenous antibiotics
- ☐ E None of the above

7.14 A 29-week gestation baby on the neonatal intensive care unit is 8/52 old. With regard to childhood immunisations, what is the BEST advice to give to parents?

- ☐ A Immunise at term
- ☐ B Immunise now
- ☐ C Immunise just before discharge from neonatal unit
- ☐ D Warn parents of the increased risk of side effects from immunisations in preterm infants
- ☐ E Immunise at corrected gestational age of 2 months

7.15 A 1-year-old boy from eastern Europe emigrates to the UK. He is suspected of exposure to mumps. He is otherwise well and thriving. Parents are unsure about his MMR status. What is the next BEST step?

- ☐ A Vaccinate with the MMR immunisation
- ☐ B Vaccinate with the single measles and rubella immunisations
- ☐ C Check mumps serology
- ☐ D Advise against the MMR immunisation
- ☐ E None of the above

7.16 A 6-year-old boy is seen at his GP surgery with a rapidly spreading non-blanching rash, fever of 38°C, heart rate 170 beats/min, central refill time 4 seconds. He is given intramuscular benzylpenicillin by his GP before being brought into hospital by an ambulance. Which investigation is most likely to lead to a diagnosis?

- ☐ A Lumbar puncture sending CSF off for microscopy, culture and sensitivity (MC&S)
- ☐ B Blood culture for MC&S
- ☐ C Pneumococcal urinary antigen
- ☐ D Meningococcal PCR (polymerase chain reaction)
- ☐ E None of the above

7.17 A 10-year-old girl is brought into hospital after a camping trip in the New Forest. She has developed a ring-like rash on her leg. What is the next best step?

- ☐ A Take blood for borrelia serology
- ☐ B Prescribe amoxicillin (if she is not penicillin allergic)
- ☐ C Prescribe an antihistamine
- ☐ D Prescribe doxycyline
- ☐ E Take acute and convalescent borrelia serology and arrange outpatient follow-up

7.18 A 3-year-old boy develops chickenpox. He complains of severe and increasing pain in his leg. There is rapidly developing erythema and discoloration of the skin. What is the most likely aetiology?

- ☐ A *Staphylococcus aureus*
- ☐ B Group A streptococcus
- ☐ C Staphylococcal toxin
- ☐ D Disseminated intravascular coagulation
- ☐ E *Staphylococcus epidermidis*

7.19 A 12-year-old girl presents with upper respiratory tract symptoms and a high fever for 3 days followed by erythema and swelling around the left eye. She complains of double vision. What is the next BEST step?

- ☐ A Commence oral antibiotics
- ☐ B Prescribe oral antihistamines
- ☐ C Commence intravenous antibiotics and organise urgent CT scan of head
- ☐ D Refer for ophthalmology outpatient assessment
- ☐ E Reassess after 48 hours of intravenous antibiotics

7.20 A 7-year-old child with sickle cell disease develops a painful limp with restriction of hip movement. Two days previously he had a sore throat and fever. He now has a normal hip ultrasound scan.

WBC 26 × 10^9/l

Neutrophils 24.9 × 10^9/l

Hb 9.7 g/dl

ESR 87

CRP 110

What is the MOST likely diagnosis?

- ❑ A Septic arthritis
- ❑ B Avascular necrosis of femoral head
- ❑ C Post-streptococcal arthritis
- ❑ D Irritable hip
- ❑ E Salmonella osteomyelitis

7.21 A 7-year-old develops a fever with sore throat, cervical lymphadenopathy and palatal petechiae. The monospot test is negative. Which investigation is most likely to lead to a diagnosis?

- ❑ A CMV (cytomegalovirus) in urine
- ❑ B Blood film
- ❑ C EBV (Epstein–Barr virus) serology
- ❑ D Throat swab for MC&S
- ❑ E Blood culture for MC&S

7.22 A 16-year-old girl develops tender, raised, purple lesions on her shins in addition to persistent cervical lymphadenopathy. She has a new kitten. She is on the oral contraceptive pill. What is the most likely cause of her lesions?

- ❑ A Streptococcal infection
- ❑ B Epstein–Barr virus
- ❑ C Oral contraceptive pill
- ❑ D *Bartonella henselae*
- ❑ E Tuberculosis

7.23 An otherwise healthy 3-year-old developed a persistent submandibular swelling with no systemic symptoms or fever and has a normal white count. Treatment with co-amoxiclav was not beneficial. Needle aspiration resulted in formation of a fistula. What is the most likely diagnosis?

- ☐ A *Mycobacterium tuberculosis*
- ☐ B Cat-scratch disease
- ☐ C Lymphoma
- ☐ D Atypical mycobacterial infection
- ☐ E Adenovirus

7.24 A baby is born with growth retardation, microcephaly, hepatosplenomegaly and petechiae. Cranial ultrasound scan demonstrates hydrocephalus. What is the most likely diagnosis?

- ☐ A Congenital rubella
- ☐ B Congenital syphilis
- ☐ C Congenital toxoplasmosis
- ☐ D Congenital CMV
- ☐ E Congenital herpes simplex virus

7.25 A toddler presents with a 3-day history of high fever. He develops a truncal rash that appears when the fever settles. He has a simple febrile convulsion. What is the MOST likely diagnosis?

- ☐ A Meningococcal septicaemia
- ☐ B Parvovirus B19
- ☐ C Human herpesvirus 6 (HHV-6)
- ☐ D Adenovirus
- ☐ E Enterovirus

7.26 A 5-year-old child presents with chronic diarrhoea, generalised lymphadenopathy, oral candida infection and bilateral parotitis. What is the MOST likely diagnosis?

- ☐ A Acute leukaemia
- ☐ B Chronic granulomatous disease
- ☐ C Di George syndrome
- ☐ D HIV
- ☐ E Wiscott–Aldrich syndrome

7.27 A mother who is hepatitis B positive asks you about the risk of vertical transmission. She is HBsAg positive, HBeAg negative and anti-e antibody positive. What is the best advice?

- ❑ A The risk of transmission is 90%
- ❑ B The baby should receive both the hepatitis B immunisation (at birth, 1 and 6 months) and hepatitis B immunoglobulin
- ❑ C The baby should receive only hepatitis B immunoglobulin at birth
- ❑ D The baby should receive only hepatitis B immunisation (at birth, 1 and 6 months)
- ❑ E Hepatitis B immunoglobulin should be given within 72 hours of birth

7.28 After travel to India, a child develops massive splenomegaly, pancytopenia and hepatic failure. She has very dry skin and her skin is dark in places. What is the MOST likely diagnosis?

- ❑ A Schistosomiasis
- ❑ B Malaria
- ❑ C Epstein–Barr virus
- ❑ D Brucellosis
- ❑ E Visceral leishmaniasis

7.29 A primary school trip is planned to a petting farm. Many parents have expressed concerns about farm-related infections. What is the BEST advice to give after handling animals at the farm?

- ❑ A Hand gels alone are adequate protection
- ❑ B Handwashing with water is sufficient
- ❑ C Handwashing with hot running water and soap is sufficient
- ❑ D Handwashing with hot running water and soap, drying followed by sanitising hand gels may provide extra benefit
- ❑ E Hand wipes alone are adequate protection

7.30 A 13-year-old girl returns from a holiday to Africa. She has a fever, lethargy, headache, myalgia and diarrhoea. What is the best NEXT investigation?

- ❑ A Throat swab for MC&S
- ❑ B Stool for microscopy, culture, ova, cysts and parasites
- ❑ C Rapid influenza diagnostic test (RIDT)
- ❑ D Lumbar puncture
- ❑ E Thick and thin films

7.31 A 7-year-old Indian child is confirmed as having vivax malaria. What is the BEST next step?

- ❑ A Contact a specialist for advice (Tropical Disease Centre or Infectious disease unit)
- ❑ B Start intravenous quinine as sole therapy
- ❑ C Start chloroquine as sole therapy
- ❑ D Start chloroquine and then test for G6PD before starting an appropriate treatment course
- ❑ E Start chloroquine and primaquine treatment

7.32 A 2-year-old child with hypopigmented skin and photosensitivity has recurrent skin abscesses and bruises. What may be seen on ophthalmological examination that confirms the diagnosis?

- ❑ A Bilateral ptosis
- ❑ B Partial oculocutaneous albinism
- ❑ C Glaucoma
- ❑ D Macular degeneration
- ❑ E Cherry-red spot

7.33 A 3-year-old boy presents with a persistent fever and right upper quadrant pain. He previously had osteomyelitis aged 6 months. Ultrasonography confirms a liver abscess. Which investigation is MOST likely to lead to the diagnosis?

- ❑ A Liver aspirate/biopsy for histological analysis
- ❑ B Immunoglobulin quantification
- ❑ C Nitroblue tetrazolium test (NBT)
- ❑ D Magnetic resonance imaging (MRI) of the liver
- ❑ E Aspiration of abscess with culture of aspirate

7.34 A 15-year-old patient with Crohn disease is about to start infliximab (Remicade) treatment. What is the BEST advice to give about the drug?

- ❑ A It is a type of protein that recognises, attaches and blocks a substance in your body called tumour necrosis factor (TNF) Blocking TNF may reduce inflammation but may also reduce the body's ability to fight infection
- ❑ B Common side effects include sinus infection and sore throat
- ❑ C It is given by subcutaneous injection
- ❑ D It is given by intravenous injection
- ❑ E If you develop a fever, bruise or bleed easily or look very pale call a doctor urgently

7.35 A 9-year-old girl complains of fever, weight loss and lack of appetite. She complains of lethargy and aches for months. Her school performance has deteriorated. She develops a photosensitive rash and presents to outpatients. Which investigation is MOST likely to lead to the diagnosis?

- ❑ A Thyroid function test
- ❑ B Upper and lower endoscopy with biopsy
- ❑ C Anti nuclear antibodies (ANAs)
- ❑ D Anti-double-stranded DNA
- ❑ E Coeliac screen

7.36 A child is at a birthday party when she suddenly complains of an itchy tongue, starts scratching her throat, sneezes, develops lip swelling, difficulty swallowing and urticaria. On arrival of the paramedics, what is the next BEST step?

- ❑ A Give oral piriton
- ❑ B Give intramuscular antihistamine
- ❑ C Give subcutaneous adrenaline
- ❑ D Give intravenous adrenaline
- ❑ E Give intramuscular adrenaline

7.37 A child has recurrent staphylococcal infections, an eczema-like rash, a history of staphylococcal lung infections and two sets of teeth simultaneously. What is the MOST likely diagnosis?

- ❑ A Chronic granulomatous disease
- ❑ B Wiscott–Aldrich disease
- ❑ C Hyper-IgE syndrome
- ❑ D Severe combined deficiency disease (SCID)
- ❑ E X-linked agammaglobulinaemia

7.38 A sibling of an inpatient on a ward with several immunosuppressed children visits and plays with the other patients. The following day she develops the first crop of chickenpox lesions. What is the BEST management?

- ❑ A Varicella zoster immunoglobulin (VzIg) to the high-risk contacts
- ❑ B Immunise the child herself
- ❑ C Immunise the at-risk children
- ❑ D Oral aciclovir to the high-risk children
- ❑ E No immediate action needed; observe for signs in the high-risk children

Extended Matching Questions

7.39–7.41 Theme: Primary immunodeficiencies

- ☐ A C1–4 complement deficiency
- ☐ B Chronic granulomatous disease (CGD)
- ☐ C Chronic mucocutaneous candidiasis
- ☐ D Common variable immunodeficiency (CVID)
- ☐ E Di George syndrome
- ☐ F Leukocyte adhesion deficiency
- ☐ G Selective Ig A deficiency
- ☐ H Severe combined immunodeficiency (SCID)
- ☐ I Wiscott–Aldrich syndrome
- ☐ J X-linked agammaglobulinaemia (Bruton disease)

Choose the most likely diagnosis from the list above for each of the three descriptions below. Each option may be used once, more than once or not at all.

7.39

A 2-month-old baby presents with chronic diarrhoea and failure to thrive. A chest radiograph is indicative of a viral pneumonitis and the thymus is absent.

7.40

A 4-month-old boy develops a staphylococcal pneumonia. The thymus is present.

7.41

A 4-year-old child with recurrent pneumococcal chest infections, chronic diarrhoea and malabsorption with lymphadenopathy and splenomegaly; reduced IgA and IgG, normal IgM.

7.42–7.44 Theme: Respiratory infections

- ❑ A *Chlamydia trachomatis*
- ❑ B Group B streptococcus
- ❑ C *Haemophilus influenzae*
- ❑ D *Mycoplasma pneumoniae*
- ❑ E Parainfluenza
- ❑ F Pertussis
- ❑ G *Pneumocystis jiroveci* (PCP – formerly named *P carinii*)
- ❑ H Respiratory syncytial virus (RSV) bronchiolitis
- ❑ I *Streptococcus pneumoniae* (pneumococcus)
- ❑ J Tuberculosis

Choose the most appropriate diagnosis from the list above for each of the three scenarios described below. Each option may be used once, more than once or not at all.

7.42

A 6-month-old ex preterm born at 29 weeks' gestation infant develops shortness of breath, recession and poor feeding over Christmas. On auscultation there are bilateral crackles and wheeze.

7.43

A 3-week-old baby with conjunctivitis presents with a paroxysmal cough and tachypnoea. She is afebrile and has scattered crackles but no wheeze.

7.44

A 4-month-old baby has respiratory distress. Temperature 37.5°C, respiratory rate 70, saturations in air 80%. Lactate dehydrogenase (LDH) is elevated. Mother is receiving medical treatment.

7.45–7.47 Theme: Rashes

- ☐ A Adenovirus
- ☐ B Cytomegalovirus (CMV)
- ☐ C Coxsackie virus
- ☐ D Epstein–Barr virus (EBV)
- ☐ E Herpes simplex virus (HSV)
- ☐ F Measles
- ☐ G Parvovirus
- ☐ H Rubella
- ☐ I Toxoplasmosis
- ☐ J Varicella virus

Choose the most appropriate diagnosis from the list above for each of the three scenarios described below. Each option may be used once, more than once or not at all.

7.45

A 3-year-old has a generalised maculopapular rash with conjunctivitis, rhinorrhoea, red lips and lesions on his inner cheeks.

7.46

A neonate develops a vesicular rash over her fetal scalp sampling area. She then feeds poorly and becomes lethargic.

7.47

A 2-day-old baby develops a vesicular rash. Her mother has had a recent febrile illness and crops of papules that are now forming blisters.

7.48–7.50 Theme: Fever

- ❑ A Adenovirus
- ❑ B Cytomegalovirus (CMV)
- ❑ C Epstein–Barr virus (EBV)
- ❑ D Scarlet fever
- ❑ E Influenza B
- ❑ F Juvenile idiopathic arthritis
- ❑ G Kawasaki disease
- ❑ H Measles
- ❑ I Rubella
- ❑ J Rheumatic fever

Choose the most appropriate diagnosis from the list above for each of the three scenarios described below. Each option may be used once, more than once or not at all.

7.48

A 14-year-old has a high fever, cough, muscle aches, sudden onset of extreme fatigue and diarrhoea.

7.49

An 18-month-old child who has not been immunised develops a rash starting on her face. which then spreads to the rest of her body. She is febrile with painful lymphadenopathy including suboccipital nodes.

7.50

A 7-year-old has a high fever, a strawberry tongue and a sandpaper-like rash on her trunk and upper arms.

7.51–7.53 Theme: Treatments

- ❑ A Aciclovir
- ❑ B Amoxicillin or doxycycline depending on age
- ❑ C Amphotericin
- ❑ D Chloroquine followed by primaquine
- ❑ E Co-trimoxazole
- ❑ F Ganciclovir
- ❑ G Isoniazid, rifampicin, ethambutol, pyrazinamide
- ❑ H Praziquantel
- ❑ I Quinine
- ❑ J Sodium stibogluconate

Choose the most appropriate treatment from the list above for each of the three scenarios described below. Each option may be used once, more than once or not at all.

7.51

A neonate is born with microcephaly, periventricular calcification and chorioretinitis. Which treatment option should be considered?

7.52

A 7-year-old presents with fevers, night sweats and unexplained weight loss. He visited his family in Pakistan in the summer.

7.53

A 15-year-old presents with dysuria, frequency and gross haematuria. Her symptoms have not improved on admission. She has been on a watersports holiday in Malawi.

7.54–7.56 Theme: Investigations

- ☐ A Blood culture for microscopy, sensitivity and culture
- ☐ B Bronchoscopy
- ☐ C Coagulation studies
- ☐ D HIV antibody test
- ☐ E Immunoglobulins
- ☐ F Meningococcal PCR
- ☐ G Oral fluid (saliva) swab for serology/PCR
- ☐ H Sweat test
- ☐ I Viral culture of urine
- ☐ J None of the above

Choose the most discriminating investigation to aid diagnosis from the list above for each of the three scenarios described below. Each option may be used once, more than once or not at all.

7.54

A 3-year-old with three episodes of right-sided pneumonia over the previous year. The original presentation occurred after a choking episode.

7.55

A 9-year-old boy with bilateral parotid swelling that is painful on chewing.

7.56

A 3-year-old child with fever and spreading purpuric rash who has been given intramuscular penicillin by his GP before arrival at hospital.

7.57–7.59 Theme: Diagnosis

- ❑ A *Campylobacter* spp
- ❑ B EBV virus
- ❑ C Hepatitis A
- ❑ D Kawasaki disease
- ❑ E Lyme disease
- ❑ F Malaria
- ❑ G Measles
- ❑ G *Streptococcus pneumoniae*
- ❑ H *Streptococcus pyogenes*
- ❑ I Typhoid

Choose the most likely diagnosis from the list above for each of the three scenarios described below. Each option may be used once, more than once or not at all.

7.57

A 13-year-old returns from an unplanned trip to Africa with fever and gastroenteritis symptoms.

7.58

A 5-year-old child with diarrhoea, lethargy, low-grade fever who then develops jaundice.

7.59

A 3-year-old with a fever for 5 days, sore throat, cervical lymphadenopathy, a maculopapular rash, misery and anti-streptolysin O titre (ASOT) >200.

CHAPTER 8

Neonatology

Multiple True–False Questions

8.1 Polyhydramnios is a feature of

- ☐ A Renal agenesis
- ☐ B Oesophageal atresia
- ☐ C Duodenal atresia
- ☐ D Anencephaly
- ☐ E Coarctation of the aorta

8.2 Nitric oxide

- ☐ A It is a pulmonary vasodilator
- ☐ B It often causes systemic hypotension
- ☐ C It is synthesised from L-arginine and oxygen
- ☐ D It is released from vascular walls during stress
- ☐ E It causes contraction of gastrointestinal sphincters

8.3 The following are useful in the assessment of gestational age in pre-term infants.

- ☐ A The presence of palmer creases
- ☐ B Breast size
- ☐ C Sacral oedema
- ☐ D The scarf sign
- ☐ E Posture and muscle tone

8.4 Infants of mothers with diabetes

- ☐ A They usually develop hypoglycaemia on the second day of life
- ☐ B They are always large for gestational age
- ☐ C Sacral agenesis is one of the congenital anomalies seen
- ☐ D They are at increased risk of developing a transient hypertrophic cardiomyopathy
- ☐ E They have an increased incidence of respiratory distress syndrome

8.5 Problems associated with preterm gestation include:

- ❑ A Pulmonary haemorrhage
- ❑ B Hyperglycaemia
- ❑ C Jaundice
- ❑ D Metabolic acidosis
- ❑ E Periventricular leukomalacia

8.6 Chickenpox in the neonate

- ❑ A This is a contraindication to breastfeeding
- ❑ B It should be treated with intravenous aciclovir
- ❑ C It is prevented by varicella-zoster immunoglobulin (VZIg) given postnatally
- ❑ D It has a mortality rate untreated of 90%
- ❑ E It is suggestive of an underlying immunodeficiency

8.7 Which of the following are associated with neonatal cataracts?

- ❑ A Galactosaemia
- ❑ B Congenital cytomegalovirus infection
- ❑ C Myotonic dystrophy
- ❑ D Hurler syndrome
- ❑ E Gilbert syndrome

8.8 The following are associated with an increased risk of sudden infant death syndrome.

- ❑ A Maternal smoking antenatally
- ❑ B Paternal smoking postnatally
- ❑ C Lower parental age
- ❑ D Prone sleeping position
- ❑ E Maternal drug abuse in pregnancy, if the child is removed at birth

Best of Five Questions

8.9 Which of the following statements about hypoxic ischaemic encephalopathy (HIE) of the newborn is most factually correct?

- ❑ A Neonatal cooling acts to prevent primary neuronal injury caused by perinatal hypoxia
- ❑ B Hypothermia is indicated for treatment of neonates of all gestational age within 6 hours of delivery for suspected HIE
- ❑ C Inclusion criteria for treatment with hypothermia are based entirely on blood gas analysis taken within 60 minutes of delivery on cord, arterial, venous or capillary samples
- ❑ D Hypothermia has been shown to improve neurological outcome in neonates after moderate hypoxic ischaemic injury
- ❑ E Prompt resuscitation of neonates after hypoxic ischaemic insults results in the prevention of the secondary neuronal injury that would otherwise occur

8.10 Which of the following statements about massive pulmonary haemorrhage in the neonate is most factually correct?

- ❑ A Massive pulmonary haemorrhage is commonly caused by traumatic suctioning of the endotracheal tube (ETT) in a ventilated neonate
- ❑ B Massive pulmonary haemorrhage is common in term babies with meconium aspiration syndrome
- ❑ C Surfactant treatment has been implicated in the aetiology of massive pulmonary haemorrhage and is therefore always contraindicated in neonates with this condition
- ❑ D Acute mortality rate associated with massive pulmonary haemorrhage is approximately 90%
- ❑ E Treatments used in this condition include adrenaline via the ETT and high-frequency oscillatory ventilation

8.11 Which of the following statements with regard to retinopathy of prematurity is the most factually correct?

- ❑ A Retinal detachment is a potentially sight-threatening consequence of the neovascularisation occurring in retinopathy of prematurity
- ❑ B Laser treatment is necessary in almost all cases of retinopathy of prematurity to preserve sight
- ❑ C Drug treatment has proved effective in the prevention and treatment of retinopathy of prematurity (ROP)
- ❑ D The most significant risk factor for the development of severe ROP is gestational age
- ❑ E Hypoxia is the most important factor in the development of stage I ROP

8.12 Which of the following statements about meconium aspiration syndrome (MAS) is most factually correct?

- ❑ A Decreasing gestational age is associated with increasingly severe consequences from MAS
- ❑ B Meconium aspiration is associated with the deactivation of endogenous surfactant
- ❑ C Treatment with antibiotics is essential due to the high rate of primary bacterial infection
- ❑ D Long-term pulmonary complications persisting into childhood are common in this population
- ❑ E The incidence of MAS is decreased by expectant management of post-date pregnancies compared with induction of labour

8.13 Which of the following statements about immunisation in preterm infants is the most factually correct.

- ❑ A It is recommended that all preterm infants be immunised according to the UK childhood immunisation schedule, starting at 8 weeks' corrected gestational age
- ❑ B It is recommended that all preterm (<34 weeks) and small-for-gestational-age (<1500 g) infants should have their immunisations as inpatients, under physician supervision, due to the increased incidence of apnoea and bradycardia seen in this group of babies after immunisation
- ❑ C There is no need to consider additional vaccines in the preterm or low-birthweight infant because the current UK schedule should lead to adequate protection to this group of children
- ❑ D Influenza vaccine is recommended for all preterm infants with chronic lung disease once they have reached 6 months of age
- ❑ E There is good evidence to show that the preterm and low-birthweight children in the UK get their immunisations in good time due to the widely recognised vulnerability of this group and the good levels of protection afforded by immunisation

8.14 Which of the following statements about persistent pulmonary hypertension (PPHN) is most accurate?

- ❑ A PPHN is most commonly a problem affecting infants born at very low gestations (<25 weeks) and is rare in babies >34 weeks' gestation
- ❑ B The first-line treatment for confirmed PPHN is intravenous pulmonary vasodilators
- ❑ C Mortality rate associated with PPHN is approximately 40%
- ❑ D Most cases of PPHN are associated with obvious and defined risk factors
- ❑ E Treatment with minimal handling, paralysis, sedation and nitric oxide is useful in this population

8.15 Which of the following statements with regard to pulmonary air leaks in the neonate is the most factually correct?

- ❑ A An underwater seal drain is generally not required for ventilated babies
- ❑ B The use of high rates (>60 beats/min) during conventional ventilation increases the risk of air leaks in neonates
- ❑ C Air leaks in term babies are invariably associated with significant mortality and morbidity
- ❑ D The treatment of choice for a minimally symptomatic air leak regardless of gestation of the child is 100% inspired oxygen to help hasten absorption
- ❑ E Surfactant use decreases the risk of developing an air leak in a preterm baby

8.16 Which of the following statements about neonates who are small for gestational age is most factually correct?

- ❑ A Of those neonates born small for gestational age 75% have an identified pathological cause for their size at gestation
- ❑ B Neonates who are growth restricted will be born weighing less than the 10th percentile for weight at their gestational age
- ❑ C Retrolental fibroplasia is commonly seen in children born small for gestational age
- ❑ D Growth hormone is licensed for the treatment of continued short stature (>4 years) in children born small for gestational age
- ❑ E Being born small for gestational age does not seem to produce consequences for the child beyond puberty

8.17 Which of the following statements about corticosteroid use in neonates is the most factually correct?

- ❑ A Courses of steroids given early (<92 h) are associated with improved neurodevelopmental outcomes compared with delayed courses (>3 weeks)
- ❑ B Dexamethasone is believed to have a decreased neurotoxic effect when compared with hydrocortisone
- ❑ C There is clear evidence that postnatal administration of corticosteroids produces acute improvement in respiratory mechanics and therefore facilitates extubation
- ❑ D The neurotoxic effects of dexamethasone do not appear to be dose dependent
- ❑ E The weight of evidence of poor neurological outcomes after postnatal administration of corticosteroids for bronchopulmonary dysplasia means that corticosteroid use is no longer acceptable in treatment of neonatal bronchopulmonary dysplasia

8.18 Which of the following statements concerning necrotising enterocolitis (NEC) is the most factually correct?

- ❑ A Standardising feeding regimens in neonatal units had no effect in decreasing the incidence of NEC within those units
- ❑ B NEC is a diagnosis exclusive to preterm babies
- ❑ C Infective organisms are identified in 80% of cases of NEC
- ❑ D Breast milk and to a lesser extent donor breast milk decrease the probability of developing NEC in high-risk neonates when compared with formula-fed control infants
- ❑ E Probiotics have no role in the prevention of NEC in very-low-birthweight neonates

8.19 Which of the following statements concerning birth injuries is the most factually correct?

- ❑ A Fracture of the cervical spine sustained at delivery will be evident on radiograph
- ❑ B Waiter's tip positioning of the arm is seen with Klumpke paralysis
- ❑ C Phrenic nerve palsy with diaphragmatic weakness associated with Erb palsy generally needs surgical intervention as an emergency to improve respiratory function
- ❑ D Caput succedaneum is limited by suture lines
- ❑ E The clavicle is the most common bone to fracture during labour and delivery

8.20 Which of the following statements about recurrent apnoeas in preterm neonates is most factually correct?

- ☐ A Primary apnoea of prematurity is common, affecting approximately 40% of neonates between 34 and 35 weeks' gestation
- ☐ B Gastro-oesophageal reflux is the leading cause of apnoeas in preterm babies and so the most commonly used pharmacological treatment for apnoeas is infant Gaviscon
- ☐ C Treatment of apnoea of prematurity with caffeine is associated with a decrease in the frequency of episodes and a decrease in the need for ventilation; however, current data suggest that this treatment is not associated with long-term improvement in the mortality and morbidity associated with this condition
- ☐ D Theophylline is superior to caffeine in the treatment of recurrent apnoeas of prematurity
- ☐ E Nasal CPAP is an effective treatment for recurrent apnoeas in preterm neonates that do not respond to medical treatment

8.21 Which of the following statements concerning respiratory distress syndrome (RDS) is most factually correct?

- ☐ A Radiant heat sources and the use of occlusive plastic bags to decrease the incidence of hypothermia are advantageous strategies to help to prevent/reduce the severity of RDS
- ☐ B Resuscitation of the preterm neonate should use 100% oxygen from the start
- ☐ C All babies less than 30 weeks' gestation should be electively intubated and given exogenous surfactant at birth
- ☐ D The prognosis of RDS is generally better in male infants
- ☐ E Antenatal steroids given to the mother within 4 hours of delivery will reduce the incidence of RDS and neonatal death

8.22 Which of the following statements about phototherapy is the most factually correct?

- ☐ A Phototherapy reduces serum conjugated bilirubin levels
- ☐ B Phototherapy is a substitute for exchange transfusion in small preterm infants
- ☐ C Phototherapy is less effective in dark-skinned infants
- ☐ D Clinical detection of jaundice can be difficult in children, especially those with increased skin pigmentation, so a low threshold for measuring serum bilirubin is essential
- ☐ E Phototherapy is known to cause dehydration and supplementary fluids/feeds should be used in all children undergoing this treatment

8.23 Which of the following statements about neonatal polycythaemia is most factually correct?

- ❑ A Polycythaemia is defined as a haemoglobin level ≥180 g/l
- ❑ B Trisomy 21 is a predisposing factor for developing polycythaemia
- ❑ C The risk of necrotising enterocolitis associated with polycythaemia is reduced by treatment with umbilical exchange transfusion
- ❑ D The optimum fluid for exchange transfusion for the treatment of polycythaemia is 45% human albumin solution
- ❑ E There is good evidence to support the treatment of all polycythaemic infants with partial exchange transfusion with 09% saline due to the associated decrease in long-term complications

8.24 Which of the following statements about perinatal hypoxic ischaemic insult is most factually correct?

- ❑ A Of those children graded as suffering from HIE grade III about 30% survive, the vast majority with neurological impairment
- ❑ B HIE is the most common cause of cerebral palsy in the UK
- ❑ C Of those suffering long-term neurodevelopmental consequences of HIE, diplegia is the most common form of cerebral palsy
- ❑ D Persistent fetal circulation is a recognised complication of HIE
- ❑ E Seizures occur in the vast majority of patients with grade I HIE

8.25 Which of the following statements about intestinal obstruction/bile-stained vomit on the first day of life is most factually correct?

- ❑ A Most cases of duodenal atresia occur as isolated abnormalities
- ❑ B A history of meconium-stained amniotic fluid rules out intestinal obstruction as a cause for vomiting in a neonate
- ❑ C Non-bile-stained vomiting on the first day of life suggests a diagnosis of hypertrophic pyloric stenosis
- ❑ D Bile-stained vomiting in a neonate requires a barium enema to rule out malrotation
- ❑ E Distal intestinal obstruction in the neonate most commonly presents with vomiting within the first 24 hours of life

8.26 Which of the following statements about neonatal anaemia is most factually correct?

- ☐ A Anaemia due to reduced red cell production rarely becomes clinically evident before 3–4 months of age
- ☐ B Fetal haemoglobin consists of two α and two β chains
- ☐ C β Thalassaemia commonly presents with anaemia in the neonatal period
- ☐ D There is no clear evidence that using a restrictive red blood cell (RBC) transfusion policy to manage neonates on the neonatal intensive care unit (NICU) leads to an increased length of admission to NICU or an increase in rates of intraventricular haemorrhage, NEC or chronic lung disease
- ☐ E The Coombs test differentiates fetal from maternal haemoglobin

8.27 Which of the following statements about seizures in neonates is most factually correct?

- ☐ A The overall prognosis of neonatal seizures in term babies is poor, with approximately 30% achieving a good long-term outcome
- ☐ B Neonatal seizures are twice as common in the preterm neonate as in the term neonate
- ☐ C Infection is the second most common cause of seizures in the neonatal period
- ☐ D Anticonvulsants in the neonatal period achieve good seizure control in 80% of patients
- ☐ E There is evidence that anticonvulsive medication commonly used to control neonatal seizures may have detrimental effects on developmental outcome when used in neonates; however, the balance of risks is still in favour of treating seizures to try to get the best outcome possible for the patient

8.28 Which of the following statements about congenital dislocation of the hip is the most factually correct?

- ☐ A Congenital dislocation of the hip is more common in females and more commonly affects the right hip
- ☐ B Outcome is improved with early detection because early surgical intervention is possible
- ☐ C If a Pavlik harness can be fitted before 6 weeks of age, the treatment will be successful in approximately 90% of patients
- ☐ D Avascular necrosis of the femoral head is a recognised complication of corrective surgery but not Pavlik harness treatment of developmental dysplasia of the hip
- ☐ E The Pavlik harness is most commonly worn for 6 months, followed by a weaning period of a further 6 months

8.29 In a well, thriving, breastfed, 14-day-old term baby with jaundice, what is the most appropriate investigation?

- A α_1-Anti-trypsin phenotype
- B Urine amino acids
- C Thyroid function tests
- D Blood culture
- E Conjugated and unconjugated bilirubin

8.30 Which of the following statements about oxygen transfer across the placenta *in utero* is most factually correct?

- A Oxygen transfer from the placenta to fetus is possible because of relative left shift of the oxygen dissociation curve in haemoglobin F
- B Oxygen transfer from the placenta to fetus is possible because of relative right shift of oxygen dissociation curve in HbF
- C Oxygen transfer from the placenta to fetus is possible because of relative polycythaemia of fetal compared with adult blood
- D Oxygen transfer from the placenta to fetus is possible because of the osmotic gradient across the placental membrane
- E Oxygen transfer from the placenta to fetus is possible because of higher fetal stroke volume/kg

8.31 You are asked to review a 2-day-old baby with poor feeding. On examination the baby is floppy with absent reflexes although appearing otherwise well and alert. She is admitted and undergoes a full septic screen and treated with antibiotics. There is no change in her condition and the septic screen is negative. Which of the following investigations is most likely to yield a definitive diagnosis for this infant's presenting features?

- A Creatine kinase
- B Muscle biopsy
- C Nerve conduction studies
- D Lumbar puncture
- E Genetic testing for deletion on chromosome 5q

8.32 A systolic murmur is heard in an asymptomatic, pink, term baby with normal pulses and otherwise normal examination, with no dysmorphic features on the routine first day neonatal check. The MOST appropriate action to take immediately is:

- ☐ A Four limb saturations
- ☐ B Four limb blood pressure
- ☐ C Echo same day
- ☐ D Chest radiograph
- ☐ E Discharge with written advice about possible symptoms of heart disease and clinical review in one week

Extended Matching Questions

8.33–8.35 Theme: Differential diagnosis of shock presenting in the neonatal period

- ☐ A Group B streptococcal sepsis
- ☐ B Pneumococcal pneumonia
- ☐ C Malrotation and volvulus
- ☐ D Persistent pulmonary hypertension of the newborn
- ☐ E Congenital hypothyroidism
- ☐ F Duct dependent cardiac lesion
- ☐ G Atrioventricular septal defect (AVSD)
- ☐ H Pyloric stenosis
- ☐ I Congenital adrenal hyperplasia
- ☐ J Galactosaemia

For each of the clinical scenarios below choose the most likely pathological process from the list above. Each option may be used once, more than once or not at all.

8.33

A 10-day-old baby is admitted from home with short (24 h) history of poor feeding and cool peripheries. She was born at term after an uncomplicated pregnancy with normal antenatal care and screening. She was 3.5 kg at birth and was discharged after a normal neonatal examination at 24 hours of age, feeding well. She had regained her birthweight but has had a rapid deterioration of feeding, associated with breathlessness, over the last 24 hours. On examination she appears unwell with an apex rate of 190 beats/min, a respiratory rate of 80 beats/min and a temperature of 36.8°C. It is difficult to feel her femoral pulses and she has an enlarged liver palpable per abdomen.

8.34

A 4-day-old baby girl is admitted with a 6-hour history of decreased feeding and lethargy, with associated increased rate of breathing and decreased temperature. She was born at term after an uneventful pregnancy and is the first child of unrelated parents. She had been feeding well at home since discharge before her rapid deterioration. On examination she is lethargic and mottled with an tachycardia of 190 beats/min and increased respiratory rate of 80 beats/min, associated with intercostal and subcostal recession. She is relatively hypothermic with a temperature of 35.5°C and saturations of 88% in air, which rapidly improve on administration of 100% oxygen by re-breathe mask.

8.35

A 3-week-old baby boy presents to the emergency department with 72 hours of progressive vomiting. He is unsettled but is not pyrexial and has no symptoms of diarrhoea. His birthweight was 3.3 kg and he has not settled into a good feeding pattern since birth. On examination he appears unwell and wasted with tachycardia and a delayed capillary refill time of 2.5 seconds centrally. His weight on admission is 3.0 kg. Initial blood investigations are as follows:

- Na^+ 120 mmol/l
- K^+ 6.1 mmol/l
- Urea 10 mmol/l
- Creatinine 47 mmol/l
- Bicarbonate 18 mmol/l
- CRP <2 mg/l
- Glucose 2.8 mmol/l

8.36–8.38 Theme: Syndromes associated with congenital heart disease

- ❑ A VSD
- ❑ B ASD
- ❑ C Coarctation of the aorta
- ❑ D Transposition of the great arteries
- ❑ E Total anomalous pulmonary venous connection
- ❑ F Hypoplastic left heart
- ❑ G Pulmonary valve stenosis
- ❑ H Tetralogy of Fallot
- ❑ I Truncus arteriosus
- ❑ J AVSD

Choose from the list above the most commonly associated cardiac abnormality found in children with the following recognised syndromes. Each option may be used once, more than once or not at all.

8.36

A child born with trisomy 21.

8.37

Noonan syndrome.

8.38

A child born with trisomy 18.

8.39–8.41 Theme: Conjugated hyperbilirubinaemia

- ❑ A Biliary atresia
- ❑ B Inspissated bile syndrome
- ❑ C Postnatal cytomegalovirus (CMV) infection
- ❑ D Cystic fibrosis
- ❑ E Choledochal cyst
- ❑ F Galactosaemia
- ❑ G Alagille syndrome
- ❑ H Neonatal haemochromatosis
- ❑ I Hypothyroidism
- ❑ J Congenital CMV infection

Choose the most likely condition from the list above for each of the three scenarios described below. Each option may be used once, more than once or not at all.

8.39

A term baby presents at birth with jaundice (conjugated hyperbilirubinaemia), petechiae, hepatosplenomegaly and microcephaly, having a birthweight below the 0.4th centile for age.

8.40

A baby is seen at 14 days of age due to prolonged conjugated jaundice. On examination he has pale stools and dark urine, but otherwise appears well, feeds vigorously and is growing along the 25th centile for weight.

8.41

A term baby is born to a mother with a triangular face, prominent forehead and small chin. The baby is well but is referred for routine assessment of prolonged jaundice and is found to have a conjugated hyperbilirubinaemia. On auscultation a loud murmur is heard and hepatosplenomegaly is present on abdominal palpation.

8.42–8.44 Theme: Neonatal meningitis

- ❑ A Group A streptococcus
- ❑ B *Neisseria meningitidis*
- ❑ C *Escherichia coli*
- ❑ D *Haemophilus influenzae*
- ❑ E *Listeria monocytogenes*
- ❑ F Group B streptococcus
- ❑ G *Staphylococcus aureus*
- ❑ H *Streptococcus pneumoniae*
- ❑ I *Enterobacter cloacae*
- ❑ J Herpes simplex virus

For each of the clinical scenarios below choose the most likely pathogen from the list above. Each option may be used once, more than once or not at all.

8.42

A 29-week gestation baby is delivered after prolonged rupture of membranes of 4 days. Green-stained liquor is present at delivery. At 2 hours of age the baby is grunting and poorly perfused.

8.43

A term baby born by forceps delivery with fetal scalp monitoring in labour presents in the second week of life with a 6-hour history of temperature instability, decreased feeding and irritability. He develops seizures while being assessed in the accident and emergency department. His lumbar puncture shows a haemorrhagic lymphocytosis.

8.44

A baby born at 34 weeks' gestation presents with pyrexia, tachypnoea and a bulging fontanelle at 12 hours of age. She was born after her mother's membranes ruptured 36 hours before the onset of preterm labour. She is irritable and will not feed and has tachycardia and poor peripheral perfusion.

8.45–8.47 Theme: Neonatal presentation of congenital abnormalities

- ❑ A Beckwith–Weidemann syndrome
- ❑ B Trisomy 13
- ❑ C Prader–Willi syndrome
- ❑ D Turner syndrome
- ❑ E Trisomy 18
- ❑ F Di George syndrome
- ❑ G Hypothyroidism
- ❑ H VATER association
- ❑ I Crigler–Najjar syndrome
- ❑ J Trisomy 21

Choose the most likely diagnosis from the list above for each of the three scenarios described below. Each option may be used once, more than once or not at all.

8.45

Antenatal scan showing horseshoe kidney and pedal oedema and fetal growth within normal limits.

8.46

A term baby boy of appropriate birth weight is floppy and feeding poorly, with cryptorchidism on examination.

8.47

An antenatal scan of a term baby shows duplex kidney. The first feed is very 'gurgly'.

8.48–8.50 Theme: Neonatal thrombocytopenia

- ❑ A Neonatal alloimmune thrombocytopenia (NAIT)
- ❑ B Maternal drugs
- ❑ C TORCH infection
- ❑ D Sepsis
- ❑ E α Thalassaemia
- ❑ F Rhesus disease
- ❑ G Renal vein thrombosis
- ❑ H Maternal systemic lupus erythematosus
- ❑ I Maternal idiopathic thrombocytopenic purpura
- ❑ J Necrotising enterocolitis

Choose the most likely condition from the list above for each of the three scenarios described below. Each option may be used once, more than once or not at all.

8.48

A 1-day-old well-looking baby with platelet count 30 × 10^9/l, petechial rash and a cephatohaematoma. Maternal platelet count is normal.

8.49

A baby with intrauterine growth retardation with platelets 20 × 10^9/l and with lens opacities.

8.50

A well baby presents on day 7 of life with petechial rash, platelets 20 × 10^9/l and bradycardia of 60/min. The maternal platelet count is normal.

CHAPTER 9

Nephrology Questions

Multiple True–False Questions

9.1 Angiotensin II

- ❑ A Increases renin production
- ❑ B Stimulates catecholamine release
- ❑ C Increases aldosterone synthesis
- ❑ D Reduces after load on the heart
- ❑ E Is synthesised solely in the kidneys

9.2 Causes of inappropriate antidiuretic hormone (ADH) secretion include:

- ❑ A Hib meningitis
- ❑ B Pneumococcal pneumonia
- ❑ C Vincristine
- ❑ D Renal tubular acidosis
- ❑ E Phenytoin

9.3 The following are used in the emergency treatment of hyperkalaemia.

- ❑ A Physiological (09%) saline infusion
- ❑ B Intravenous salbutamol
- ❑ C Nebulised salbutamol
- ❑ D Intravenous adenosine
- ❑ E Intravenous hydrocortisone

9.4 Renal osteodystrophy

- ❑ A Is a complication of chronic renal failure
- ❑ B Is characterised by an increased plasma phosphate
- ❑ C Is characterised by a reduced serum alkaline phosphatase
- ❑ D Is characterised by a normal parathyroid hormone level
- ❑ E Is familial

9.5 Metabolic acidosis occurs in association with which of the following conditions?

- ❑ A Pyloric stenosis
- ❑ B Cystinuria
- ❑ C Bartter syndrome
- ❑ D Cystinosis
- ❑ E Pseudohypoaldosteronism

9.6 Orthostatic proteinuria

- ❑ A Is benign
- ❑ B Is present only when the patient is upright
- ❑ C Can be large
- ❑ D Is commonly familial
- ❑ E Can be precipitated by upper respiratory tract infection

9.7 Chloride

- ❑ A Is a cation
- ❑ B Serum levels are high in pyloric stenosis
- ❑ C Serum levels are high in renal tubular acidosis
- ❑ D Serum levels may rise if normal saline is infused
- ❑ E Is lost in the stool in chloridorrhoea

9.8 Membranous glomerulonephritis

- ❑ A Accounts for 20–40% of adult nephrotic syndrome
- ❑ B Can be associated with hepatitis A infection
- ❑ C Is commoner in males than in females
- ❑ D Is not improved by steroids
- ❑ E Can be secondary to systemic lupus erythematosus

Best of Five Questions

9.9 Which of the following statements about the principles of managing chronic kidney disease is most factually correct?

- ☐ A Cadaveric renal transplants have equitable long-term graft survival when compared with a related live donor
- ☐ B It is important to treat anaemia with blood transfusion in order to maximise learning potential and quality of life in children with chronic kidney disease
- ☐ C Haemodialysis is the preferred method of renal replacement therapy in the vast majority of children
- ☐ D Early recognition and treatment of chronic kidney disease can delay progression of the disease and improve long-term outcome
- ☐ E Poor nutrition is a significant problem in children with chronic kidney disease, and high calorie feeds with calcium and phosphate supplements can improve both growth and underlying bone disease in this population

9.10 Which of the following statements about scrotal pain is most factually correct?

- ☐ A It is impossible to differentiate between testicular torsion and torsion of the hydatid of Morgagni
- ☐ B Most torted testes remain viable up to 18 hours after the onset of symptoms
- ☐ C If torsion of the testis cannot be excluded clinically exploration of the scrotum is the only safe management of an acutely inflamed scrotum
- ☐ D Testicular torsion accounts for just over 50% of the cases of acute scrotum presenting in childhood
- ☐ E Postoperatively a previously torted viable testis will go on to display completely normal spermatogenesis in adult life

9.11 Which of the following statements about cranial diabetes insipidus is most factually correct?

- ☐ A Cranial diabetes insipidus is usually an inherited disorder that is inherited in an X-linked recessive fashion
- ☐ B Irritability, growth retardation, hyperthermia and weight loss may be the presenting features of the disorder in infancy
- ☐ C Water deprivation test is the gold standard of diagnosing this disorder and is positive if it shows an increased serum (>290 mosmol/kg) and renal osmolality (>800 mosmol/kg)
- ☐ D Secondary causes of cranial diabetes insipidus include chronic renal insufficiency, lithium toxicity, tubulointerstitial disease, and hypercalcaemia and hypokalaemia
- ☐ E The most common aeticlogy of cranial diabetes insipidus is, postmeningitis, most commonly pneumococcal disease

9.12 Which of the following statements about nocturnal enuresis is most factually correct?

- ☐ A Behavioural strategies such as star charts are not beneficial in the management of nocturnal enuresis because the symptoms are beyond cognitive control
- ☐ B Nocturnal enuresis in children under the age of 10 years has equal sex distribution with increasing proportions of males affected after 13 years of age
- ☐ C Increasing day-time fluid intake can be an effective intervention in helping to decrease the symptom of nocturnal enuresis in some children
- ☐ D Nocturnal enuresis is a primary condition (the child never having achieved dryness for 6 consecutive months) in 90% of cases
- ☐ E Longstanding day-time symptoms of urinary urgency, incontinence, frequent (over seven) or infrequent (fewer than four) episodes of urination can be associated with enuresis in patients with diabetes mellitus

9.13 Which of the following statements about Berger disease (mesangial IgA nephritis) is most factually accurate?

- ☐ A There is a female predominance in cases of IgA nephropathy
- ☐ B In 90% of cases patients present with proteinuria and microscopic haematuria
- ☐ C Exacerbations associated with macroscopic haematuria typically present 10 days after an upper respiratory infection
- ☐ D Overall 20–30% of patients diagnosed with IgA nephropathy will develop end-stage renal failure 15–20 years after the onset of the disease
- ☐ E Investigations typically reveal an elevated serum IgA and a decreased serum C3

9.14 In a 2-year-old prerenal rather than renal failure is most accurately suggested by which one of the following?

- ☐ A A fractional excretion of sodium of 4%
- ☐ B Urinary sodium 10 mmol/l
- ☐ C Urine osmolality 250 mmol/l
- ☐ D A urine:plasma creatinine ratio of 5
- ☐ E A preceding history of diarrhoea

9.15 Which of the following statements about renal involvement in Henoch–Schönlein purpura (HSP) is most factually correct?

- ☐ A Renal involvement in HSP occurs in 20–50% of cases
- ☐ B Renal involvement in HSP is always present within 4 weeks of the onset of the rash
- ☐ C Renal involvement in HSP usually manifests itself as an nephrotic syndrome
- ☐ D Renal involvement in HSP is usually associated with a low serum C3 and C4
- ☐ E Renal involvement in HSP is usually progressive

9.16 Which of the following statements about the inheritance patterns of these renal syndromes is most factually correct?

- ☐ A Nephrogenic diabetes insipidus is inherited in an autosomal recessive pattern
- ☐ B Alport syndrome is inherited in an X-linked dominant pattern
- ☐ C Hartnup disease is inherited in an X-linked recessive pattern
- ☐ D Vitamin D-resistant rickets (hypophosphataemic rickets) is inherited in an autosomal dominant pattern
- ☐ E Cystinosis is inherited in an X-linked recessive pattern

9.17 Which of the following statements about minimal change nephrotic syndrome is most factually correct?

- ☐ A Minimal change nephrotic syndrome has a peak incidence in children <2 years of age
- ☐ B Minimal change nephrotic syndrome is commonly associated with macroscopic haematuria
- ☐ C Minimal change nephrotic syndrome has a male predominance
- ☐ D Minimal change nephrotic syndrome is usually associated with low serum C3
- ☐ E Minimal change nephrotic syndrome does not occur in adults

9.18 Which of the following statements about urinary tract infection (UTI) in children is most factually correct?

- ❑ A The degree of scarring found on a DMSA scan is proportional to the number of previous episodes of upper urinary tract infections
- ❑ B Treatment with a 3-day course of oral antibiotics is appropriate in a 2-year-old child with proven UTI and symptoms of a lower UTI
- ❑ C Prophylaxis for recurrent UTIs is no longer indicated according to NICE guidelines for the management of UTIs in children
- ❑ D Pseudomonas UTIs are associated with renal stones
- ❑ E All upper renal tract infections in children <3 years old should be treated initially with intravenous antibiotics

9.19 Which of the following statements about haemolytic uraemic syndrome is most factually correct?

- ❑ A In children with haemolytic uraemic syndrome the C3 is usually low
- ❑ B In children with diarrhoea-associated haemolytic uraemic syndrome, the acute mortality rate is approximately 20%
- ❑ C Treatment of *E coli* O157 diarrhoea with antibiotics decreases the risk of developing HUS
- ❑ D CNS involvement is a rare complication of HUS and occurs in less than 5% of cases
- ❑ E Pneumococcal pneumonia and meningitis are implicated in the development of HUS

9.20 Which of the following statements about hypertension in childhood is most factually correct?

- ❑ A The use of a small blood pressure cuff will produce a falsely low reading of blood pressure
- ❑ B Hypertension in childhood is defined as a systolic blood pressure (BP) >120 mmHg
- ❑ C The vast majority of cases of hypertension in children are secondary to endocrine disease
- ❑ D Ambulatory BP measurements are not acceptable in the vast majority of children due to discomfort
- ❑ E The vast majority of children are asymptomatic but hypertensive encephalopathy presenting as severe hypertension with headache, vomiting, hyperreflexia and seizures is a medical emergency requiring admission to hospital for a controlled gradual decrease in BP

9.21 Which of the following statements concerning post-streptococcal glomerulonephritis is most factually correct?

- ☐ A It is characterised by a low C4 and normal C3 in the acute phase
- ☐ B It follows non-haemolytic streptococcal infection in 50% of cases
- ☐ C Hypertensive encephalopathy is a recognised complication
- ☐ D Treatment with 10 days of phenoxymethylpenicillin reduces the time course of the nephritis
- ☐ E It is most common in children under the age of 2 years

9.22 Which of the following statements concerning undescended testis is most factually correct?

- ☐ A Undescended testes are less common in the low-birthweight and preterm infants
- ☐ B By 12 months of age 8% of previously undescended testes remain outside the scrotum
- ☐ C Early orchidopexy has been shown to reduce infertility in later life
- ☐ D It is essential to perform a karyotype to exclude mixed gonadal dysgenesis and disorders of sex differentiation in all cases of undescended testes and retractile testes
- ☐ E Cases of retractile testes should undergo orchidopexy to decrease the associated risk of testicular torsion

9.23 Which of the following statements about Wilms tumours is most factually correct?

- ☐ A Forty per cent of cases of Wilms tumours are bilateral
- ☐ B Wilms tumours account for approximately 50% of abdominal masses in childhood
- ☐ C There has been no genetic basis for Wilms tumour identified to date but in some families there is a very high incidence of Wilms tumour
- ☐ D Hemihypertrophy, genitourinary abnormalities and aniridia are all associated with an increased risk of developing Wilms tumours
- ☐ E The most common presentation of Wilms tumour is with painful haematuria

9.24 Which of the following statements about paediatric hyponatraemia is the most factually correct?

- ❑ A Diabetes insipidus is a well-recognised cause for hyponatraemia
- ❑ B Hyponatraemia and low urinary sodium <20 mmol/l is indicative of SIADH
- ❑ C Acute hyponatraemic encephalopathy is potentially life-threatening event that requires urgent treatment with isotonic saline in the first instance
- ❑ D Severe gastroenteritis is a cause of the syndrome of inappropriate ADH secretion (SIADH)
- ❑ E Fluid restriction is appropriate treatment for hyponatraemia when SIADH is suspected to be the cause

9.25 Which of the following statements about polycystic kidney disease is most factually correct?

- ❑ A Polycystic kidney disease presenting in childhood is X linked in 80% of cases
- ❑ B Autosomal dominant polycystic kidney disease typically present in the neonatal period
- ❑ C Adult presentation of polycystic kidney disease is associated with progression to renal failure in 90% of cases by the seventh decade
- ❑ D Congenital hepatic fibrosis is strongly associated with autosomal recessive polycystic kidney disease and portal hypertension can be the presenting feature
- ❑ E Hypertension is a rare complication of polycystic kidney disease

9.26 Which of the following statements concerning vesicoureteric reflux is most factually correct?

- ❑ A Vesicoureteric reflux occurs in less than 5% of children who present with a confirmed urinary tract infection
- ❑ B The aim of prophylactic antibiotics in children with vesicoureteric reflux is to minimise the harmful consequences of renal scarring and progression towards renal impairment and subsequent failure
- ❑ C The damage caused by vesicoureteric reflux can be reversed with the use of corrective surgery
- ❑ D Spontaneous remission of vesicoureteric reflux is rare
- ❑ E Vesicoureteric reflux can most accurately be diagnosed using a DMSA scan

9.27 Which of the following statements about hypercalciuria is most factually correct?

- ❑ A Thiazide diuretics are a recognised cause of hypercalciuria
- ❑ B The only way to investigate the renal excretion of calcium is with a 24-hour collection of urine
- ❑ C Hypoparathyroidism is a well-recognised cause of hypercalciuria
- ❑ D Hypercalciuria is an important cause in the differential of any child presenting with haematuria
- ❑ E Vitamin D deficiency is a well-recognised cause of hypercalciuria

9.28 Which of the following statements about congenital nephrotic syndrome is most factually correct?

- ❑ A Infants with congenital nephrotic syndrome have a raised serum α-fetoprotein
- ❑ B Congenital nephrotic syndrome usually presents between 6 and 12 months of age
- ❑ C Most cases of congenital nephrotic syndrome are associated with a good prognosis
- ❑ D Steroids are useful in the treatment of Finnish-type congenital nephrotic syndrome
- ❑ E Congenital syphilis is a cause of congenital nephrotic syndrome

9.29 A 2-year-old girl is admitted after a short diarrhoeal illness with irritability.

Parents have noticed that she looks 'puffy' and that she has not passed urine for 24 hours. On examination she is apyrexial but irritable. She has pedal oedema and is pale.

The MOST appropriate initial management is:

- ❑ A Transfusion of packed cells
- ❑ B Start diuretics and iron supplements
- ❑ C Start antidiarrhoeals and arrange outpatient review
- ❑ D Admit for investigation and fluid balance
- ❑ E Arrange to start peritoneal dialysis

9.30 A 2-week-old baby boy whose mother had no antenatal care is referred for assessment of failure to thrive.

History gives few clues but he has a rather poor urine stream. On examination he is scrawny with a preauricular tag and has palpable loin masses.

The NEXT step should be:

- ❑ A Start antibiotics and arrange review
- ❑ B Urgent renal ultrasonography
- ❑ C Catheterisation
- ❑ D Renal biopsy
- ❑ E Intravenous urography

9.31 A 5-year-old boy is referred with a 2-week history of general malaise and facial swelling.

There is a history of recent upper respiratory tract infection. On examination, he has generalised oedema with shifting dullness on abdominal percussion. He has 4+ proteinuria and BP 140/100 mmHg. His initial investigations show an albumin of 18 g/l normal renal function and a normal C3 and C4.

The BEST initial management is:

- ❑ A Start high-dose prednisolone
- ❑ B Infusion of 20% human albumin solution
- ❑ C Immediate transfer to paediatric nephrology service
- ❑ D High-dose oral furosemide
- ❑ E Dietary review and start high protein diet

9.32 A 4-year-old girl is referred with periumbilical pain and urinary frequency for some months.

Multiple MSUs have been negative. She has regressed behaviourally with frequent temper tantrums at home, but is well behaved at nursery school. Other members of her family have been well. She has a new baby sister who is 6 months old. Examination including BP is normal.

The MOST appropriate approach would be:

- ☐ A Start antibiotic prophylaxis for possible missed urinary tract infections while arranging a renal isotope scan and cystogram
- ☐ B Arrange a screen of blood tests and abdominal ultrasonography
- ☐ C Arrange to be seen jointly with social services on suspicion of abuse
- ☐ D Surgical opinion
- ☐ E Reassure that this is a normal reaction to new siblings and that no investigation is needed

Extended Matching Questions

9.33–9.35 Theme: Causes of acute kidney injury (previously known as acute renal failure)

- ☐ A Intrinsic renal failure secondary to postinfective glomerulonephritis
- ☐ B Prerenal failure secondary to intravascular depletion
- ☐ C Intrinsic renal failure secondary to Henoch–Schönlein purpura
- ☐ D Intrinsic renal failure secondary to haemolytic uraemic syndrome
- ☐ E Acute tubular necrosis secondary to inadequate renal perfusion
- ☐ F Intrinsic renal failure secondary to nephrotoxic effects of drugs
- ☐ G Prerenal failure secondary to sepsis
- ☐ H Intrinsic renal failure secondary to SLE nephritis
- ☐ I Renal injury secondary to obstructive uropathy
- ☐ J Renal injury secondary to renal vein thrombosis

Choose the most likely diagnosis from the list above for each of the three following clinical scenarios. Each of the options may be used once, more than once or not at all.

9.33

A 4-year-old boy presented with a 3-day history of diarrhoea and vomiting. He had passed multiple watery stools per day and night and had vomited seven times in the 6 hours before admission. There was no blood in his stools. On examination he was lethargic with a pulse rate of 120 beats/min at rest and a capillary refill time of 5 s peripherally and 3.5 s centrally. His initial blood results are listed below. He was catheterised and passed < 0.5 ml/kg of urine over the first 3 hours of admission.

Na^+ 148 mmol/l

K^+ 6.0 mmol/k

Urea 28 mmol/l

Creatinine 80 mmol/l

Urinary Na^+ <10 mmol/l

9.34

A 2-year-old girl was admitted after a 3-day history of diarrhoea and vomiting. Her stools were initially loose and watery and then developed blood in the last 12 hours. The family had visited a petting zoo 2 days before the onset of symptoms; no other member of her family had developed symptoms. She had not passed urine for 24 hours before admission. On admission her temperature was 38.9°C and her pulse rate was 162 beats/min. Her blood pressure measured 100/60 mmHg with a manual mercury sphygmomanometer. Her admission investigation results are listed below:

Hb 7.1 g/dl

WBC 16.2 × 10^9/l

Neutrophils 10.1 × 10^9/l

Platelets 115 × 10^9/l

Na^+ 145 mmol/l

K^+ 5.5 mmol/l

Urea 11.7 mmol/l

Creatinine 125 mmol/l

C-reactive protein (CRP) 37 mg/dl

9.35

A 4-year-boy presented with a 3-day history of facial and scrotal swelling. He had been reported to have had a rash over his legs 3 weeks before admission and had swelling and pain in his ankles associated with this. His rash was fading but was still palpable and around his ankles. On examination he had moist mucous membranes, a normal pulse rate, and swelling around his eyes, ankles and obviously involving his scrotum. His blood pressure on manually measurement with a mercury sphygmomanometer was 110/68 mmHg. On dipstick of his urine he had 3+ of blood, 3+ of protein and urinary sodium of 35 mmol/l. He had increased his weight by 4 kg over the 3 weeks of his illness. His admission investigations were as follows:

Hb 9.0 g/dl

Na^+ 136 mmol/l

Urea 12.5 mmol/l

Creatinine 130 mmol/l

Albumin 22 mmol/l

9.36–9.38 Theme: Biochemistry investigations

- ❑ A Coeliac disease
- ❑ B Pyloric stenosis
- ❑ C Diabetes mellitus
- ❑ D Acute gastroenteritis
- ❑ E Distal renal tubular acidosis type I
- ❑ F Congenital adrenal hyperplasia
- ❑ G Fanconi syndrome
- ❑ H Cows' milk protein intolerance
- ❑ I Gastro-oesophageal reflux disease
- ❑ H Distal renal tubular acidosis type IV

Choose the most likely diagnosis from the list above for each of the three following clinical scenarios. Each of the options may be used once, more than once or not at all.

9.36

A 16-month-old boy presents to the paediatric assessment unit with a history of a month of weight loss and vomiting. On examination he was dehydrated, apyrexial and tachycardic, with a central and peripheral capillary refill time of 3 s. Despite this he continued to void good volumes of urine. On further examination he also had swollen wrists and ankles and swollen costochondral junctions. His height and weight had both tracked the 0.4th centile and had over the last 2 months drifted below these centile lines.

His initial biochemical investigations showed:

Venous blood	**pH 7.21**
Na^+	**125 mmol/l**
K^+	**1.9 mmol/l**
HCO_3^-	**17 mmol/l**
Urea	**8.2 mmol/l**
Creatinine	**89 µmol/l**
Calcium	2.32 mmol/l
PO_4^{3-}	0.70 mmol/l
Blood glucose	6.0 mmol/l
Urinalysis	glucose 3+
	proteinuria 2+
	pH 6.0

9.37

A 3-year-old boy with recurrent urinary tract infections secondary to severe vesicoureteric reflux is reviewed in paediatric clinic. He is found to have poor growth; having been born on the 25th centile he has drifted down to below the 0.4th centile over the preceding 3 months with reasonable growth along the 25th centile before this. He has had three separate urinary tract infections proven on urine culture over the previous 6 months. On blood and urine biochemical investigation the following results are obtained:

Urine MC&S	no growth
Venous blood gas	pH 7.21
Anion gap	8 mmol/l (normal range)
Bicarbonate	16 mmol/l
Serum sodium	122 mmol/l
Serum potassium	2.3 mmol/l
Serum urea	5.4 mmol/l
Serum creatinine	42 mmol/l
Urinalysis	glucose negative
	protein negative
	pH 7.0

9.38

A 3-week-old boy presents with 3 days of progressively worsening vomiting described by his parents as projectile. He is apyrexial and has decreased frequency of stooling since the onset of his vomiting. He is the firstborn child to his non-consanguineous white parents. He was born at term with a birthweight of 3.85 kg; he initially appeared to maintain his weight but presents to the assessment unit weighing 3. 65 kg, with obvious wasting. On examination he is tachycardic and tachypnoeic, with a decreased capillary refill time both centrally and peripherally.

Investigations on presentation:

Venous pH	7.51
Serum sodium	118 mmol/l
Serum potassium	7.3 mmol/l
Urea	12.2 mmol/l
Creatinine	54 mmol/l
Chloride	90 mmol/l
Bicarbonate	48 mmol/l
Glucose	4.5 mmol/l
CRP	<2 mg/l
Urinary dipstick	NAD
	pH 3.8

9.39–9.41 Theme: Haematuria

- ❑ A Urinary tract infection
- ❑ B Mesangiocapillary glomerulonephritis
- ❑ C Shunt nephritis
- ❑ D Renal calculi
- ❑ E Renal vein thrombosis
- ❑ F Fabricated or fictitious illness
- ❑ G Wilms tumours
- ❑ H Poststreptococcal glomerulonephritis
- ❑ I Alport syndrome
- ❑ J Haemolytic uraemic syndrome

Choose the most likely diagnosis from the list above for each of the following three scenarios described below. Each option may be used once, more than once or not at all.

9.39

A 10-year-old girl presents with frank haematuria and recurrent episodes of colicky loin pain and vomiting, and is apyrexial.

9.40

A 6-year-old girl with known nephrotic syndrome presents with flank pain and macroscopic haematuria and increased severity of proteinuria.

9.41

A 4-year-old boy presents with an episode of macroscopic haematuria and has a normal urine culture and ultrasound scan. On follow-up is found to have persistent microscopic haematuria. There is a family history of male deafness and his maternal grandfather had renal failure.

9.42–9.44 Theme: Blood pressure

- ❑ A Renal artery stenosis
- ❑ B Acute glomerulonephritis
- ❑ C Poststreptococcal glomerulonephritis
- ❑ D Henoch–Schönlein purpura
- ❑ E Nephrotic syndrome
- ❑ F Haemolytic uraemic syndrome
- ❑ G Wilms tumour
- ❑ H Renal tubular acidosis
- ❑ I Vesicoureteric reflux with scarring in infancy

Choose the most likely diagnosis from the list above for each of the three scenarios described below. Each option may be used once, more than once or not at all.

9.42

A 2-year-old boy is admitted with diarrhoea. On examination he is pale with pedal oedema. His blood pressure is 140/100 mmHg and platelet count is 70×10^9/l.

9.43

A 13-year-old girl complains of headaches over the preceding several months. Her blood pressure is 150/110 mmHg. An ultrasound scan shows bilaterally small kidneys.

9.44

A 3-year-old with one 'thin arm' since birth presents with intermittent haematuria. On examination he is pale with abdominal mass and hemihypertrophy. His blood pressure is 90/60 mmHg.

9.45–9.47 Theme: Investigations

- ❑ A Micturating cystourethrography
- ❑ B MAG-3 scan
- ❑ C DMSA isotope scan
- ❑ D DTPA scan
- ❑ E Renal tract ultrasonography
- ❑ F Abdominal computed tomography (CT)
- ❑ G Abdominal magnetic resonance imaging (MRI)
- ❑ H Renal angiography
- ❑ I Renal biopsy
- ❑ J None of the above

Choose the most useful investigation from the list above for each of the three requirements described below. Each option may be used once, more than once or not at all.

9.45

Assessment of degree of renal scarring post confirmed UTI.

9.46

At the initial presentation of nephrotic syndrome.

9.47

Assessment of suspected perinephric abscess.

9.48–9.50 Theme: The kidney in systemic disease

- ❑ A Systemic lupus erythematosis
- ❑ B Diabetes
- ❑ C Congenital hypothyroidism
- ❑ D Rheumatic fever
- ❑ E Scleroderma
- ❑ F Duchenne muscular dystrophy
- ❑ G Asthma
- ❑ H Hyperparathyroidism
- ❑ I Amyloidosis
- ❑ J TB

Choose the most likely diagnosis from the list above for each of the three conditions described below. Each option may be used once, more than once or not at all.

9.48

Renal failure with longstanding juvenile chronic arthritis and more recent development of hepatosplenomegaly.

9.49

Renal involvement (nephritis) at outset of illness, accompanied by fever, fatigue, erythematous malar rash and arthritis.

9.50

Microalbuminuria.

CHAPTER 10

Neurology

Multiple True–False Questions

10.1 The following are risk factors for SUDEP (sudden unexplained death in epilepsy)

- ❑ A Poorly controlled epilepsy
- ❑ B Focal epilepsy
- ❑ C Being a child
- ❑ D Sudden and frequent changes in anticonvulsants
- ❑ E Nocturnal seizures

10.2 Carpal tunnel syndrome

- ❑ A It is more common in females
- ❑ B It is due to entrapment of the ulnar nerve
- ❑ C Pain is rarely a symptom
- ❑ D Sensation over the thenar eminence is not affected
- ❑ E Therapeutic options include diuretics

10.3 Nystagmus

- ❑ A It may be inherited as an X-linked dominant condition
- ❑ B In cerebellar nystagmus the direction of the fast phase is contralateral to the lesion
- ❑ C In vestibular nystagmus the direction of the rapid phase is ipsilateral to the lesion
- ❑ D It may be caused by phenytoin toxicity
- ❑ E If vertical suggests that a cataract is possible

10.4 The following are causes of cerebral palsy

- ❑ A Hypothyroidism
- ❑ B Preterm delivery
- ❑ C Werdnig–Hoffmann disease
- ❑ D Neonatal meningitis
- ❑ E Congenital cytomegalovirus infection

10.5 The following conditions are inherited as autosomal dominant

- ☐ A Tuberous sclerosis
- ☐ B Ataxia telangiectasia
- ☐ C Colour blindness
- ☐ D Haemophilia
- ☐ E Myotonic dystrophy

10.6 Myoclonic jerks are commonly seen in

- ☐ A Lennox–Gastaut syndrome
- ☐ B Juvenile myoclonic epilepsy
- ☐ C Landau–Kleffner syndrome
- ☐ D West syndrome
- ☐ E Gilbert syndrome

10.7 The following statements are true concerning primitive reflexes

- ☐ A It is normal for the Moro reflex to be present at 8 months of age
- ☐ B The palmar grasp reflex usually disappears by 3 months of age
- ☐ C Persistence of the asymmetrical tonic neck reflex is an early sign of cerebral palsy
- ☐ D The parachute reflex is present at birth
- ☐ E The plantar reflex is normally flexor by 4 weeks

10.8 The following conditions are associated with hydrocephalus

- ☐ A Anaemia
- ☐ B Klippel–Feil syndrome
- ☐ C Choroid plexus papilloma
- ☐ D Dandy–Walker malformation
- ☐ E Mucopolysaccharidoses

10.9 Recognised causes of microcephaly include

- ☐ A Chickenpox in the third trimester
- ☐ B Dandy–Walker syndrome
- ☐ C Myotonia congenita
- ☐ D Neurofibromatosis type 1
- ☐ E Maternal phenylketonuria

Best of Five Questions

10.10 A 15-year-old girl with juvenile myoclonic epilepsy is being routinely followed up in clinic. She has had good seizure control on sodium valporate for the last 6 months. Select the BEST advice to give her about contraception and pregnancy.

- ❑ A No advice because she is 15 years old and under the legal age to have sexual intercourse
- ❑ B If in the future she wants to become sexually active, discuss the issues around anticonvulsant medication and contraception further as it is important for patients with epilepsy to have pre-pregnancy advice
- ❑ C If she were to become pregnant she should stop taking her medication, because sodium valporate is teratogenic
- ❑ D She should seek medical advice when she becomes pregnant because they will change her anticonvulsants to one that will not harm her baby
- ❑ E To avoid oral contraception while on anticonvulsant medication because their interactions can be complex

10.11 Concerning narcolepsy, select the MOST appropriate statement.

- ❑ A It typically starts in the early childhood years
- ❑ B It is familial
- ❑ C Psychiatric problems are uncommon
- ❑ D Rapid eye movement (REM) sleep does not occur
- ❑ E Associated cataplexy is unusual

10.12 A 12-year-old boy was knocked unconscious while playing football; on arrival to the emergency department he had a GCS score of 15.

He complains of a headache and vomits. While in the department he has a generalised tonic–clonic seizure. The seizure self-terminates after 3 minutes; after this the boy is drowsy.

Select the BEST next step given this clinical scenario.

- ❑ A Intravenous lorazepam
- ❑ B Urgent EEG
- ❑ C Urgent CT scan
- ❑ D Intravenous phenytoin
- ❑ E Intravenous fluids

10.13 Concerning Gilles de la Tourette syndrome, select the MOST appropriate statement.

- ☐ A It has a characteristic abnormal EEG
- ☐ B Learning difficulties are rare
- ☐ C Symptoms disappear during sleep
- ☐ D It may be triggered by haloperidol,
- ☐ E It may be treated by methylphenidate,

10.14 Concerning head injuries, select the MOST appropriate statement.

- ☐ A They are an uncommon cause of death in children
- ☐ B Conscious level should be assessed using the full Glasgow Coma Scale score in all children
- ☐ C Raised intracranial pressure is less common in infants
- ☐ D All children with a GCS of less than 13 should be intubated and ventilated
- ☐ E Analgesia should not be given in order to allow continuous assessment of the patient's neurological status

10.15 Concerning Guillain–Barré syndrome, select the MOST appropriate statement.

- ☐ A Implicated infectious agents include Coxsackievirus
- ☐ B Sensory loss does not occur
- ☐ C Increased reflexes are present
- ☐ D Weakness is usually asymmetrical
- ☐ E Autonomic involvement does not occur

10.16 The following statements refer to spinal muscular atrophy type I (Werdnig–Hoffmann disease). Select the MOST appropriate statement.

- ☐ A It presents in late childhood
- ☐ B The genetic abnormality is localised to chromosome 5
- ☐ C The usual presentation is with delayed walking
- ☐ D Creatine phosphokinase is always raised
- ☐ E Survival beyond 3 months is rare

10.17 Concerning epilepsy, select the MOST appropriate statement.

- ❑ A In a complex seizure consciousness is retained
- ❑ B Simple refers to short duration
- ❑ C Partial seizures begin focally
- ❑ D Epilepsy that is difficult to control is classified as symptomatic
- ❑ E An aura is necessary to make a diagnosis

10.18 A 7-month-old child attends an assessment unit with a 1-week history of episodes of twitching.

Her mum described how her arms would rise into the air and jerk, with jerking of her head; these episodes would occur in clusters.

What is the next BEST step?

- ❑ A Genetic testing
- ❑ B Start prednisolone
- ❑ C Start anticonvulsants
- ❑ D A CT scan
- ❑ E An urgent EEG

10.19 The following statements refer to tuberous sclerosis. Select the MOST appropriate.

- ❑ A There is no increased recurrence risk in offspring
- ❑ B Adenoma sebaceum is a feature
- ❑ C Classic EEG findings are 3 Hz/s spike and wave
- ❑ D Good response of seizures to treatment with topiramate
- ❑ E There is frequent occurrence of malignant tumours

10.20 The following statements refer to cerebral palsy. Select the MOST appropriate statement.

- ❑ A It is more prevalent in girls
- ❑ B Birthweight <1500 g is a risk factor
- ❑ C Severe learning difficulties occur in more than 50% of cases
- ❑ D Perinatal asphyxia accounts for more than 50%
- ❑ E Prevalence is 1%

10.21 Which of the following is MOST likely to cause hypotonia in infancy?

- ❑ A Becker muscular dystrophy
- ❑ B Crohn disease
- ❑ C Subacute sclerosing panencephalitis
- ❑ D Duchenne muscular dystrophy
- ❑ E Down syndrome

10.22 Which of the following symptoms are MOST likely to be caused by a frontal lobe lesion?

- ❑ A Contralateral homonymous hemianopia
- ❑ B Impaired memory
- ❑ C Impaired spatial orientation
- ❑ D Receptive dysphasia
- ❑ E Apraxia

10.23 The following statements refer to Duchenne muscular dystrophy. Select the MOST appropriate statement.

- ❑ A Inheritance is X linked
- ❑ B Creatine phosphokinase is low
- ❑ C Muscle biopsy is unhelpful
- ❑ D The defect is on chromosome 6
- ❑ E Cardiac involvement is rare

10.24 Which of the following statements is most likely to be a risk factor for a simple febrile convulsion.

- ❑ A Age <6 months
- ❑ B Family history of epilepsy
- ❑ C Family history of febrile convulsions
- ❑ D Past history of asthma
- ❑ E Developmental delay

10.25 The following statements refer to temporal lobe epilepsy. Select the MOST appropriate statement.

- ☐ A It can present with feelings of déjà vu
- ☐ B Ethosuximide is the drug of first choice
- ☐ C The EEG shows 3/s spikes
- ☐ D It can present as brief loss of vision
- ☐ E It is the most common form of childhood epilepsy

10.26 The following statements refer to the radial nerve. Select the MOST appropriate statement.

- ☐ A It supplies the small muscles of the hand
- ☐ B The nerve root is T1
- ☐ C It is responsible for elbow flexion
- ☐ D The lesion is called Klumpke paralysis
- ☐ E Palsy causes wrist drop

10.27 Which of the following is the MOST likely cause of primary microcephaly?

- ☐ A Holoprosencephaly
- ☐ B Meningitis
- ☐ C Hypoxic ischaemic encephalopathy
- ☐ D Thyrotoxicosis
- ☐ E Intrauterine infection

10.28 With regard to brain tumours, select the MOST appropriate statement.

- ☐ A Medulloblastomas are the most common brain tumours in adolescence
- ☐ B Craniopharyngiomas can present with a visual field defect
- ☐ C Metastatic tumours are common in childhood
- ☐ D Oligodendrogliomas are the most common brain tumours in childhood
- ☐ E Brain tumours are the most common malignancy in childhood

10.29 On admission of a 3-year-old child with a first afebrile tonic–clonic seizure, select the MOST appropriate investigation.

- ☐ A Computed tomography (CT) head scan
- ☐ B Serum calcium
- ☐ C Blood culture
- ☐ D ECG
- ☐ E EEG

10.30 With regard to Horner syndrome, select the MOST appropriate statement.

- ❑ A Pupillary dilatation is a feature
- ❑ B It is a cause of facial weakness
- ❑ C Middle-ear infection is a cause in children
- ❑ D It causes proptosis
- ❑ E It is caused by a deficiency of parasympathetic activity

10.31 With regard to EEG, select the MOST appropriate statement.

- ❑ A A sufficiently abnormal EEG alone can be enough make a diagnosis of epilepsy
- ❑ B EEG should be preformed in cases of probable syncope to ensure that a diagnosis of epilepsy is not being missed
- ❑ C EEG can help in providing likely prognosis in patients in whom an epilepsy syndrome is suspected
- ❑ D A sleep EEG is no better than a standard EEG in providing diagnostic information; however, it makes it easier to place the electrodes on children
- ❑ E EEG should be used to exclude the diagnosis of epilepsy in patients in whom the clinical presentation supports a diagnosis of a non-epileptic event

10.32 A previously fit and well 8-year-old child presents with irregular jerky movements of her limbs which have come on over a few days; before this her parents had noted her to be generally more agitated.

The movements reduce and sometimes disappear on sleep. Several weeks previously she had had a sore throat.

Select the MOST appropriate advice to give the parents.

- ❑ A This may be epilepsy and she will need an EEG to confirm
- ❑ B These episodes are being fabricated by the patient, otherwise they would not terminate with sleep
- ❑ C This may be choreoathetoid cerebral palsy and she will need an urgent MR scan
- ❑ D This may be Sydenham chorea, which would be treated with antibiotics and has an overall good prognosis but may take several weeks to recover
- ❑ E This may be Gilles de la Tourette syndrome and she will need referral to a psychiatrists

10.33 With regard to paediatric stroke, select the MOST appropriate statement.

- ❑ A The majority of paediatric strokes are haemorrhagic
- ❑ B Approximately half of children presenting with an arterial ischaemic stroke have a known predisposing condition
- ❑ C Most childhood strokes occur in neonates
- ❑ D CT is not able to exclude haemorrhage
- ❑ E Dehydration predisposes to haemorrhagic stroke

10.34 Select the MOST appropriate statement with regard to craniosynostosis.

- ❑ A In posterior plagiocephaly due to positional moulding, the ear position is more anterior on the side of the flattening, whereas, in that due to synostosis of the lambdoid suture, the ear position is more posterior
- ❑ B Secondary craniosynostosis caused by primary failure of brain growth is approximately twice as common as primary craniosynostosis caused by premature suture fusion
- ❑ C The major morbidity associated with primary craniosynostosis affecting one or two sutures is raised intracranial pressure
- ❑ D Normal skull growth occurs parallel to each suture
- ❑ E In order to prevent the need for multiple surgical procedures in children with multiple suture craniosynostosis, surgical intervention is best delayed until after age 6 months

10.35 Select the MOST appropriate of the following statements with regard to performing a lumbar puncture.

- ❑ A A lumbar puncture is always required to confirm the diagnosis of meningococcal meningitis
- ❑ B A lumbar puncture can be safely performed in the presence of a Glasgow Coma Scale score of 12 in an adolescent
- ❑ C Normal findings on CT or MR scan of the brain confirm that it is safe to perform a lumbar puncture
- ❑ D Abnormal posturing is a contraindication to performing a lumbar puncture
- ❑ E Delaying lumbar puncture until after the administration of antibiotics results in negative CSF cultures and should therefore be avoided

10.36 The following statements refer to migraine in childhood. Select the MOST appropriate.

- ❑ A Girls are more commonly affected than boys throughout childhood
- ❑ B Pre-school children are not affected
- ❑ C They are preceded by auras – most commonly visual
- ❑ D When complicated by hemiplegia, the headache precedes the onset of the neurological weakness
- ❑ E Propranolol and sodium valproate can be used as prophylaxis

10.37 The following statements refer to juvenile myoclonic epilepsy (JME). Select the MOST appropriate.

- ❑ A Myoclonic jerks, generalised tonic–clonic seizures and absence seizures may all feature
- ❑ B Seizure control is usually possible with low-dose anticonvulsant therapy, and successful drug withdrawal is possible after a suitable seizure-free interval has been achieved
- ❑ C Myoclonic jerks are typically experienced at night
- ❑ D Sodium valproate, lamotrigine and carbamazepine can all be used successfully as monotherapy to control seizure activity
- ❑ E JME is frequently associated with learning difficulties

10.38 A 3-year-old African–Caribbean boy develops an acute onset right-sided hemiplegia after a fall. Select the MOST appropriate of the following statements.

- ❑ A The most likely cause of the hemiplegia is an ischaemic stroke secondary to arterial dissection caused by the fall
- ❑ B The boy should be screened for sickle cell disease because this is associated with a significantly increased risk of cerebrovascular events
- ❑ C A haemorrhagic event is more likely to be the cause than an ischaemic event
- ❑ D Aspirin at a dose of 5 mg/kg per day should be commenced if the diagnosis of stroke is confirmed
- ❑ E Most children with a stroke survive without long-term neurological or cognitive sequelae

Extended Matching Questions

10.39–10.41 Theme: Neurocutaneous syndromes

- ❑ A Sturge–Weber syndrome
- ❑ B Hypomelanosis of Ito
- ❑ C Ataxia–telangiectasia
- ❑ D Neurofibromatosis type 1
- ❑ E Neurofibromatosis type 2
- ❑ F Tuberous sclerosis
- ❑ G Von Hippel–Lindau disease
- ❑ H Incontinentia pigmenti
- ❑ I Ether–Danlos syndrome

Choose the most likely diagnosis from the list above for each of the three cases described below. Each option may be used once, more than once or not at all.

10.39

A 6-month-old child presenting with right focal seizures who is noted to have a left facial haemangioma..

10.40

A 8-year-old boy who has had a number of afebrile seizures; on examination he has seven café-au-lait patches. His father also has a large number of café-au-lait patches.

10.41

A 2-year-old child who at birth had a blistering rash presents with developmental delay. She has small teeth and brown swirl-like patches on her skin.

10.42–10.44 Theme: Cranial nerve palsies

- ❑ A Nerve III palsy
- ❑ B Nerve VI palsy
- ❑ C Nerve V palsy
- ❑ D Nerve IV palsy
- ❑ E Nerve VII palsy
- ❑ F Nerve X palsy
- ❑ G Nerve XII palsy
- ❑ H Nerve II palsy
- ❑ I Nerve IX palsy

Choose the most likely diagnosis from the list above for each of the three cases described below. Each option may be used once, more than once or not at all.

10.42

Complete ptosis and downward lateral gaze of the affected eye.

10.43

Paralysis of muscles of facial expression.

10.44

Diplopia and inability to abduct affected eye.

10.45–10.47 Theme: Epilepsy

- ❑ A Juvenile myoclonic epilepsy
- ❑ B Severe myoclonic epilepsy of infancy
- ❑ C Childhood absence epilepsy
- ❑ D Benign rolandic epilepsy
- ❑ E Panayiotopoulos syndrome
- ❑ F Frontal seizures
- ❑ G Temporal lobe seizures
- ❑ H Febrile convulsion
- ❑ I West syndrome
- ❑ J Non-epileptic seizures

Choose the most likely diagnosis from the list above for each of the three cases described below. Each option may be used once, more than once or not at all.

10.45

An 8-year-old boy woke from sleep with tingling feeling of his lips and tongue on the right side of his face. His parents heard him making gurgling noises in his room. When they found him he was conscious but had twitching down the right side of his body; this lasted several seconds and then he seemed to lose consciousness and all four limbs started to shake. This lasted a few minutes after which he was sleepy. He recovered fully from this episode. His parents describe two other similar episodes. An EEG performed after this shows centrotemporal spike wave discharges.

10.46

A 5-year-old boy attends a paediatric outpatient clinic. His schoolteachers had raised concern that he had been noticed to be 'day dreaming' on several occasions during the day. During these episodes they have noticed he tends to pick at his clothes. His EEG shows 3 Hz/s spike–wave discharges.

10.47

A 3-year-old boy who has had a number of typical episodes; during these episodes he has woken from sleep, becomes pale and feels sick. His eyes and subsequently head turn to the right. The episodes last about 15 minutes then he vomits. His eyes and head slowly return back to the midline but he is drowsy for 30 minutes after. In between episodes he has a normal neurological examination, a normal ECG and normal MR brain scan. An EEG showed occipital and frontal spike wave discharges.

10.48–10.50 Theme: Anticonvulsant treatment

- ❑ A Carbamazepine
- ❑ B Sodium valporate
- ❑ C Ethosuximide
- ❑ D Lamotrigene
- ❑ E Levetiracetam
- ❑ F Phenytoin
- ❑ G Phenobarbital
- ❑ H Lorazepam
- ❑ I Topiramate

Choose the most appropriate treatment from the list above for each of the three cases described below. Each option may be used once, more than once or not at all.

10.48

A 17-year-old girl with difficult to control migraine.

10.49

An 8-day-old baby with seizures secondary to hypoxic ischaemic injury.

10.50

A 1-year-old with left focal seizures secondary to an *in utero* infarction.

10.51–10.53 Theme: Ataxia

- ❑ A Genetic studies for ataxia–telangiectasia
- ❑ B CSF microscopy
- ❑ C Genetic analysis of the frataxin gene on chromosome 9
- ❑ D 24-hour urinary copper
- ❑ E Very-long-chain fatty acids
- ❑ F Urinary catecholamine metabolities
- ❑ G Carbamazepine level
- ❑ H Blood alcohol level
- ❑ I CSF protein

Choose the most likely diagnostic investigation from the list above for each of the three cases described below. Each option may be used once, more than once or not at all.

10.51

A 12-year-old boy with a year's history of becoming increasingly clumsy. Initially he had noticed that he was stumbling and falling more than previously, but lately he has had some trouble with his handwriting. He continues to do well academically and, although frustrated at times at his own clumsiness, there has been no change in his personality. On examination he has ataxia worse in his lower limbs than upper limbs and early signs of pes cavus in both his feet. He has absent ankle jerks but bilateral extensor plantars.

10.52

A 4-year-old girl with an unsteady gait. She has only been walking for just under 2 years but her mother feels that her walking has not improved as she would have expected and she still remains quite unsteady. On examination her tone and reflexes are normal but she has a wide-based gait and is reluctant to walk without her mother's supportive hand. She has a small collection of prominent blood vessels on her eye and her mother reports that she has a number of these on her back and legs.

10.53

A 6-year-old boy with a month's history of being more unsteady on his feet. His mother also tells of a marked change in behaviour, becoming withdrawn and aggressive at times. His teachers remark that he isn't concentrating or academically doing as well.

10.54–10.56 Theme: Hypotonia

- ❑ A Muscle biopsy for congenital myopathy
- ❑ B Serum creatine kinase for Duchenne muscular dystrophy
- ❑ C Genetic studies for 22q11 deletion
- ❑ D Thyroid function tests
- ❑ E Urine toxicology screen
- ❑ F Plasma very-long-chain fatty acids
- ❑ G Urinary reducing substances
- ❑ H Chromosomal analysis for Down syndrome
- ❑ I Genetic studies for cri-du-chat syndrome

Choose the most likely diagnostic investigation from the list above for each of the three cases described below. Each option may be used once, more than once or not at all.

10.54

A hypotonic baby boy with large anterior fontanelle, hepatomegaly and seizures.

10.55

A hypotonic female neonate of low birthweight with high-pitched cry, microcephaly, round face and full cheeks, heart murmur, epicanthal folds and short fingers.

10.56

A hypotonic male infant with generalised hyporeflexia and reduced muscle bulk. Mother reports reduced fetal movements *in utero*.

10.57–10.59 Theme: Meningitis

- ❑ A Group B streptococcus
- ❑ B *Listeria monocytogenes*
- ❑ C Pneumococcus
- ❑ D *Escherichia coli*
- ❑ E *Haemophilus influenzae* type b
- ❑ F Herpes simplex virus
- ❑ G *Neisseria meningitidis*
- ❑ H *Pseudomonas aeruginosa*
- ❑ I *Staphylococcus epidermidis*
- ❑ J *Mycobacterium tuberculosis*

Choose the most likely infecting organism from the list above for each of the three scenarios described below. Each option may be used once, more than once or not at all.

10.57

A 6-week-old baby with fever and irritability has the following lumbar puncture result:

- appearance: cloudy
- red cell count (RBC): 5/mm³
- white cell count (WCC): 1407/mm³ (polymorphs 70%)
- protein: 1 g/l
- CSF glucose: 2.1 mmol/l
- blood glucose: 5.6 mmol/l
- Gram stain: Gram-negative bacilli.

10.58

A 5-year-old girl with known sickle cell disease who has had a recent upper respiratory tract infection treated with amoxicillin presents with headache and vomiting. The lumbar puncture result is as follows:

- appearance: turbid
- RBC: 2/mm³
- WCC– 3589/mm³ (lymphocytes 62%)
- protein: 0.7 g/l
- CSF glucose: 2.8 mmol/l
- blood glucose: 7.4 mmol/l
- Gram stain: no organisms seen.

10.59

A 33-week preterm neonate born 72 hours after rupture of membranes develops seizures on day 5. After stabilisation, a lumbar puncture is performed with the following results:

- appearance: blood stained
- RBC: 137/mm^3
- WCC: 11 247/mm^3 (lymphocytes 80%)
- protein: 2.4 g/l
- CSF glucose: 1.8 mmol/l
- blood glucose: 3.6 mmol/l
- Gram stain: Gram-positive bacilli.

CHAPTER 11

Respiratory

Multiple True–False Questions

11.1 The following cause the oxyhaemoglobin dissociation curve to shift to the right:

- ❑ A Alkalosis
- ❑ B High altitude
- ❑ C Increased PCO_2
- ❑ D Increased temperature
- ❑ E low concentration of 2,3-diphosphoglycerate (2,3-DPG)

11.2 Lymphocytic intestinal pneumonitis

- ❑ A Has an insidious onset in most cases
- ❑ B Usually presents in the first year of life
- ❑ C Has a mortality rate of more than 50%
- ❑ D Is due to *Pneumocystis jiroveci* infection
- ❑ E Responds to oral steroids

11.3 Pulmonary hypoplasia of the newborn

- ❑ A Is most commonly a primary condition
- ❑ B Is associated with oligohydramnios
- ❑ C Is seen in 1 in 10 000 births
- ❑ D Can be unilateral
- ❑ E Occurs in Potter syndrome

11.4 The following are characteristic of type II respiratory failure:

- ❑ A Hyperventilation
- ❑ B Hypoxia
- ❑ C Ventilation–perfusion mismatch
- ❑ D Raised $PaCO_2$
- ❑ E Head injury as a possible cause

11.5 Rigid bronchoscopy is generally required to

- ❑ A Remove a foreign body
- ❑ B Exclude vocal cord paralysis
- ❑ C Diagnose TB
- ❑ D Assess persistent atelectasis
- ❑ E Remove a blood clot

11.6 Which of the following conditions may cause a false-positive sweat test?

- ❑ A Ventricular septal defect
- ❑ B Adrenal insufficiency
- ❑ C Pseudohypoaldosteronism
- ❑ D Asthma
- ❑ E Chronic renal failure

11.7 Which of the following are present in the lung in their adult quota at birth?

- ❑ A Alveoli
- ❑ B Goblet cells
- ❑ C Terminal bronchioles
- ❑ D Pulmonary vessels
- ❑ E Acini

11.8 The peak expiratory flow rate:

- ❑ A Is increased in obstructive airway disease
- ❑ B Is effort independent
- ❑ C Is a suitable measure to attempt on a 3-year-old child
- ❑ D Is diagnostic of asthma if the value increases by 20% after administration of bronchodilators
- ❑ E Is influenced by airway diameter

Best of Five Questions

11.9 A 3-year-old boy presented to hospital with a 2-day history of cough, fever, anorexia and malaise, complaining of abdominal pain.

On admission he was noted to have a temperature of 39.5°C, a respiratory rate of 65 beats/min and oxygen saturations of 91% in air. Clinically he had reduced air entry and crepitations in his right lower zone. His chest radiograph revealed consolidation in his right lower zone and he was admitted for intravenous antibiotics and supportive oxygen therapy. Over the next 72 hours his temperature continued to fluctuate and his symptoms persisted. He was re-examined and found to have become dull to percussion in the right lower zone of his chest. Repeat chest radiograph revealed a 'white-out' of the right side of his chest and demonstrated a new scoliosis not present on his presenting radiograph.

Which of the following investigations would be the most important next step in this child's management?

- ❑ A CT scan of the chest
- ❑ B Ultrasound scan of the chest
- ❑ C Repeat blood cultures
- ❑ D Diagnostic pleural tap
- ❑ E Sputum culture

11.10 A 4-month-old baby is admitted with a 2-week history of cough and low-grade fever not responding to treatment with oral amoxicillin.

On examination the baby is tachycardic and tachypnoeic but has a clear chest on auscultation. His saturations are 86% in air but improve with supplementary oxygen. It is noted on admission that, despite being born on the 50th centile for weight the child has gradually drifted down to the 2nd centile over the preceding 3 months, and has had recurrent bouts of diarrhoea over this time. He has also suffered in the past with recurrent oral candidiasis. During his admission he clinically deteriorates despite intravenous antibiotics and requires ventilation to maintain adequate oxygenation.

What is the most important investigation after intubation to aid diagnosis for this child's condition?

- ❑ A Respiratory viral screen
- ❑ B Bronchoalveolar lavage (BAL) polymerase chain reaction (PCR) for *Pneumocystis jiroveci* (formerly known as *P carinii*)
- ❑ C Sweat test
- ❑ D Respiratory sample for *Aspergillus* spp
- ❑ E Anti-HIV IgG

11.11 Which of the following signs is MOST helpful in showing that a 2-year-old child presenting with asthma has had a severe attack?

- ❑ A Pulsus paradoxus >20 mmHg
- ❑ B Confusion/agitation
- ❑ C PEFR (peak expiratory flow rate) <60% of predicted
- ❑ D Saturations of 90% in air
- ❑ E Pyrexia

11.12 An 18-month-old boy is brought to the accident and emergency department by ambulance at 3am.

He has been relatively well over the last week with mild coryzal symptoms over the last 24 hours. He woke his parents 30 minutes before admission with an abrupt onset of a barking cough and severe difficulty in breathing. His symptoms are mildly improved on admission but he still has obvious respiratory distress with a respiratory rate of 50 beats/min and oxygen saturations of 98% in air, intercostal recession and obvious stridor at rest in a non-distressed state. He has a mild temperature of 37.9°C.

What is the most appropriate first step in the management of this child?

- ❑ A Lateral neck radiograph
- ❑ B Nebulised adrenaline (5 ml of 1:1000)
- ❑ C Nebulised budesonide (2 mg in 4 ml water)
- ❑ D Oral dexamethasone (no dosage)
- ❑ E Humidified oxygen via facial mask

11.13 A 7-month-old baby was seen in the emergency department.

She has a 2-day history of coryza followed by a 2-day history of increasing coughing and rapid breathing. She has stopped tolerating her feeds, has only taken a third of her usual volume over the last 24 hours, and has vomited after every feed. On examination she has intercostal recession but no nasal flaring. She has bilateral inspiratory crepitations and polyphonic wheeze, a temperature of 37.6°C 3 hours after her last dose of Calpol and a respiratory rate of 65 beats/min. She has a heart rate of 130 beats/min and saturations of 93% in air.

What should your next step in her management be? Choose the best answer from those listed below.

- ❑ A Discharge home with advice to return if patient deteriorates over the next 24 hours
- ❑ B Admit and commence oral antibiotics
- ❑ C Admit and commence intravenous antibiotics and intravenous fluids
- ❑ D Admit and obtain intravenous access and initiate treatment with intravenous fluids at 75% of maintenance fluid
- ❑ E Admit for assessment and commence nasogastric feeding if not tolerating >50% of maintenance requirement during the next feed

11.14 Which of the following treatments would be your drug of choice for use immediately before starting exercise in a child who suffers from exercise-induced asthma?

- ❑ A Sodium cromoglicate
- ❑ B Salbutamol
- ❑ C Fluticasone propionate
- ❑ D Monteleukast
- ❑ E Salmeterol

11.15 Which of the following statements best describes the likely feeding outcome of a child born with a previously undiagnosed isolated cleft lip and palate?

- ❑ A The child will not be able to breastfeed and mothers should be dissuaded from trying because failure will contribute to bonding problems
- ❑ B The child will not be able to bottle feed and so a nasogastric tube should be sited initially
- ❑ C Specialist bottles and teats are essential to feed this child so intravenous fluids should be started until specialist help is available
- ❑ D Mothers with babies born with cleft lip and palate should be offered support and specialist advice to feed their child by their chosen method
- ❑ E Specialist feeding advice is very difficult to obtain in the first couple of days of life because there are so few centres specialising in cleft lip and palate management

11.16 A 2-year-old boy was admitted to accident and emergency with a 2-hour history of high temperature and noisy breathing.

On examination he was quiet and very pale, sitting up with his neck extended and drooling, he had obvious stridor and increased work of breathing. He was from a travelling community and had not completed his childhood immunisation schedule. He had no significant past medical history of note.

What is the most likely diagnosis in this child?

- ❑ A Acute tonsillitis with peritonsillar abscess
- ❑ B Foreign body aspiration
- ❑ C Severe viral croup
- ❑ D Epiglottitis
- ❑ E Bacterial tracheitis

11.17 Which of the following methods of administration of β_2 agonist is the best choice for a 4-year-old with an acute exacerbation of chronic asthma not requiring hospital admission?

- ❑ A Home nebuliser
- ❑ B Pressurised MDI (metered dose inhaler) plus spacer device
- ❑ C Turbohaler
- ❑ D Breath-actuated device
- ❑ E Oral syrup solution

11.18 A 4-year-old Asian boy is referred from his GP to paediatric outpatients for assessment due to chronic cough.

He was born at term but required an admission to the neonatal intensive care unit for respiratory distress. He has suffered from chronic ear infections over the last year and has also had three courses of antibiotics for chest infections that have not required hospital admission. He is small for his age and plots just above the 0.4th centile, having been born on the 50th centile and having a midparental height just above the 50th centile. He has also had concerns raised by his preschool about his ability to hear; neonatal screening test for hearing was normal. He does not have any gastroenterological complaints and in clinic – 4 weeks after his last course of antibiotics – his examination is entirely normal He previously had a negative immunoreactive trypsin on newborn screening.

What is the most likely diagnosis in this young boy?

- ❑ A Cystic fibrosis
- ❑ B Poorly controlled asthma
- ❑ C Primary ciliary dyskinesia
- ❑ D Recurrent bronchiolitis
- ❑ E TB

11.19 A 14-year-old girl presents to her local paediatric department with abdominal distension, nausea and cramping abdominal pain increasing over the last week. She has cystic fibrosis and open access to the department as a consequence.

She was diagnosed in the neonatal period presenting with meconium ileus and required a laparotomy. She has recently had a 'vomiting bug' that had affected her entire family, and had decreased frequency of bowel motions along with a decreased oral intake over the last few days. She ordinarily has good compliance with her medications, including enzyme replacement. She is well grown with height and weight following the 25th centile for age, with her midparental centile between the 25th and 50th centiles. On examination she was relatively comfortable at rest with a normal heart rate and temperature; she had mild tachypnoea and some mild intercostal recession. Her chest was clear on auscultation and her oxygen saturations were 99% in air. Her abdominal examination revealed a mildly distended but soft abdomen with a mass in the right iliac fossa that was tender on palpitation.

What is the most likely diagnosis?

- ❑ A Chronic constipation
- ❑ B Acute appendicitis with appendix mass
- ❑ C Intestinal obstruction secondary to adhesions from her previous surgery
- ❑ D Infective colitis
- ❑ E Distal intestinal obstruction syndrome

11.20 A 3-year-old girl presents to the paediatric assessment unit with a history of recurrent chest infections; she is currently unwell with cough, fever and vomiting.

She is an only child of non-consanguineous white parents. She has had a 'wet' cough off and on over the past year, showing improvement with courses of oral antibiotics but subsequent deterioration off antibiotics. She has a steroid inhaler and reliever for symptoms of recurrent wheeze. She has no family history of atopy. She is not well grown with a height and weight less than the 0.4th centile, and midparental centile just above the 50th. She has had a decreased oral intake associated with her current illness but normally has a very good appetite and eats as well as her 10-year-old half-brother.

What is the most likely diagnosis in this case?

- ❑ A Community-acquired pneumonia
- ❑ B Poorly controlled atopic asthma
- ❑ C IgA deficiency
- ❑ D Cystic fibrosis
- ❑ E Pertussis infection

11.21 A 7-year-old boy presented to a paediatric outpatient clinic with a 2-year history of recurrent chest infections and persistent cough responsive to multiple courses of antibiotics.

He had dyspnoea on exertion and had symptoms of wheeze responsive to bronchodilators but not controlled by regular inhaled steroids at moderate dosage. He had a family history of mild atopy and had mild infantile eczema himself. He was reported to have good technique and compliance with his inhaled medications by his local respiratory nurse who had personally assessed his inhaler technique and monitored his repeat prescription rates.

On examination his height and weight were just above the 0.4th centile. His midparental height plotted above the 50th percentile and his younger brother, who was 2 years his junior, was 3 cm taller than him. On examination of his chest he was mildly tachypnoeic and had mild intercostal recession at rest. On auscultation he had course crepitations and wheeze heard throughout the right lower zone. His oxygen saturations were 97% in room air. He was clubbed.

He had a sweat test performed and his sweat sodium was 39 mmol/l in an adequate sample.

He had a positive skinprick tests to tree pollen and cat.

What is the most likely explanation of the symptoms of this young man from the list below?

- ☐ A Under-treated atopic asthma
- ☐ B Cystic fibrosis
- ☐ C Community-acquired pneumonia
- ☐ D Bronchiectasis
- ☐ E Congenital heart disease

11.22 A 5-year-old boy presents to his GP with an 8-month history of hyperactivity, inattentiveness and aggressive behaviour since starting school.

On further questioning his mother says that he has very disturbed sleep with snoring, frequent waking, and pronounced tossing and turning during the night. He has also become enuretic at night having been previously dry since the age of 3. He is otherwise well but does tend to mouth breathe most of the time. His examination including fundoscopy, detailed neurological examination and BP are all normal. His height plots on the 75th centile and his weight is above the 99th centile. What are the most appropriate referral and investigation for this young man?

- ❑ A Referral to a general paediatrician for MRI of the head to exclude space-occupying lesion
- ❑ B Referral to a community paediatrician for assessment and management of attention-deficit hyperactivity disorder
- ❑ C Referral to community enuresis clinic for assessment and treatment of his secondary enuresis
- ❑ D Referral to ENT surgeon for pharyngolaryngoscopy
- ❑ E Referral to respiratory paediatrician for a sleep study

11.23 A 9-year-old boy presents to his GP with a 3-day history of temperature – spiking up to 39.3°C, headache, sore throat and dry cough.

The cough has increased in frequency and severity over a 3-day period. He had symptoms of shortness of breath that were limiting his normal activities and new-onset wheeze associated with the cough; he had not previously had recurrent chest infections and had no background or family history of asthma. He was lethargic and looked unwell at review. He had a temperature of 38°C and a respiratory rate of 55 beats/min at rest; his oxygen saturations in air were 94% and he had slight intercostal recession. On auscultation of his chest he had right lower zone crepitations and widespread wheeze bilaterally.

What is the most appropriate treatment for this young man?

- ❑ A Oral amoxicillin
- ❑ B Salbutamol and prednisolone
- ❑ C Oral erythromylin
- ❑ D Salbutamol and amoxicillin
- ❑ E Erythromycin and salbutamol

11.24 A 7-year-old child presents to the GP with a 24-hour history of sore throat and cough. She is drinking a little fluid but has not eaten for the last 24 hours.

On examination she has a mild fever of 37.5°C and is not tachycardic. She has a capillary refill time of <2 s. She has enlarged erythematous tonsils without obvious exudate and a few petechiae on her soft palate. She has enlarged cervical lymphadenopathy that is not tender to touch.

What is the BEST management plan for this girl?

- ❑ A Give a prescription for phenoxymethylpenicillin and advise the use of the prescription in 48 hours if symptoms continue to increase or there is no sign of settling within this time frame Advise to re-present if child looks severely unwell at any time
- ❑ B Commence treatment with oral amoxicillin for 5 days
- ❑ C Commence treatment with penicillin for 10 days
- ❑ D Advise parents about the importance of pain relief and fluid intake in the acute illness and send them home
- ❑ E Give a prescription for amoxicillin and advise to start antibiotics if symptoms are not entirely better within the next 24 hours

11.25 A 5-year-old girl presented to A&E with a history of rapid onset of wheeze, increased work of breathing, urticaria and facial swelling after her first ingestion of peanuts at a birthday party.

She had a previous history of recurrent wheeze with exercise and a family history of atopy. She lives with her parents on a farm 35 minutes from the nearest hospital.

What is the best strategy for managing this child post discharge?

- ❑ A Refer to allergist for further investigation and management
- ❑ B Refer to GP and asthma nurse for optimisation of asthma management
- ❑ C Prescription of EpiPen if further reactions occur
- ❑ D Advise to avoid peanuts in the future
- ❑ E Prescription of EpiPen, education re its use and referral to allergist

11.26 Which of the statements regarding TB is most accurate?

- ☐ A *Mycobacterium tuberculosis* is commonly found in the soil
- ☐ B A positive Mantoux test is diagnostic of infection with *Mycobacterium tuberculosis*
- ☐ C A strongly positive Mantoux test (>15 mm) is suggestive of a diagnosis of TB even if the patient has been immunised with BCG
- ☐ D NICE guidelines recommend treatment with triple therapy for 6 months in all cases of confirmed TB
- ☐ E QuantiFERON-TB is now the first-line investigation of choice for all suspected cases of fulminant TB

11.27 A 1-year-old child is admitted unwell. The following arterial blood gas is taken on arrival in the unit while the child is on 10 l/min oxygen via a facemask.

pH 7.13

PCO_2 4.2 kPa

PO_2 11 kPa

HCO_3^- 10 mmol/l

Base excess −10

Blood glucose 10 mmol/l

What is the most likely cause for this child's acute presentation?

- ☐ A Bronchiolitis
- ☐ B Pneumonia
- ☐ C Sepsis
- ☐ D Diabetic ketoacidosis
- ☐ E Severe croup

11.28 Which of the following statements BEST describes congenital lobar emphysema?

- ☐ A Commonly affects the lower lobes
- ☐ B If symptomatic, will usually present with tachypnoea and signs of respiratory distress in the neonatal period
- ☐ C It is associated with a cardiac abnormality in less than 5% of cases
- ☐ D It should be treated by lobectomy in order to prevent secondary bacterial infection or pneumothorax
- ☐ E It is most commonly secondary to an intrinsic deficiency of bronchial cartilage

11.29 Select the MOST appropriate statement from the following, with respect to monoclonal antibody (palivizumab) to respiratory syncytial virus (RSV).

- ❑ A Reduces admission rates to hospital and intensive care units in infants with bronchopulmonary dysplasia (BPD) when compared with placebo
- ❑ B It is licensed for preventing RSV infection if given to children aged <3 years with congenital heart disease
- ❑ C It is licensed for children aged <2 years who are born at less than 35 weeks' gestation
- ❑ D It can be given annually to protect the at-risk infant throughout the RSV season
- ❑ E It can be administered as an alternative to ribavirin to reduce the duration of mechanical ventilation for the treatment of babies with BPD

11.30 Which of the following statements about whooping cough is MOST accurate?

- ❑ A It is caused by infection with Gram-positive bacillus *Bordetella pertussis*
- ❑ B Immunisation has controlled the spread of disease in the developed world and it is no longer a public health concern in the UK
- ❑ C The initial catarrhal phase is indistinguishable from common upper respiratory tract infections
- ❑ D During the paroxysmal stage, patients have evidence of lower respiratory tract disease on examination
- ❑ E Macrolide antibiotics are helpful in altering the clinical course throughout the illness and should be given whenever the diagnosis is made, as long as the patient is still symptomatic

11.31 A 4-year-old boy presents to A&E with a 3-day history of cough and fever.

On examination his respiratory rate is 30/min and oxygen saturations are 97% in air. There is no evidence of dehydration. He has course crackles at the right base. He has right lower lobe pneumonia on chest radiograph with no associated collapse.

What would the most appropriate treatment be?

- ❑ A Admission for broad-spectrum intravenous antibiotics for 48 hours or until fever settles
- ❑ B Supportive treatment only as the most likely causative agent is viral
- ❑ C Treatment with a macrolide antibiotic orally with follow-up chest radiograph in 6–8 weeks
- ❑ D Treatment with oral amoxicillin
- ❑ E Chest physiotherapy together with oral antimicrobial therapy

11.32 A 5-year-old boy with asthma is having frequent exercise-induced and nocturnal symptoms despite good compliance with his current prescribed regimen of inhaled steroids (fluticasone 125 µg twice daily) and long-acting β agonist (salmeterol 50 µg twice daily) taken via a large volumatic spacer without facemask. Which would be the MOST appropriate alteration to his therapy?

- ☐ A Change his inhaled steroids to budesonide 200 µg twice daily
- ☐ B Add monteleukast at a dose of 4 mg once daily
- ☐ C Change to dry powder device because drug delivery will be improved
- ☐ D Advise administration of short-acting bronchodilator before exercise
- ☐ E Increase dose of inhaled fluticasone to 250 µg twice daily

Extended Matching Questions

11.33–11.35 Theme: Chronic cough

- ☐ A Asthma
- ☐ B Inhaled foreign body
- ☐ C Cystic fibrosis
- ☐ D Primary ciliary dyskinesia
- ☐ E Protracted bacterial bronchitis
- ☐ F *Mycoplasma pneumoniae*
- ☐ G Pertussis
- ☐ H Bronchiolitis
- ☐ I Lobar sequestration
- ☐ J Persistent isolated chronic cough

Choose the most likely diagnosis from the list above for each of the three scenarios described below. Each option may be used once, more than once or not at all.

11.33

A 4-year-old girl has been referred to a paediatric outpatient clinic with a history of chronic cough query asthma by her GP. Her symptoms started around the time of a viral infection 12 months ago and at that time her coughing was present through the day and night, and associated with vomiting at times. Her symptoms improved over a period of 4–6 weeks but a persistent night-time cough has remained. She has some coughing associated with running about during the day and the coughing will limit her activity but she is not otherwise short of breath. She has a family history of maternal childhood eczema but had no eczema herself. She has had a 2-month trial of beclometasone 100 μg twice daily via MDI with spacer with no relief in symptoms. On examination she is well grown with her height and weight plotting on the 75th centile – appropriate for her midparental height. She has no wheeze to hear in her chest and no increased work of breathing or chest deformity. She is not clubbed.

11.34

A 3-year-old boy was referred to the paediatric outpatient clinic with a history of chronic cough. His cough was described as wet, but was not productive of sputum. He had had symptoms of coughing both at night and during the day for over 6 months. He had partially responded to a course of 5 days of amoxicillin but had relapsed into chronic cough again within a week of completion of the course. His mother had had mild childhood asthma, but he had no personal history of atopy. His symptoms seemed to fluctuate in severity, increasing with viral infections but had not resolved for more than 2 weeks since the start of the condition. On examination he was well grown on the 75th centile for height and weight and this was appropriate for his midparental centile just below the 75th. His chest was clear with no added sounds, no signs of chronic lung disease or increased work of breathing. There was no finger clubbing.

11.35

A 2-year-old child was seen in the outpatient clinic after an 8-week history of cough. The cough had started abruptly one evening and had persisted day and night despite a week's course of Amoxil and a trial of salbutamol inhaler via a spacer with a mask. She has no family or personal history of atopy. She is well grown and has no signs of chronic lung disease on examination. She has a few crepitations in the right middle zone of her chest and chest radiograph shows signs of isolated right middle lobe collapse/consolidation.

11.36–11.38 Theme: Cervical lymphadenopathy

- ❑ A Acute myeloid leukaemia
- ❑ B Non-TB mycobacterial infection
- ❑ C Tuberculosis
- ❑ D Kawasaki disease
- ❑ E Cat-scratch disease
- ❑ F Lymphoma
- ❑ G Juvenile systemic arthritis
- ❑ H CMV
- ❑ I Group A haemolytic streptococcal lymphadenitis
- ❑ J Viral upper respiratory tract infection

Choose the most likely diagnosis from the list above for each of the three scenarios described below. Each option may be used once, more than once or not at all.

11.36

A 3-year-old girl presents with a week's history of fever, fatigue and a single enlarged cervical lymph node. She complained of pain associated with the lump. On close examination she has a small fading pustule on the base of her neck and multiple fading scratch marks over her hands and arms. The gland itself is 3 cm in diameter and hot, and the overlying skin is erythematous with some induration. She is not clinically anaemic and has no palpable organomegaly.

11.37

A 2-year-old girl presents to outpatients with a 4-week history of a painless enlargement of a cervical lymph node. There is a slight violaceous discoloration of the skin overlying the node. She has no clinical anaemia, no fever, no other lymphadenopathy or organomegaly palpable, and her node has failed to respond to 2 weeks' treatment with broad-spectrum antibiotics by her GP. She has no personal history of contact with cats or anybody known to be high risk of having or being diagnosed with TB.

11.38

A 6-year-old child presents to the accident and emergency department with a 24-hour history of high fever up to 39.0°C, and a painful, enlarged (3 cm diameter), firm, hot and erythematous cervical lymph node. There were no other skin lesions within the region of the enlarged lymph node. He had been relatively well for the 24 hours before admission but had complained of a sore throat and had not eaten his tea the previous night.

11.39–11.41 Theme: Diagnosis of asthma in children

- ☐ A Trial of salbutamol MDI plus volumatic spacer device and planned review with GP
- ☐ B Trial of inhaled steroid MDI plus spacer at standard dose with defined reassessment and follow-up
- ☐ C Trial of oral course of prednisolone with follow-up if symptoms do not resolve
- ☐ D Spirometry investigation with assessment of reversibility and treatment with salbutamol MDI plus spacer if reversibility demonstrated
- ☐ E Spirometry investigation; if shows obstructive picture proceed to a trial of inhaled steroid MDI plus spacer at standard dose with defined reassessment and follow-up
- ☐ F Chest radiograph and sweat test
- ☐ G Referral to respiratory paediatrician for further assessment
- ☐ H Flexible bronchoscopy
- ☐ I Treatment with oral course of azithromycin
- ☐ J Management of acute symptoms followed by discharge advice to avoid trigger factors and treat exacerbations with salbutamol MDI plus volumatic spacer with planned follow-up

For each of the following clinical scenarios, choose from the above options the best course of action to be taken for the ongoing management or investigation of the patient. Each option may be used once, more than once or not at all.

11.39

A 5-year-old girl presents to the GP with a 3-month history of recurrent wheeze, cough and shortness of breath. Symptoms occur multiple times a day, most days, and are increased at night and in association with exertion/exercise. She is limited in her exercise tolerance compared with her peers. She has eczema and her mother had treatment for childhood asthma. On examination she has widespread wheeze on auscultation and mild tachypnoea. She has no chest deformity and no clubbing.

11.40

An 18-month-old child is admitted to the paediatric assessment unit with cough, wheeze and shortness of breath. His symptoms started 6 hours earlier and he has a 24 hour history of runny nose. He has had a similar episode 6 weeks ago and was admitted at the age of 6 months to hospital with RSV bronchiolitis. He has no history of eczema and no family history of atopy. On examination he has widespread wheeze bilaterally with intercostal recession and saturations of 97% in air.

11.41

A 6-year-old girl, AP, presents to the A&E with a 6-hour history of wheeze and shortness of breath. Symptoms started when she visited a friend's house for tea. The friend's parents were heavy smokers and had three longhaired cats. She had a similar exacerbation 3 months previously when she had her first horse-riding lesson but has not experienced wheeze or shortness of breath between these episodes. She has a history of infantile and childhood eczema and her brother was diagnosed with asthma the year before. On examination she has widespread wheeze and is too breathless to talk in entire sentences. Her wheeze settles with a 5 mg salbutamol nebuliser.

11.42–11.44 Theme: Abnormalities of the airway

- ❑ A Inhaled foreign body
- ❑ B Unilateral vocal fold paralysis
- ❑ C Bilateral vocal fold paralysis
- ❑ D Unilateral choanal atresia
- ❑ E Bilateral choanal atresia
- ❑ F Laryngomalacia
- ❑ G Acquired subglottic stenosis
- ❑ H Congenital subglottic stenosis
- ❑ I Vascular ring
- ❑ J Subglottic haemangioma

For each of the following clinical scenarios pick the most appropriate diagnosis from the list above, each option can be used once more than once or not at all.

11.42

A 4-week-old baby is admitted to the paediatric department with a history of increasingly noisy breathing. His mother states that his breathing has been noisy since day 3 of life. She describes the noise as 'snuffly', and over the last couple of days it has become more persistent. It is now present when he is feeding, crying and most recently when he is sleeping. His cry is normal. He is managing feeds equivalent to 150 ml/kg per day. He recovered birthweight at day 10 and is gaining weight along the 50th centile. On examination he is bright and alert, apyrexial, with a heart rate of 140 beats/min, a respiratory rate of 40/min and saturations of 98%; he has no signs of increased work of breathing but has a moderate audible inspiratory stridor at rest in a supine position.

11.43

An 18-month-old boy was seen in paediatric clinic due to continued symptoms of wheeze. He was born at term with an unremarkable neonatal history. He was admitted twice during his first winter with feeding difficulties and had always had what his mother described as recurrent episodes of wheeze and cough. He had had treatment with two courses of oral antibiotics for chest infections over the previous 8 weeks and had been treated for recurrent wheeze with a spacer and salbutamol inhaler, with no improvement of symptoms. He had no family history of atopy and he had not had infantile eczema. He was thriving along the 75th centile for height and weight. On examination he was apyrexial, with no signs of respiratory distress. On auscultation of his chest there was a fixed biphasic stridor and bilateral wheeze. His heart sounds were normal and there were no audible murmurs. The stridor had no variability with position and he had normal saturations in air. He had no other abnormalities on examination of his skin, cranial nerves or fingernails.

11.44

A baby was admitted to the neonatal unit after she was noted to have recurrent dusky episodes associated with feeding on the postnatal ward. She was 30 minutes' old at the time of admission having been born at term weighing 2.5 kg. Mother had had an uneventful pregnancy and only routine antenatal care. The baby looked pink and was vigorously crying on admission but was observed to desaturate down to 69% with obvious cyanosis on feeding. She had marked signs of respiratory distress associated with her cyanosis and was mildly dysmorphic, with slightly low-set simple ears. Cardiovascular examination revealed a soft systolic murmur but peripheral pulses were present and normal in volume.

11.45–11.47 Theme: Respiratory diseases

- ❑ A Bronchiolitis obliterans
- ❑ B α_1-Antitrypsin deficiency
- ❑ C Tracheo-oesophageal fistula
- ❑ D Cystic fibrosis
- ❑ E Pulmonary haemosiderosis
- ❑ F Bronchomalacia
- ❑ G Lobar sequestration
- ❑ H Cystic adenomatoid malformation
- ❑ I Asthma
- ❑ J Bronchiolitis

Choose the most likely diagnosis from the list above for each of the three scenarios described below. Each option may be used once, more than once or not at all.

11.45

A 10-month-old child with a history of progressive tachypnoea, cough, wheeze and faltering growth is found to have patchy perihilar changes on chest radiograph. He is jaundiced with hepatosplenomegaly. He has a microcytic anaemia and his stools are positive for faecal occult bloods.

11.46

A previously well 3-year-old girl is seen in outpatient clinic with a history of dry cough and being generally run down for the last 4 months. Mum reports that she appears more breathless on exertion than previously. Symptoms appeared to develop after a flu-like illness. Inhaled steroids (fluticasone 125 μg twice daily) have had no effect on symptoms. She has an elevated respiratory rate at rest. Chest radiograph shows hyperinflation with some patchy lower lobe infiltrates bilaterally.

11.47

A 10-year-old boy is seen in clinic for follow-up 2 months after a recent admission to hospital with a left-sided pneumonia. Parents report that he is now back to normal but they are concerned because, in the last few years, he has required a number of courses of antibiotics from the GP for recurrent episodes of chest infection. A follow-up chest radiograph shows persisting shadowing in the left lower zone. He is well grown and otherwise healthy.

11.48–11.50 Theme: Management of acute respiratory illness

- ❑ A Intravenous cefotaxime
- ❑ B Nebulised adrenaline and supplementary oxygen
- ❑ C Oral azithromycin
- ❑ D Intravenous hydrocortisone
- ❑ E Supplementary oxygen and nasogastric enteral fluids
- ❑ F Oral dexamethasone
- ❑ G Intravenous benzylpenicillin
- ❑ H Oral amoxicillin
- ❑ I Regular nebulised salbutamol
- ❑ J Regular 10 puffs of salbutamol via a volumatic spacer

Choose the most appropriate INITIAL treatment from the list above for each of the three scenarios described below. Each option may be used once, more than once or not at all.

11.48

A 3-year-old girl whose family have recently arrived in the UK seeking asylum presents to A&E with stridor. You are unable to take a history because the family cannot speak English and an interpreter is not available. On examination, she is febrile (38°C), quiet, drooling and pale, and has poor peripheral perfusion with oxygen saturations of 92% in air. She is tachypnoeic (respiratory rate 50/min) and has continuous soft stridor with evidence of tracheal tug and intercostals recession.

11.49

A 4-month-old baby (who was born at 32 weeks' gestation) is admitted to the paediatric ward on Christmas Day with a 3-day history of being off feeds, snuffly and coughing. On examination he has a temperature of 37.5°C and oxygen saturations of 89% in air, with marked subcostal recession and a respiratory rate of 60/min. He has fine inspiratory crackles bilaterally and diffuse wheeze.

11.50

A 7-year-old boy who has been previously fit and well is seen on the paediatric assessment unit with a 5-day history of being generally unwell. He has had a wheezy cough and intermittent headache helped by paracetamol. Examination reveals that his oxygen saturations are 97% in air with no evidence of increased work of breathing. His right tympanic membrane is moderately inflamed. He has occasional wheeze and crackles mainly on the right and his chest radiograph shows patchy interstitial shadowing on this side.

CHAPTER 1

Cardiology Answers

MTF Answers

1.1 Neonatal cyanosis

Answers: B C D E

Eisenmenger syndrome is an acquired defect secondary to pulmonary hypertension. Cyanosis occurs in the hypoplastic left heart syndrome secondary to circulatory failure and worsens when the duct closes. Severe (critical) aortic stenosis can present in the neonatal period with cyanosis by the same mechanism.
Cardiac conditions presenting with neonatal cyanosis:

- Decreased pulmonary flow
  - pulmonary atresia
  - tetralogy of Fallot
  - Ebstein anomaly (abnormality of tricuspid valve position and function)
- Increased pulmonary flow
  - hypoplastic left heart
  - tricuspid atresia
  - truncus arteriosus
  - total anomalous pulmonary venous drainage
  - double-outlet ventricle
  - single ventricle
  - poor mixing
    - transposition of the great arteries.

1.2 Paediatric ECGs

Answers: A B C E

Mean QRS

- At birth – 125°
- 1 month – 90°
- 3 years – 50°.

The right axis deviation seen in newborns is due to right ventricular dominance in the fetus. Right ventricular deviation in older children implies right ventricular hypertrophy. Left axis deviation (superior axis) in the neonatal period is seen in the following cardiac lesions:

- Tricuspid atresia
- AVSD
- Pulmonary stenosis.

Right bundle-branch block

Right bundle-branch block is the most common conduction disturbance seen in children. The abnormality is usually due to right ventricular overload prolonging right ventricular depolarisation as a result of lengthening of the conduction pathway.

Criteria for right bundle-branch block include:

- prolonged QRS
- right axis deviation
- terminal slurring of the QRS over the right ventricular leads V3R, V4R and V1
- ST depression and T-wave inversion in adults (rarely in children).

Causes of right-bundle branch block include:

- AVSD
- Ebstein anomaly
- coarctation of the aorta (infants)
- endocardial cushion defects
- post right ventriculotomy
- partial anomalous pulmonary venous drainage
- normal variant.

Congenital heart block

Congenital complete heart block (complete atrioventricular dissociation) occurs in infants of mothers with systemic lupus erythematosus (SLE), particularly those with anti-Ro (SS-A) and anti La (SS-B) antibodies. The damage to the conduction pathway is irreversible. Antenatal diagnosis is possible because of persistent fetal bradycardia; 50% have an associated structural defect, usually congenitally corrected transposition. The condition is usually well tolerated and often does not require a pacemaker.

Heart rate

Heart rate varies with the age and status of the patient. A rate of 110–150 is normal in the newborn and the adult rate of 60–100 is achieved by the age of 6 years.

QT interval

Romano–Ward is a congenital long QT syndrome.

1.3 Chest radiographs

Answers: C D E

Coeur en sabot (heart in a boot)

Seen in tetralogy of Fallot; due to hypoplasia of the main pulmonary artery and the consequent upturning of the apex away from the diaphragm. A right-sided aortic arch is seen in 25%.

Rib notching

A feature of coarctation of the aorta; it occurs as a consequence of the increase in size of the intercostal vessels which function as collaterals. The upper two or three ribs are spared because their posterior intercostal arteries do not arise from the aorta. It is rarely seen in children aged <5 years.

Other chest radiograph changes of coarctation

- Dilatation of the ascending aorta, descending aorta (post-stenotic dilatation)
- Cardiomegaly
- Increased pulmonary vascular shadowing.

Truncus arteriosus

The features on the chest radiograph include a right-sided aortic arch, absent thymus (30% of cases have Di George syndrome), cardiomegaly and a prominent ascending aorta.

Total anomalous pulmonary venous drainage

There are two types:

1. Unobstructed – cardiomegaly, increased pulmonary vascular markings
2. Obstructed – normal heart size, increased pulmonary vascular markings (severe pulmonary oedema).

The lesion may be supracardiac, cardiac, infracardiac or mixed. Obstructed lesions are usually infracardiac. In the supracardiac lesion, unobstructed total anomalous pulmonary venous drainage, and dilatation of the left and right superior vena cavas and the left innominate vein give rise to a 'cottage loaf' or 'snowman' appearance on the chest radiograph.

Scimitar syndrome

This is a form of partial anomalous pulmonary venous drainage whereby the veins from the right lung drain directly into the inferior vena cava (IVC). The right lung is hypoplastic as a consequence and this allows movement of the heart to the right (dextroposition). The single vein draining the right lung produces a (scimitar) shape on the posteroanterior (PA) chest radiograph as it heads towards the right cardiodiaphragmatic angle.

1.4 Conditions associated with an increased risk of heart disease

Answers: A B C D

Kawasaki disease

The cardiac lesions appear in the second week of the illness as proximal coronary artery aneurysms healing by fibrosis and thrombosis. Lesions are most common on the left side. Protection is offered by the early administration of intravenous immunoglobulin. Other cardiac lesions can occur including aortic and mitral regurgitation, myocarditis, pericarditis, pericardial effusion and myocardial infarction.

Congenital rubella

Infection with rubella during the first trimester causes the classic triad of sensorineural deafness, ophthalmological defects (cataracts, infantile glaucoma and pigmentary retinitis) and cardiac anomalies. Cardiac defects include PDA (patent ductus arteriosus) and peripheral pulmonary artery stenosis most commonly, and are present in 50% of babies infected in the first 10 weeks of pregnancy. Rarer cardiac manifestations of first trimester infection include coarctation of the aorta, myocarditis, VSD and ASD. Other abnormalities seen in the congenital rubella syndrome include microcephaly and learning disability, microphthalmia, intrauterine growth retardation, hepatitis and neonatal thrombocytopenia.

Marfan syndrome

This is an inherited disorder of connective tissue. Cardiac manifestations include:

- mitral valve prolapse
- dilatation/dissection of the ascending aorta
- aortic regurgitation
- pulmonary artery aneurysm
- mitral valve prolapse.

Turner syndrome

The most common cardiac lesion is coarctation of the aorta (15–30%). Other cardiac lesions seen include aortic stenosis, AVSD (atrioventricular septal defect) and bicuspid aortic valves. Hypertension is not uncommon. Lesions commonly seen in Noonan syndrome include pulmonary stenosis and obstructive cardiomyopathy. For examination purposes it is worth remembering that, in Noonan syndrome, right-sided heart lesions are seen and, in Turner syndrome, left-sided heart lesions.

There is no increase in the incidence of congenital heart disease in petit mal epilepsy.

1.5 Congenital heart disease

Answers: C E

The most common form of congenital heart disease is a VSD.

The lung fields are oligaemic in tetralogy of Fallot as a consequence of the pulmonary stenosis.

Blalock–Taussig shunt

This is an anastomosis between the subclavian artery and the pulmonary artery and is used for palliation in conditions with severe restriction pulmonary blood flow, e.g. pulmonary atresia and tetralogy of Fallot. The murmur is continuous. Continuous murmurs characteristically pass through the second heart sound into diastole.

Ebstein anomaly

The tricuspid valve is malformed and leaks. The septal and posterior leaflets of the tricuspid valve are set further into the right ventricle, causing atrialisation of part of the right ventricle. In severe cases, children can present with cyanosis and cardiac failure in the neonatal period. Arrhythmias are common including Wolff–Parkinson–White syndrome. Lithium during pregnancy is a risk factor.

Nitric and not nitrous oxide is used to treat persistent pulmonary hypertension.

Causes of plethoric lung fields

Acyanotic

- AVSD
- VSD
- PDA
- Endocardial cushion defect
- Partial anomalous pulmonary venous drainage.

Cyanotic

- Single ventricle
- Truncus arteriosus
- Hypoplastic left heart
- Transposition of the great arteries
- Total anomalous pulmonary venous drainage.

Causes of continuous murmurs

- Blalock–Taussig shunt
- AV malformation
- Aneurysm
- Collateral vessels
- PDA
- Venous hum
- Peripheral pulmonary stenosis.

1.6 Fetal circulation

Answer: none correct

Oxygenated blood from the placenta returns to the fetus via the umbilical vein: 50% enters the hepatic circulation and 50% bypasses the liver via the ductus venosus. As it enters the right atrium most of the inferior caval blood is directed through the foramen ovale into the left atrium. The right atrium contains blood from the superior vena cava (SVC), coronary sinus and some from the IVC. Right atrial blood enters the right ventricle, and 85% of right ventricular blood passes into the descending aorta via the ductus arteriosus and 15% enters the fetal lungs.

Changes in the fetal circulation occur at birth: the ductus venosus closes and loss of the low-resistance placenta results in an increase in systemic vascular resistance. There is a functional closure of the foramen ovale. Lung expansion results in a fall in pulmonary vascular resistance, increased pulmonary blood flow and increased delivery of blood to the left atrium. Flow through the ductus arteriosus changes from the pulmonary to the systemic circulation to the systemic to the pulmonary circulation. The high concentration of oxygen in the blood causes smooth muscle contraction of the duct and closure.

1.7 Congenital heart disease

Answers: C E

Poor growth (height and weight) is common in children with cyanotic congenital heart disease. Catch-up growth after corrective surgery is common. Failure to thrive and feeding difficulties are common in infants with a symptomatic congenital heart disease. The contraindications to immunisation are as for the normal population; immunisation should be encouraged to prevent potentially serious and/or deadly diseases. The oral contraceptive pill is contraindicated in girls with cyanotic congenital heart disease due to the risk of thrombosis. The coil is also contraindicated because it is a potential focus of infection predisposing to endocarditis. Unplanned pregnancy for those with congenital heart disease can be disastrous, so informed and appropriate advice for this population is vital. A chromosomal abnormality is present in 6–10% of children with congenital heart disease and 30% of newborn infants with chromosomal abnormalities have heart defects.

1.8 Teratogens

Answers: A B D E

The following are teratogens for the defects shown.

Alcohol	ASD, VSD, PDA, TGA
Amphetamines	ASD, VSD, PDA, TGA
Lithium	Ebstein anomaly
Oestrogens/progesterones	VSD, TGA, TOF
Phenytoin	Pulmonary stenosis, aortic stenosis, PDA, coarctation, ASD, VSD
Thalidomide	TOF, truncus arteriosus
Sodium valproate	TOF, VSD, coarctation
Warfarin	TOF, VSD

ASD, atrial septal defect; VSD, ventricular septal defect; PDA, patent ductus arteriosus; TGA, transposition of the great arteries; TOF, tetralogy of Fallot.

Maternal diseases linked to an increased risk of congenital heart disease include:

- Diabetes – transposition, septal defects, coarctation, transient cardiomyopathy
- Phenylketonuria – tetralogy of Fallot
- SLE – congenital heart block.

1.9 Circulatory failure in the neonatal period

Answers: A B C D E

Acute circulatory failure (shock) is characterised by inadequate tissue and organ perfusion. Organ perfusion relies on a functioning pump (heart), an adequate delivery system (integrity of structure and vasomotor tone of all vascular beds – venous, arterial and capillary) and an adequate substrate delivering nutrients and removing toxins and waste. Failure of any of the three components in isolation or in combination will lead to shock.

Cardiogenic causes of neonatal shock:

- Critical aortic stenosis
- Hypoplastic left heart
- Coarctation
- Myocardial ischemia (hypoxic ischaemic encephalopathy, hypoglycaemia)
- Cardiomyopathy
- Arrhythmia
- Arteriovenous fistula
- Obstructed pulmonary venous drainage
- TGA with VSD.

By the end of the first week, when pulmonary vascular resistance falls, left-to-right shunts become an important cause of heart failure including VSD, PDA, AVSD and truncus arteriosus.

Non-cardiogenic causes of neonatal shock:

- Hypovolaemia (blood, fluid or electrolyte losses)
- Dissociative shock (severe anaemia or methaemoglobinaemia)
- Distributive (sepsis, vasodilators, myocardial depression or endothelial injury)
- Obstructive shock (tension pneumothorax or cardiac tamponade).

The treatment of neonatal circulatory failure depends on identifying the cause and treating accordingly.

BOF Answers

1.10 Cardiac arrest

Answer A: Basic life support with high concentration oxygen should be continued throughout any resuscitation with the minimum of interruptions

In all states of cardiac arrest the establishment and continuity of basic life support (BLS) should take precedence over any advanced management.

Asystole

This is the most common arrest rhythm in children:

1. Clear airway
2. Ventilation with high-concentration oxygen and cardiac massage (15:2)
3. Attach monitor
4. Adrenaline dose every 4 minutes (avoid higher doses as associated with poorer outcomes) intravenously or intraosseously (10 µg/kg = 0.1 ml/kg of 1 in 10 000) plus flush! (ETT dose is 10×)
5. Intubate and proceed with uninterrupted CPR (cardiopulmonary resuscitation)
6. Consider reversible causes (pulseless electrical activity or PEA).

Pulseless electrical activity (including electro-mechanical dissociation)

It should be treated as asystole. It can be secondary to a treatable cause:

- Severe hypovolaemia
- Tension pneumothorax
- Pericardial tamponade
- Hypothermia
- Hypoxia
- Acidosis
- Toxic
- Hypocalcaemia/hyperkalaemia/hypokalaemia
- Pulmonary thromboembolus.

Ventricular fibrillation

This is rare in childhood. Suspect in cases of sudden collapse or with underlying cardiac disease, hypothermia and/or overdose with a tricyclic antidepressant.

- BLS with high-flow oxygen should be established straightaway and continued throughout the resuscitation with the minimum pauses possible.
- A single asynchronous DC shock (4 J/kg) is given at 2-minute intervals throughout the resuscitation with immediate resumption of CPR after each shock, and a short pause for rhythm reassessment immediately before the next shock is delivered.
- Intubation and the establishment of vascular access should be secured as soon as possible without compromising CPR or the DC shocking protocol.
- Adrenaline is given immediately before the third shock (10 µg/kg).
- Amiodarone 5 mg/kg is given before the fourth DC shock at 5 mg/kg.
- Further adrenaline can be given every other shock (every 4 minutes) and reversible causes should be sought.

Pulseless VT should be treated as VF. Prolonged resuscitation may be indicated in hypothermia.

1.11 Palpitations

Answer C: Reassurance that her palpitations do not have a significant cause, advice about relaxation and stress control during exam season, and discharge to follow-up from clinic

This young girl has got physiological tachycardia associated with situation-specific stress and requires strong reassurance not further investigation or referral.

Palpitations are common in paediatrics. A minority will have true arrhythmias (13%).

Differential diagnosis includes:

- Cardiac conditions
- Potentially life threatening:
  - SVT – WPW syndrome
  - prolonged QT syndrome
  - hypertrophic cardiomyopathy
  - myocarditis
  - sick sinus syndrome
  - arrhythmias associated with congenital heart disease
- Not immediately/non-life-threatening cardiac causes:
  - premature atrial contractions
  - premature ventricular contractions
  - acute rheumatic fever with valvular disease
- Non-cardiac conditions
  - potentially life threatening
  - hypoglycaemia
  - drug/toxin exposure
  - phaeochromocytoma
- Not immediately/non-life threatening
  - fever
  - anaemia
  - exercise
  - emotional arousal
  - anxiety/hyperventilation/panic attacks
  - drug ingestion
  - past orthostatic tachycardia syndrome
  - hyperthyroidism.

A careful history and examination are essential to correctly identify the aetiology:

- Cardiac arrhythmias are often described as having abrupt onset and offset.
- Children with premature atrial or ventricular beats may describe a flip-flop feeling when the heart stops and then compensates with a larger stroke volume on the following beat.
- Palpitations associated with excessive periodic sweating, headaches and

hypertension may suggest the rare underlying diagnosis of phaeochromocytoma.

- Palpitations with heat intolerance, sweating and weight loss may suggest hyperthyroidism.
- Syncope (with injury), exercise intolerance, and a past history or family history of cardiac disease, sudden death or deafness (PQT) may indicate significant underlying cardiac pathology.
- Tachycardia out of proportion to fever may indicated myocarditis.

A thorough systemic examination is vital in all cases and a 12-lead ECG should be performed.

Consider referral tc cardiologist plus 24-hour ECG or event monitor may help to clarify aetiology in concerning cases.

1.12 New onset cardiac failure

Answer C: Viral myocarditis

This baby presents with a short history of new onset cardiac failure associated with faltering growth at 18 months of age following shortly after a viral illness. This is consistent with an acquired cardiac failure not a congenital cause:

- Myocarditis – inflammation of the heart muscle
- Cause of sudden death in previously healthy children
- Can lead to acute dilated cardiomyopathy
- Viral myocarditis is the leading cause in the western world:
  - adenovirus (up to 39% of cases)
  - Coxsackievirus (Coxsackie B enterovirus)
- Other causes include:
  - toxins
  - autoimmune processes
  - other infection (viral, bacterial, protozoal, parasitic)
- Clinical presentation: prodromal viraemia (70–90%) – fever, myalgia, coryzal and/or gastroenteritis
- ECG changes:
  - non-specific ST-segment and T-wave abnormalities
  - pathological Q waves
  - T-wave inversion
  - low QRS voltages (<5mm in any precordial leads)
  - VT and frequent ventricular ectopics can be seen
- Symptoms and signs accompanying ECG abnormalities:
  - asymptomatic
  - palpitations
  - presyncope/syncope
- Symptoms and signs (heart failure):

- dyspnoea
- sweating
- poor feeding
- orthopnoea/PND (paroxysmal nocturnal dyspnoea)
- faltering growth
- tachypnoea
- tachycardia (out of proportion to fever)
- gallop rhythm
- murmur of mitral regurgitation
- hepatomegaly
- peripheral oedema
- raised JVP (jugular venous pressure)

Natural history of the disease depends on severity of presentation

- Asymptomatic patients/ECG changes generally recover completely
- Mild left ventricular systolic impairment generally recover within weeks to months
- Severe left ventricular dysfunction:
  - 25% recover
  - 25% progress to transplantation
  - 50% develop chronic dilated cardiomyopathy (DCM)

Diagnosis

- Needs high index of suspicion
- ECG
- Echocardiography
- Troponin T/I level
- Viral serology and PCR (polymerase chain reaction)
- Endomyocardial biopsy:
  - histological
  - viral PCR
  - immunohistochemistry

Management

- Supportive: ionotropic support, anticoagulation, afterload reduction and diuresis
- Assist devices or ECMO in severe cases
- Specific heart failure treatments: ACE (angiotensin-converting enzyme) inhibitors, β blockers
- Immune-mediated therapy
  - IVIG (intravenous immunoglobulin)
  - immunosuppression with prednisolone in immune-mediated disease.

1.13 ECG changes in electrolyte disturbances

Answer A: ECG changes associated with hyperkalaemia are progressive with the severity of hyperkalaemia leading to the absence of p waves, broadening of QRS complexes, and VF or VT

Hypokalaemia

ECG changes

- ST depression
- Flattened or inverted T waves
- U waves
- Cardiac arrhythmias, atrial and ventricular ectopics, atrial tachycardia, heart blocks, VF and VT
- Increased P-wave amplitude and duration
- QRS prolongation.

Hyperkalaemia

ECG changes occur in a sequence associated with progression on hyperkalaemia:

- Early ECG changes include:
  - peaked T waves,
  - decreased QT interval
  - ST-segment depression/elevation
- Progression of hyperkalaemia leads to:
  - widening of QRS complex 2° to bundle-branch blocks
  - increased PR interval (first-degree heart block)
  - decreased amplitude of P wave
- Without treatment further progression leads to:
  - P waves disappearing
  - QRS widening to a sine wave morphology
  - VF or asystole follows
- These ECG changes generally correct with potassium
- Potentially life-threatening arrhythmias can occur at almost any level of hyperkalaemia without the warning sequence of ECG changes described above.

Hypomagnesaemia (ECG changes resemble hypokalaemia)

- May be associated with non-specific ECG changes including:
  - ST depression
  - flattening T waves
  - prominent U waves
  - loss of voltage
- Severe magnesium deficiency may cause:
  - PR prolongation
  - widening of QRS complex
  - tachycardia

– rarely premature ventricular contraction and fibrillation.

Hypermagnesaemia (ECG changes may resemble hyperkalaemia)

- Prolonged PR interval
- Widened QRS (intraventricular conduction delay).

Hypercalcaemia

- Reduced QT interval on ECG
- T-wave duration unaffected
- ST-segment duration shortened
- May present with a variety of arrhythmias
- Significant hypercalcaemia may present with ECG changes mimicking myocardial ischaemia.

Hypocalcaemia

- The main ECG change is a prolonged QT interval
- No change in T-wave duration but ST segment is prolonged.

Hyper-/hyponatraemia

- No significant ECG abnormalities are associated

1.14 Aortic stenosis

Answer E: There is an association with sudden death in patients with aortic stenosis

Aortic valve stenosis

This accounts for 5% of congenital heart defects. It is more common in males.

Associations of aortic stenosis

- Turner syndrome
- Williams syndrome
- Coarctation of the aorta
- Other cardiac abnormalities, e.g. hypoplastic left ventricle, mitral valve abnormalities.

The stenosis can be either supravalvular, valvular or subvalvular. There is often an associated bicuspid valve. Aortic stenosis is usually asymptomatic but in its most severe form can cause congestive cardiac failure, arrhythmias and sudden death in infancy (rare). The murmur is best heard in the aortic area (upper left sternal edge) and radiates to the neck. An ejection click suggests valvular stenosis. A palpable thrill is usually present in the suprasternal notch. A2 (the aortic component of the second heart sound) is quiet. Although left ventricular hypertrophy is common the ECG can be normal.

Assessment of severity

- Symptoms – angina-like pain
- Syncope/dizziness on exertion
- Palpitations on exertion

- ECG evidence of left ventricular strain
- Exercise test positive
- ST and T-wave changes on the ECG during exercise.

Treatment

Treatment is conservative in most cases avoiding valve replacement in the young patient. If the gradient across the valve is >60 mmHg treatment is indicated. This is usually in the form of a balloon valvoplasty at cardiac catheter, or surgical valvuloplasty.

1.15 Williams syndrome

Answer C: Diagnosis of Williams syndrome can be confirmed by fluorescence in situ hybridization (FISH) studies

Williams syndrome is a neurodevelopmental disorder. It is caused by a micro deletion involving the elastin gene on the long arm of chromosome 7. Diagnosis can be confirmed by FISH studies.

Features

- Characteristic elfin facies (which may be difficult to detect in young babies):
  - stellate iris
  - flattened nasal bridge with small upturned nose
  - long philtrum
  - wide (carp-shaped) mouth
  - partially missing teeth, defective tooth enamel or small, widely spaced teeth
- Characteristic affect – over-friendly with better verbal than visuospatial skills
- Behavioural problems with poor concentration and distractibility
- Normal birth weight with post-natal growth retardation secondary to poor feeding (failure to thrive)
- Neurodevelopmental delay with delayed motor milestone and IQ of 50–60
- Idiopathic hypercalcaemia in approximately 15% (presents as irritability, vomiting and constipation in babies) – resolves at age 2 years; management is with low calcium and vitamin D intake, and aetiology unknown
- Hypercalciuria (nephrocalcinosis)
- Squints
- Hernia
- Rectal prolapse
- Cardiovascular abnormalities (75%):
  - supravalvular aortic stenosis
  - peripheral pulmonary artery stenosis
  - others including valvular and septal defects have been reported
  - hypertension.

1.16 Down syndrome

Answer B: Echocardiography is indicated in all cases of Down syndrome for identification of congenital cardiac disease even if a murmur is not present

Cardiac lesions in Down syndrome

Cardiac lesions are present in 40–50% of children with Down syndrome. Forty-five per cent are AVSDs and 35% are isolated ventricular septal defects (VSDs). Others commonly seen include tetralogy of Fallot, PDA and secundum ASDs. Of all children with an AVSD, 25% have Down syndrome. All children with Down syndrome should have an echocardiogram to detect congenital heart disease (CHD). The symptoms associated with a right-to-left cardiac shunt can be delayed in children with Down syndrome due to the persistence of high pulmonary vascular resistance.

Atrioventricular septal defect

Partial AVSD refers to an ostium primum ASD and is present with or without a cleft in the mitral valve. Complete AVSD refers to a common atrioventricular valve with clefts in both the pulmonary and the mitral valves. Treatment of AVSD and large VSD includes:

- diuretics to control heart failure
- nutritional support to maximise growth
- delayed closure at 3–6 months.

Upper airway obstruction

Obstructive sleep apnoea is common in children with Down syndrome, affecting 30–50%. The aetiology includes hypotonic upper airway muscles, adenotonsillar hypertrophy, macroglossia, glossoptosis, flattened midface and narrowed nasopharynx. Laryngomalacia and gastro-oesophageal reflux disease (GORD) are both increased in children with Down syndrome which may worsen airway disease. Recurrent hypoxaemia is a contributing factor to the development of pulmonary arterial hypertension (PAH).

Pulmonary arterial hypertension in children with Down syndrome

There is an increased incidence of pulmonary vascular disease in children with Down syndrome, both with and without associated CHD. The principal aetiology is cardiac (increased pulmonary flow). Other contributing factors include upper airway obstruction and an increased incidence of intrinsic lung disease (pulmonary hypoplasia). When congenital cardiac defects are present, long-standing increased pulmonary vascular resistance due to a right-to-left shunt may lead to reversal of flow across the shunt and Eisenmenger syndrome.

1.17 Transposition of the great arteries

Answer B: Transposition of the great arteries is the most common cause of cyanotic congenital heart disease in the neonatal period

Transposition of the great arteries (TGA) represents about 6% of all CHD. It is the most common cause of cyanotic CHD in the neonatal period. It is more common in boys than girls (3:1). It is not usually associated with syndromes. Left untreated it is lethal in 90% of cases by age 1 year.

In TGA the aorta arises from the right ventricle and carries deoxygenated blood to the body, and the pulmonary artery arises from the left ventricle and carries oxygenated blood to the lungs. Children presenting in the neonatal period with this condition have high pulmonary blood flow and are severely cyanosed unless a lesion that mixes the two circulations is present (examples include PDA, ASD, VSD). The child is usually cyanotic from or shortly after birth. The lesion is duct dependent and the infant's condition deteriorates when the duct closes. There is usually a metabolic acidosis at presentation. If adequate mixing is possible due to one of the defects listed above, the child may present later in infancy with poor feeding and congestive cardiac failure rather than collapse, acidosis and hypoxia on duct closure in the neonatal period. Arrhythmias of all types are common. ECG shows a right-sided axis and right ventricular hypertrophy. The chest radiograph shows cardiomegaly and increased pulmonary vascularity. Antenatal diagnosis on anomaly ultrasound scanning remains difficult and so the vast majority of cases are diagnosed postnatally.

Surgical management of TGA

- Palliative – atrial septostomy
- Physiological repair (permanent palliation) – mustard, Senning; these procedures are associated with long-term complications including systemic ventricular failure, baffle leaks and stenosis, and high rates of arrhythmias including sudden death
- Anatomical:
  - – Jatene arterial switch (corrective) performed at less than 2 weeks of age, mortality rate >5%
  - – Rastelli conduit (needs replacement).

1.18 Tetralogy of Fallot

Answer B: Cyanotic spells associated with tetralogy of Fallot usually begin around 4–6 months of age

This accounts for 10% of congenital heart disease. Components of tetralogy of Fallot:

- Ventricular septal defect
- Right ventricular outflow obstruction
- Right ventricular hypertrophy
- Overriding aorta.

The severity of the right ventricular outflow obstruction will determine the clinical picture. Most cases have faltering growth and breathlessness on feeding.

- Mild obstruction: pink tetralogy of Fallot – left-to-right shunt across the VDS – murmur ejection systolic (pulmonary stenosis) – cyanotic later as the shunt reverses.
- Moderate obstruction: presents with cyanosis – right-to-left shunt across VSD – murmur is ejection systolic due to pulmonary stenosis, VSD silent.
- Severe obstruction: duct dependent, presenting with cyanosis in the neonatal period.

ECG shows right ventricular hypertrophy and right axis deviation in cyanotic tetralogy of Fallot. The ECG in acyanotic tetralogy of Fallot shows right ventricular hypertrophy because the right ventricular pressure is high. Cyanotic spells usually begin around 4–6 months of age. They are due to functional infundibular spasm and potentially fatal. Features include worsening cyanosis and a reduction in the intensity of the murmur. Associated ASDs do occur and are referred to as the quatralogy of Fallot.

Treatment of cyanotic spells is as follows:

- Bring baby's knees to chest (reduces venous return by increasing peripheral vascular resistance, decreases left-to-right shunt across the VSD)
- β Bockers
- Morphine
- Sodium bicarbonate if acidotic
- Vasoconstrictors.

Surgical management of tetralogy of Fallot is either palliative (systemic-to-pulmonary shunt) or complete. Total correction, if technically possible, is the preferred option. This is usually done at around 6 months.

Complications of tetralogy of Fallot include:

- Polycythaemia
- Subacute bacterial endocarditis
- Cerebral abscess, cerebral thrombosis
- Retardation of growth and development
- Clubbing – usually appears after age 1 year.

1.19 Atrial septal defects

Answer E: A pulmonary to systemic flow ratio of more than 2:1 is an indication for surgical or more commonly percutaneous transcatheter device closure

Isolated ASDs account for 8% of congenital heart disease. The defect is more common in girls and there are three types:

1. Ostium secundum (most common)
2. Ostium primum
3. Sinus venosus.

Ostium secundum defects are usually asymptomatic, with pulmonary hypertension and right ventricular failure occurring in the third and fourth decades. Atrial arrhythmias occur in adulthood but are rare in childhood. An ostium primum defect is likely to present earlier, usually as a component of an endocardial cushion defect. Isolated ASDs are not considered to be at high risk of developing bacterial endocarditis. Even in complex ASDs prophylactic antibiotics are no longer routinely recommended for interventional procedures in high-risk patients due their potential for harm and the lack of evidence for benefit.

ECG appearance of atrial septal defects:

- ostium primum – right bundle-branch block, left axis deviation
- ostium secundum – right bundle-branch block, right axis deviation.

The presence of right bundle-branch block is not diagnostic but its absence makes the diagnosis unlikely. A high proportion of ostium secundum ASDs close spontaneously by the age of 5 years. The risk of pulmonary hypertension and its sequelae increases with shunt size. Surgical repair is indicated if the pulmonary-to-systemic flow ratio is >2:1. High pulmonary vascular resistance is a contraindication to surgery.

Fixed splitting of the second heart sound is characteristic of an ASD. This is due to the defect producing a constantly increased right ventricular volume and prolonging ejection time. The murmur of an ASD is not due to flow across the defect but to increased flow across the pulmonary valve as a consequence of the shunt.

1.20 Ventricular septal defects

Answer D: VSDs are associated with higher oxygen content in the blood of the right ventricle than the right atrium

VSDs are the most common congenital heart defect. The defect can occur in the membranous or muscular part of the septum, although defects in the membranous septum are more common and usually single. Defects in the muscular part of the septum are usually multiple. The signs and symptoms depend on the haemodynamics of the defect, which depends on the size of the defect and the pulmonary vascular resistance. With a small defect, the murmur is rarely present at birth but appears as the pulmonary vascular resistance falls:

- Infective endocarditis occurs in less than 2% of cases.
- It is the left and not the right ventricle that is volume overloaded. The shunt occurs mainly during systole when the right ventricle is contracting, and so the shunted blood enters the pulmonary circulation.
- The right atrium contains deoxygenated blood; the right ventricle contains deoxygenated blood from the right atrium and oxygenated blood from the left ventricle.
- At cardiac catheterisation, the oxygen content of blood in the right ventricle is greater than that in the right atrium.
- Some 30–60% close spontaneously in the first 6 months and many more subsequent to that. Surgery is required if the left-to-right shunt is such (usually quoted as > 2:1) that pulmonary hypertension has or is likely to develop. Surgical closure for large defects is usually performed at around 3–5 months. The second heart sound is loud if pulmonary hypertension is present. Untreated, a large shunt will result in high pulmonary flow and can progress to pulmonary hypertension and Eisenmenger syndrome.

1.21 Eisenmenger syndrome

Answer D: Correction of the VSD before the development of pulmonary hypertension

Eisenmenger syndrome occurs as a consequence of a long-standing uncorrected congenital heart defect with intracardiac communications, leading to pulmonary hypertension with a reversed or bidirectional shunt at the atrial, ventricular or aortopulmonary level and associated cyanosis. Cardiac defects associated with the development of Eisenmenger syndrome include the following:

- Increased pulmonary arterial flow:
  - ASD
  - systemic AV fistulae
  - TAPVD (total anomalous pulmonary venous drainage)
- Increased pulmonary artery pressure and flow:
  - large VSD
  - AVSD
  - PDA
  - aortopulmonary window
  - truncus arteriosus
  - transposition of the great arteries with a VSD.

Symptoms of pulmonary vascular disease do not usually develop until the second or third decade, typically presenting between 15 and 20 years of age. Cyanosis leads to a compensatory polycythaemia which in turn causes hyperviscosity. Progression of the process often leads to early death in the second or third decade of life.

The following are risk factors for the earlier development of pulmonary hypertension:

- Cardiac defect with large shunt
- Perinatal asphyxia
- Recurrent chest infections
- Chronic upper airway obstruction
- Down syndrome
- Birth at or living at high altitude.

Symptoms and signs of Eisenmenger syndrome:

- Dyspnoea
- Syncope
- Arrhythmias
- Clubbing
- Raised jugular venous pressure
- Right ventricular heave
- Loud P2
- Hyperviscosity may lead to:
  - thromboembolic events
  - gout
  - pulmonary infarction with chest pain and haemoptysis.

Heart–lung transplantation is the only surgical option. Management with diuretics and anticoagulants may be indicated. Phlebotomy may relieve the symptoms of hyperviscosity.

Various medications including long-term prostacyclins bosentan and sildenafil, currently used to treat idiopathic pulmonary hypertension, are being investigated for their potential to treat the underlying pulmonary hypertension seen in Eisenmenger syndrome with promising initial results.

Cardiac abnormalities presenting with cyanosis and reduced pulmonary flow are protected from the development of pulmonary vascular disease. These conditions include pulmonary atresia, pulmonary stenosis and tetralogy of Fallot.

1.22 Patent ductus arteriosus

Answer E: The incidence of PDA is increased in preterm infants and those with perinatal hypoxia and/or distress

PDA is present in 40–50% of preterm infants born weighing <1750 g, 30% of whom have a significant ductus with congestive cardiac failure. The reason for the higher incidence in preterm infants is that the responsiveness of ductal smooth muscle is gestation dependent. Perinatal distress and/or hypoxia can delay the closure of the duct. If not associated with predisposing factors PDA is more common in girls (ratio 2:1). In term infants functional closure occurs within 10–15 hours of birth with complete anatomical closure by 2–3 weeks of age. A persistence of the duct for 3 months after the baby has reached term is the definition of a persistent ductus arteriosus.

Presentation of PDA in the preterm infant:

- Cardiac failure
- Apnoea
- Increased ventilatory requirements.

Presentation of PDA in the term infant or child:

- Small shunt: asymptomatic
- Large shunt:
  - poor weight gain (up to a third of children with PDA are small for age)
  - tachypnoea
  - tachycardia
  - cardiac murmur.

Findings on examination:

- Continuous machinery murmur in left infraclavicular area
- Full pulses
- Loud P2 (can be obscured by the murmur)
- In the preterm infant the murmur may be limited to systole.

Management of PDA

In the preterm infant this depends on symptoms. Spontaneous closure is likely if the duct is asymptomatic. In symptomatic infants the management is fluid restriction, diuretics, maintenance of normal haemoglobin and attempted medical closure with indometacin, ibuprofen or surgical ligation.

In the term infant indometacin is not helpful and the principal therapeutic option is surgical ligation. Catheter closure of the duct is indicated in children aged >1 year (occasionally younger). Spontaneous closure is not likely in term infants.

1.23 Coarctation of the aorta

Answer E: Adult-type coarctation of the aorta is associated with blood pressure discrepancy between the upper and lower limbs

This accounts for 5% of congenital heart disease. It is more common in boys (2:1). It can present in infancy if the coarctation is significant, making systemic perfusion duct dependent, or in late childhood or adulthood in the non-duct-dependent lesion which tends to become increasingly more severe over years.

Associated cardiac anomalies include:

- bicuspid aortic valve (70%)
- mitral valve disease
- subaortic stenosis
- VSD.

Adult-type coarctation

The coarctation is usually just after the origin of the left subclavian artery (98%) at the level of the ductus arteriosus. It can occur proximal to the origin of the left subclavian artery, in which case the blood pressure in the right arm will be higher than in the left arm, the classic discrepancy being between the upper and lower limb blood pressure. The murmur of coarctation is systolic. Continuous murmurs are occasionally heard from collaterals. Up to 10% of children with coarctation have berry aneurysms in the cerebral circulation. Rib notching does not appear until late childhood. There can be a classic '3' sign with a visible notch on the chest radiograph in the descending aorta. Treatment is surgical by balloon dilatation, graft or a subclavian flap. This is usually carried out soon after diagnosis.

Duct-dependent coarctation

This lesion is often diagnosed antenatally on screening ultrasound examinations. If not the neonate will present collapsed with absent femoral pulses at the time of the duct closure. Absence of a murmur, shortness of breath, and signs of right heart failure (hepatomegaly), breathlessness and acidosis are common at presentation. Resuscitation and urgent treatment with prostaglandin E1 or E2 is life saving in order to support the infant's circulation before urgent corrective surgery.

Associations of coarctation of the aorta include:

- trisomy 13
- trisomy 18
- Turner syndrome
- valproate toxicity.

1.24 Hypertension

Answer C: In infants the most common cause of hypertension is renal parenchymal disease

Childhood hypertension is defined as systolic or diastolic blood pressure greater than the 95th centile for age, recorded on three separate occasions. There are two types: primary (aetiology unknown) and secondary (aetiology known). Secondary hypertension is more common in infants and younger children. Primary hypertension is more common than secondary hypertension in adolescents and young adults when there is often a family history. Children with primary hypertension are rarely symptomatic. Obesity is associated with primary hypertension, and in 70–80% of children with secondary hypertension there is a renal cause. Initial investigations are aimed at detecting renal parenchymal disease.

Causes of hypertension in childhood include:

- Renal parenchymal disease:
  - renal scarring/reflux nephropathy
  - acute glomerulonephritis
  - chronic glomerulonephritis
  - chronic renal failure
  - acute renal failure
  - nephrotic syndrome
  - polycystic renal disease
- Vascular disease and renovascular disease:
  - coarctation of the aorta
  - renal artery stenosis
  - renal artery or renal vein thrombosis
- Renal tumours: Wilms tumour
- Catecholamines:
  - phaeochromocytoma
  - neuroblastoma
- Obstructive uropathy
- Corticosteroids:
  - iatrogenic
  - Cushing syndrome
- Neurological causes:
  - raised ICP (intracranial pressure)
  - seizures
  - spinal cord injury
- Drugs:
  - caffeine
  - alcohol
- Essential hypertension: significantly associated with obesity.

1.25 Infective endocarditis

Answer A: Infective endocarditis is associated with a 13-20% mortality rate

Infective endocarditis (IE) is defined as an infection of the lining of the heart, particularly affecting the heart valves.

- Associated with 20% mortality rate and considerable morbidity
- Most common organism is *Streptococcus viridians*
- Others include *Staphylococcus aureus, Enterococcus* sp. and *Streptococcus epidermidis* (on prosthetic valves).
- Lesions are usually left sided (except in intravenous drug abusers)
- Most cases have either congenital or acquired heart defects
- Increased risk with indwelling central lines and intravenous drug abuse
- Almost all congenital heart defects increase the risk of IE
- Lesions considered of no increased risk include:
  - ostium secundum ASD
  - fully repaired PDA or VSD.

The clinical manifestations are often difficult and non-specific:

- Fever in >80%
- Non-specific symptoms:
  - fatigue
  - myalgia
  - arthralgia
  - weight loss
- 50% have skin manifestations (caused by circulating antibody/antigen complexes):
  - Janeway lesions are painless haemorrhages on the soles and palms
  - Osler nodes – painful nodules in the pads of the fingers and toes
  - splinter haemorrhages in nails
- 50% have embolic phenomena; haematuria is common
- Finger clubbing in chronic cases
- Cardiac failure from valve destruction
- Murmur is universal – either a new murmur or change in character of an existing murmur.

Diagnosis is on clinical suspicion, positive blood culture (which may need to be done repeatedly – three blood cultures have a 95% pick-up rate) and by the demonstration of valvular vegetations on echocardiography. Treatment is with long-term (4–6 weeks) antibiotics. Surgery is occasionally required.

Prevention

- Good dental hygiene is essential.
- NICE (National Institute for Health and Clinical Excellence) no longer recommends prophylactic antibiotics for routine procedures.

- Antibiotics to cover IE organisms are recommended for a patient already receiving antibiotic for a gastrointestinal or genitourinary procedure who is at risk of IE.

1.26 Cardiomyopathy

Answer B: Dilated cardiomyopathy is associated with doxorubicin toxicity in children

- Common indication for cardiac transplantation
- 20% are inherited
- Peak incidence in infancy
- Second peak in adolescence (neuromuscular disorders and autosomal dominant hypertrophic cardiomyopathy or HCM).

Presentation

- Increasing effort intolerance (feeding/exercise)
- Impaired growth
- More rarely chest pain and palpitations
- Signs include dyspnoea, sweating, compromised perfusion, tachycardia, tachypnoea, hepatomegaly ± a murmur

Hypertrophic cardiomyopathy (40% overall)

- Symmetrical/asymmetrical ventricular hypertrophy without underlying structural reasons
- Atria are often enlarged.
- 60% are autosomal dominant
- Transient form seen in infants of mothers with diabetes and infants on steroids
- Syndromic associations include Beckwith–Weidemann and Noonan syndromes
- Sudden death occurs in 4–6% of cases/year
- Treatment with selective β blockers
- Anti-arrhythmics and implantable defibrillators are used in older children.

Dilated cardiomyopathy (DCM – 50% overall)

- Large, globular heart with biventricular and biatrial dilatation
- Mostly idiopathic
- Rarer X-linked adolescent presentation
- Other causes include: rate related (due to prolonged tachycardia [SVT/VT], doxorubicin toxicity, phaeochromocytoma, mitochondrial disease, vitamin D deficiency and carnitine deficiency)
- Treatment with diuretics, ACE inhibitors, non-selective β blockers and digoxin
- Endocardial fibroelastosis is a form rarely seen in childhood.

Restrictive (RCM – 3% overall)

- Rare in childhood
- Myocardium unable to relax

- Symptoms from venous congestion in the systemic and pulmonary circulations and low cardiac output
- Median age of presentation of 36 months
- Commonly idiopathic
- Rarer associations include sarcoidosis, amyloidosis, haemochromatosis, Fabry disease and Loeffler syndrome.
- Early listing for cardiac transplantation is necessary to avoid irreversible pulmonary artery damage.

Arrhythmogenic right ventricular cardiomyopathy

- This is the least common type and is exceptionally rare in young children, usually presenting in teenagers and young adults
- Right ventricular dysfunction (regional or global) + fibrofatty infiltration of the right ventricular myocardium + ECG abnormalities
- Cause of sudden death in teenagers and young adults
- A genetic cause has been identified in some cases.

1.27 Rheumatic fever

Answer C: The most commonly occurring major criterion for diagnosing rheumatic fever is polyarthritis

Rheumatic fever develops secondary to infection with group A β-haemolytic *Streptococcus* sp. It is rare in the developed world but is estimated to affect 1.3 per 1000 of all school-aged children in developing countries. It is more common in lower socioeconomic classes and the peak incidence is between the ages of 5 and 15.

Diagnosis is by the Duckett–Jones criteria:

- two major OR
- one major and two minor criteria
- **PLUS** evidence of recent streptococcal infection (raised ASO [antistreptolysin O] titres, anti-deoxyribonuclease B or positive throat swab).

Major criteria:

- Carditis: 50% (pancarditis affecting the pericardium, myocardium and endocardium)
- Chorea: 15% (a late manifestation – purposeless and involuntary movements and emotional lability, lasts >6 months but has no long-term neurological sequelae)
- Polyarthritis: 70% (migratory, involves large joints, transient with no long-term sequelae)
- Erythema marginatum: 10% (pink rings on trunk and extensor surfaces of limbs)
- Subcutaneous nodules: 1%.

Minor criteria:

- Arthralgia
- Fever

- Prolonged PR interval on ECG
- Raised erythrocyte sedimentation rate (ESR) and C-reactive protein (CRP).

Pancarditis occurs in 50%. As a consequence of this 12.4% develop dysrhythmias, and 6% develop heart block, tachycardia, cardiomegaly, congestive cardiac failure and valve disease. Its sequelae include mitral regurgitation, mitral stenosis, aortic regurgitation and tricuspid regurgitation. Aspirin is indicated in the acute phase, initially at 120 mg/kg for 14 days and then 70 mg/kg until the fever settles. Prednisolone is indicated in severe carditis. A 10-day course of penicillin is given for eradication of streptococci in the first instance and antibiotic prophylaxis should be continued long term as a 3–4 weekly intramuscular dose of benzylpenicillin. It should continue for 10 years in those with carditis or until aged 21years (whichever is longer).

1.28 Innocent murmurs

Answer E: Reassurance that the murmur is innocent and discharge from follow-up

It is essential that a paediatrician be familiar with the features of an innocent cardiac murmur. It is not appropriate for all innocent murmurs to be seen in the cardiology clinic because up to 70% of children may experience innocent murmurs at some time in childhood. Cardiac referral and echocardiogram may aggravate parental anxiety even if it is reported as normal. However, if the clinician is not confident of the diagnosis of an innocent murmur a referral to a cardiologist is essential.

Features of an innocent murmur:

- Localised
- Poorly conducting
- Musical/vibratory
- Soft grade 1–2/6*
- Systolic*
- Varies with posture
- Present in high-output states, e.g. febrile illness, during exercise
- Cardiac examination otherwise normal
- Chest radiograph, ECG normal.

*Except venous hum.

A Still's murmur

This is an early systolic murmur most commonly heard in children aged 2–6 years, resolving towards adolescence. Grades 1–3 present in early systole, heart sounds normal. Maximum intensity is at lower left sternal edge. The murmur is vibratory and best heard with the patient flat, reducing in intensity when he or she sits up.

Venous hum

This is a continuous murmur most commonly heard in children aged 2–6 years. The diastolic component is usually loudest. It is best heard over the supraclavicular fossa on the right, with the head turned to the other side. It may radiate and is often heard on both sides. It disappears on lying flat or if the neck veins are compressed.

Pulmonary flow murmur

This is a very common murmur. Characteristically it is brief and in midsystole. It is loudest with the patient supine and during expiration. Occurs in children and adolescents of all ages and is louder during hyperdynamic states such as fever and post exercise. Innocent murmurs are commonly heard in the neonatal period.

1.29 Cardiac emergencies

Answer D: Synchronous shock of 1 J/kg

Supraventricular tachycardia

The most common cardiac arrhythmia in the paediatric age group is SVT. In infants the rate is usually >220 beats/min but can be lower in older children. The QRS complex is narrow. Classically the onset is abrupt. It can last for a few minutes or several days, and is tolerated well by most children, although the majority will develop cardiac failure if the arrhythmia persists.

If haemodynamically stable:

1. Vagal stimulation – facial immersion/unilateral carotid massage
2. Adenosine into **proximal vein with flush**:
   - first dose, 100 μg/kg
   - second dose after 2 min 200 μg/kg
   - third dose 300 μg/kg after 2 min
   - consider 400–500 μg/kg (>1 month of age)
3. Synchronous DC shock or amiodarone or procainamide.

If shock present:

1. Vagal manoeuvres if no delays
2. If vascular access immediately available give adenosine
3. If not give synchronous DC shock 1 J/kg
4. Further synchronised DC shock 2 J/kg
5. Consider amiodarone

Ventricular tachycardia

If haemodynamically stable: note do not delay therapeutic intervention for long as VT can deteriorate into pulseless VT or VF.

Consider underlying causes:

- Congenital heart disease and surgery
- Poisoning: tricyclic antidepressants, procainamide, macrolide antibiotics
- Renal disease or other causes of hyperkalaemia
- Long QT syndrome
- Urgent ECG analysis by senior paediatrician with experience in cardiology and seek further advice

- Consider amiodarone 5 mg/kg over 30 min
- Consider synchronous DC shock.

Emergency treatment if shock present:

- Assess if pulse is present; if not treat as VF
- If pulse present:
  - synchronous DC shock, in the first instance 1 J/kg
  - further shocks should be asynchronous at 2 J/kg
  - consider a dose of amiodarone 5 mg/kg over a few minutes in VT if a child is in severe shock.

1.30 Wolff–Parkinson–White syndrome

Answer D: Radiofrequency ablation of the accessory pathway is potentially curable

Patients with this syndrome are prone to SVT from pre-excitation due to an anomalous atrioventricular conduction pathway bypassing the junctional tissue. The accessory pathway allows a circuit to be formed, which facilitates a re-entry tachycardia.

The ECG characteristics include:

- shortened PR interval due to rapid anterograde conduction
- prolonged QRS caused by premature action of the ventricle through the accessory pathway, followed by normal depolarisation through the AV node and the bundle of His
- delta wave – slurring of the upstroke to the QRS complex.

Wolff–Parkinson–White syndrome (WPW) syndrome is usually associated with a structurally normal heart (70–80%). It is more common in men (60–70%). There is a recognised association with Ebstein anomaly, corrected transposition and cardiomyopathy. There is a risk of sudden death of approximately 1–4%.

Patients may present with attacks of tachycardia leading to a spectrum of symptoms from mild chest discomfort or palpitations, sometimes associated with syncope, to severe shock associated with the SVT or cardiac arrest. Most patients present with tachycardia at a rate >250 beats/min and hypotension. Clinically crepitations in lung bases may coexist secondary to pulmonary vascular congestion due to rate associated cardiac compromise. Occasionally patients can present incidentally when characteristic ECG appearances are detected.

When a patient is known to have WPW syndrome, adenosine should be used only with extreme caution, having the means to perform cardioversion/defibrillation immediately available due to the risk of deterioration of the rhythm to VF as a result of blockage of the AV node and the possibility of a partial or no effect on the accessory pathway. Digoxin is contraindicated for the same reason. Appropriate anti-arrhythmics include verapamil, flecainide and procainamide. Radiofrequency ablation of the accessory pathway is a potentially curative procedure for patients with WPW syndrome.

1.31 Paediatric ECG

Answer A: The PR interval is prolonged in hyperkalaemia

The paediatric ECG is recorded at a rate of 25 mm/s.

The axis of the QRS complex is calculated by looking at the total deflection in lead 1 and AVF. The normal axis for a paediatric ECG changes with age:

- Newborn: 90–180°
- 2–5 years: 45–135°
- > 5 years: –10–100°.

Causes of a superior axis include:

- AVSD
- tricuspid atresia
- Ebstein anomaly
- Noonan syndrome
- WPW syndrome
- <1% of normal individuals.

The PR interval varies with age, normally two to four small squares (0.08–0.16 s):

- Upper limit of normal in infants – 0.14 s
- Upper limit of normal in older children – 0.16 s.

Causes of a prolonged PR interval include:

- AVSD
- atrioventricular canal defect
- Ebstein anomaly
- myocarditis
- ischaemia
- hypothermia
- hyperkalaemia
- Duchenne muscular dystrophy
- digoxin
- quinidine.

QT measurement is made from the start of the Q wave to the end of the T wave. The QT is corrected for the rate as it decreases with increased heart rate. QT corrected for rate (QTc) = QT/ √ RR in seconds. The normal range is considered to be 0.35–0.43 s (8.75–10.75 small squares).

QRS complex

- Delta wave in WPW syndrome is an upslurring of R wave
- RS progression varies with age

– neonate dominant R in V1, Dominant s in V6

– infant (1–18 months) – dominant R in V1, dominant R in V6

– adult (>18 months) – dominant S in V1, dominant R in V6

- Right ventricular hypertrophy (RVH):

  – upright T waves in V1 (abnormal from week 1 to 16 years)

  – Q in V1

  – R waves >20 mm in V1

- Left ventricular hypertrophy (LVH):

  – inverted T in V6

  – Q in V6

  – LAD

  – R waves >20 mm in V6.

1.32 Causes of QT prolongation

Answer B: Erythromycin should be avoided in patients with prolonged QT syndrome

- Prolonged QT (PQT) can be a congenital or an acquired phenomenon.
- QT prolongation can precipitate VT and VF, which may lead to syncope, cardiac arrest and sudden death.
- Torsades de pointes: a distinctive form of the ventricular tachyarrhythmia that is associated with PQT; it can degenerate into VF. Many genetic defects have been identified including:

  – autosomal dominant – Romano–Ward syndrome

  – autosomal recessive – Jervell–Lange–Nielsen syndrome (associated with congenital deafness)

  although only 50% of cases have a recognised genetic abnormality.

- Up to 30% of cases of sudden death secondary to PQT have no preceding symptoms.
- The vast majority of patients present in infancy, childhood or early adult life.
- An unexplained family death at <30 years of age may be elicited in the history
- Cardiac events may be triggered by exercise, swimming or emotional events but can occur during sleep (genetics alter the predisposition to certain triggers).
- QT (in seconds) is measured from the start of the Q wave until the end of the T wave.
- Corrected QT: measured QT/√RR.
- >0.44 is abnormal.
- Longer QT intervals have been reported in normal infants.
- A normal QTc in a patient's ECG does not exclude the diagnosis.
- Four to five per cent of cardiac events are fatal.

Management:

- β Blockers
- Left cardiac sympathetic denervation
- Occasionally pacemaker or implantable cardioverter–defibrillator device

- Avoidance of drugs that prolong QT or decrease potassium or magnesium levels
- Advice to avoid competitive sports.

Situations that prolong the QT:

- hypocalcaemia
- hypomagnesaemia
- myocarditis
- central nervous system trauma
- drugs: cisapride, quinidine, terfenadine, astemizole, amiodarone, amitriptyline, phenothiazines, antimalarials, erythromycin and trimethoprim.

1.33 Without fever there is no diagnosis

Answer B: High-grade fever for > 5 days

Kawasaki disease is an acute self-limiting systemic vasculitis with a predilection for the coronary arteries. The diagnosis is clinical. It is the leading cause of coronary vessel disease in children in the UK. Up to 25% (if untreated) will progress to develop coronary artery aneurysms; 20% of those will develop coronary artery stenosis and myocardial ischaemia, and may have a coronary thrombosis or die suddenly (mortality peaks 6 weeks post-fever onset). Most common between 6 months and 5 years (peak 9–11 months).

Definition: **fever** of 5 days' duration with no obvious underlying cause plus at least four of the following five (or **fever**, coronary aneurysms and three of the five):

- Bilateral conjunctivitis without exudate
- Oral changes (strawberry tongue, fissuring of the lips)
- Peripheral extremity changes (erythema of palms or soles, swelling, desquamation of fingers or toes [1–2 weeks after the onset of fever])
- Cervical adenopathy >1.5 cm – uncommon and may be unilateral
- Pleomorphic rash (not vesicular) generalised.

Systemic involvement is common with irritability, neurological complications, abdominal pain, vomiting, and small and large joint involvement; 15% develop hydrops of the gallbladder within the first 2 weeks.

Inflammatory markers (CRP and ESR) are raised and may take 6 weeks to normalise. A raised WBC in the acute phase (high neutrophils) is common. The platelet count often rises some 2 weeks into the illness. Derangement of serum transaminases occurs in approximately 40% and mild hyperbilirubinaemia in 10%. There is a sterile pyuria in 10% (urethritis).

Treatment:

- High-dose aspirin until fever subsides; low dose for 6 weeks (or no evidence of aneurysms on echo)
- Immunoglobulin – reduces aneurysms if given in the first 10 days
- Ten per cent do not respond to IVIG and methyl prednisolone or increasingly infliximab is used

1.34 Subacute bacterial endocarditis (SBE)

Answer A: Splinter haemorrhages

SBE is a serious systemic infection with a cardiac focus. Underlying cardiac abnormalities (of valves or septa) predispose to, but are not an imperative part of, the aetiology of this condition. Organisms include *Streptococcus viridans* and *Staphylococcus aureus*. Clinical signs include splinters, retinal haemorrhages and changing cardiac murmurs. Diagnosis rests on a positive blood culture (in practice at least three should be taken) and showing vegetations on an echo (not 100% sensitive). Treatment consists of prolonged antibiotic course (6 weeks standard), valve replacement in cases of irreversible damage and (arguably) lifelong antibiotic prophylaxis, although the NICE guidelines published in 2008 refute the value of giving routine prophylaxis to any patient with a condition that predisposes to SBE.

1.35 SVT

Answer D: Oxygen

This baby has SVT and is compromised cardiovascularly. This is more likely to be due to a re-entry phenomenon than a structural defect. As in any cardiorespiratory emergency, an ABC approach is the priority followed by management to terminate the dysrhythmia. Vagal manoeuvres such as ice packs, carotid sinus massage (hard in a baby) and ocular pressure may help to terminate the dysrhythmia. Parenteral adenosine given rapidly in escalating doses is the drug treatment of choice if vagal methods fail, followed by synchronous DC shock. Recurrent SVT may require longer-term anti-arrhythmic treatment (c.goxin, flecainide, propranolol or amiodarone). In more severe cases, pathway ablation is a final, usually successful, option.

1.36 Cyanotic congenital heart disease

Answer E: Transposition of the great arteries

This baby clinically has cyanotic congenital heart disease. The key features are deep cyanosis without major respiratory distress, indicative of a physiological right-to-left shunt. The most likely diagnosis is TGA. Until the patent ductus closes there may be no symptoms or signs, but, as the pulmonary–systemic connection reaches critical point, cyanosis becomes overt. Tetralogy of Fallot, pulmonary atresia, tricuspid atresia, anomalous pulmonary venous drainage and truncus arteriosus all give rise to a similar picture but are much less common. A VSD is unlikely to cause symptoms at this age and would manifest as heart failure without cyanosis. Persistent fetal circulation and diaphragmatic hernias present with a much 'sicker' baby who has respiratory signs and within the first few hours, if not sooner.

1.37 Barium swallow

Answer B: Barium swallow

Although 'simple' laryngomalacia is by far the most common cause of early stridor (and almost always self-resolving), the picture in this case is different. This child is failing to thrive (always significant) and has a murmur suggesting a vascular/aortic ring which is best elucidated by a barium swallow because it will compress the oesophagus. You would, of course, when presented with this clinical scenario, require an expert cardiology review and echocardiogram to evaluate the underlying cardiac signs. In addition a respiratory or ENT bronchoscopic evaluation of the upper airway may be helpful in due course.

Causes of stridor:

- Intrinsic, e.g.
  - laryngomalacia
  - cord nodules/polyps
  - haemangiomas of the cords
  - cord palsies
  - laryngeal nerve palsy
  - subglottic stenosis after prolonged intubation
  - laryngeal web
- Extrinsic, e.g.
  - vascular ring
  - right atrial enlargement
  - cystic hygroma (obvious)
  - thyroid enlargement.

1.38 Kawasaki disease

Answer C: High-dose aspirin and parenteral immunoglobulin

This child fulfils the criteria for Kawasaki disease. The rash is often confused with measles (which was rare in the UK but became more common again with the reduction in MMR vaccine uptake). However, the extreme misery, desquamation and cervical nodes point in another direction. Once suspected, treatment should be started without delay due to the risk of a coronary artery aneurysm developing or enlarging with the increased duration of the febrile phase of the illness. Meta-analyses suggest that high-dose aspirin (50 mg/kg per day in divided doses) until the fever subsides and a single dose of immunoglobulin (2 g over 12 h i.v.) is the best management pending echocardiography, and this regimen is now accepted practice.

Vitamin A at presentation is routine management of measles in developing country settings and reduces mortality by up to 50%.

EMQ Answers

1.39–1.41 Theme: Neonatal cyanosis

1.39

Answer A: Congenital pneumonia

This baby boy has risk factors for congenital pneumonia and responded to a hyperoxia test with a good increment in his saturations making a respiratory cause for his cyanosis more likely than a cardiac one.

1.40

Answer F: Transposition of the great arteries

This is the most common cyanotic congenital heart disease presenting in the neonatal period. The antenatal diagnosis on routine anomaly scan remains difficult so most of these children present postnatally despite antenatal anomaly screening. The exact presentation depends on the extent of intercirculatory mixing and the presence of associated malformations.

1.41

Answer G: Obstructed total anomalous pulmonary venous connection

This is a rare presentation (1% of all congenital heart disease); it is, however, important to consider this diagnosis in all neonates presenting with cyanosis and respiratory distress.

Differential diagnosis of cyanosis in the newborn

- Cardiac causes (cyanotic heart disease)
- Respiratory disease (structurally abnormal lung, diaphragmatic hernia, pneumothorax)
- Central nervous system depression (hypoventilation, perinatal asphyxia)
- Infective (pneumonia)
- Metabolic (lactic acidosis – shifts the oxygen dissociation curve to the right causing more cyanosis at any given arterial oxygen concentration)
- Acrocyanosis
- Methaemoglobinaemia.

Cardiac causes that are classically duct dependent:

- Transposition of the great arteries (common)
- Tetralogy of Fallot with pulmonary atresia (less common)
- Pulmonary atresia with intact ventricular septum (rare)
- Tricuspid atresia or other complex heart disease (rare)

- Ebstein anomaly (rare).

Non-duct-dependent causes of neonatal cyanosis:

- Obstructed total anomalous pulmonary venous connection (rare)
- Truncus arteriosus (rare)
- Persistent pulmonary hypertension of the newborn.

The **hyperoxia test** is used to help differentiate between cardiac and non-cardiac causes of cyanosis. Cyanosis is indicative of more than 5 g/dl of haemoglobin being in the reduced state. The test is performed as follows: once cyanosis has been confirmed by either an arterial blood gas or pulse oximetry, the infant is given 100% oxygen to inspire. The baby with a respiratory cause for cyanosis will generally show a good increment (PaO_2 >20 kPa), whereas the infant with cyanotic congenital heart disease and a right-to-left shunt will not. There are some exceptions to this including total anomalous pulmonary venous drainage (due to pulmonary oedema), in which a moderate but incomplete response to the hyperoxia test will be seen. If a duct-dependent cardiac lesion is suspected then a prostaglandin infusion should be started, which prolongs patency of the ductus arteriosus (and venosus for subdiaphragmatic TAPVC) pending transfer to a cardiac unit. Side effects of prostaglandin include apnoea, so the child needs to be ventilated.

Acrocyanosis is peripheral cyanosis of the hands, feet and occasionally the trunk. It is very common in the first 24 hours of life.

Total anomalous pulmonary venous connection is a rare form of congenital heart disease in which all four pulmonary veins drain into systemic veins (supracardiac or subdiaphragmatic) or the right atrium with or without pulmonary venous obstruction. An ASD or patent foramen ovale (PFO) is considered part of the complex because it is vital in maintaining a left ventricular output both pre- and post-delivery. Pulmonary venous obstruction leads to pulmonary venous congestion, a decrease in pulmonary blood flow and an increase in cyanosis, and therefore to an earlier presentation. Obstructed cases usually present within the first 36 hours of birth with tachycardia, tachypnoea and cyanosis. Deterioration, without intervention, is progressive with increasing pulmonary hypertension and decreasing pulmonary blood flow, with death within the first 1–4 weeks of life depending on the degree of venous obstruction. Examination reveals severe cyanosis and significant respiratory distress; a gallop rhythm may be present but a murmur is uncommon. Peripheral pulses are present at birth but decrease as heart failure progresses. Liver enlargement commonly occurs.

Infants may present later up to 6 months of age if unobstructed with a murmur or heart failure.

Management:

- Resuscitate
- Ventilate early (before transfer for definitive surgery)
- Prostaglandin may not be effective in obstructed cases but should be started; urgent surgical repair is indicated.

1.42–1.44 Theme: Illness with cardiac manifestations

1.42

Answer A: Cardiomyopathy

This boy has anthracycline cardiomyopathy. In the past these drugs were widely used but are still needed in certain malignancies. Lifelong cardiac follow-up is need with an annual echo because a proportion of these patients develop dilated cardiomyopathy, which is dose dependent. There is often a gap of many years before the signs become overt. Treatment is supportive until transplantation is possible.

1.43

Answer J: None of the above

This child has high-output failure although the underlying problem does not appear to be cardiac. Aetiology of high-output cardiac failure in this age group includes anaemia, sepsis and a vascular anomaly. Due to a normal FBC and infection screen, this picture suggests a vein of Galen aneurysm or an arteriovenous malformation. The signs will include heart failure with a cerebral bruit. The aneurysm can be delineated by magnetic resonance imaging (MRI) or angiography (MRA).

1.44

Answer C: Rheumatic fever

This boy has classic rheumatic fever with a rash, fever, arthralgia, prolonged PR interval and mitral murmur. It is post-streptococcal and the ASO titre is likely to be raised. For diagnosis, either two major criteria or one major and two minor Jones criteria plus evidence of a preceding streptococcal infection are needed (see comprehensive discussion elsewhere). Management is symptomatic. Opinions vary with regard to the need for streptococcal treatment but most would give a short course of high-dose penicillin to eradicate the infection. After rheumatic fever, long-term (at least into adulthood) 3–4 weekly intramuscular benzylpenicillin prophylaxis is recommended.

1.45–1.47 Theme: Cardiac investigations

1.45

Answer H: ECG

This has all the features of an innocent murmur: soft, systolic, positional. Up to 30% of children have such a murmur detected at some stage, often while they are being auscultated for other reasons. In this case the 'louder sitting' characteristic suggests a venous hum, as opposed to a Still's murmur or pulmonary flow (both of which are best heard lying down). No investigation is needed and only parental reassurance is necessary.

1.46

Answer A: 24-hour ECG

Although these may be simple panic attacks, the girl's complaint requires that SVT be ruled out. A 24-hour tape may show runs of SVT and it is helpful to carry this out with an event monitoring facility. A standard ECG may show signs of WPW syndrome (short PR interval with a delta wave).

1.47

Answer C: Cardiac catheter

This child's aortic valve is restenosing until proved otherwise. Doppler echo studies will be suggestive but the gold standard remains cardiac catheterisation. This child is likely to require percutaneous transluminal redilatation or an open repair should this fail.

1.48–1.50 Theme: Syncope

1.48

Answer C: 12-lead ECG with cardiac referral if abnormality is reported

This young woman is almost certainly experiencing a type of neurally mediated syncope (NMS) or vasovagal attack. However, any child experiencing syncopal events should have a 12-lead ECG as a baseline investigation, coupled with a thorough history and examination. If these were all normal, reassurance and advice with regard to avoiding exacerbating factors and strategies to abort syncopal attacks would seem the most appropriate. Advice to avoid exercise is indicated only if given by a cardiologist in specific cases of proven cardiogenic syncope, e.g. prolonged QT syndrome or hypertrophic cardiomyopathy. More complex investigations such as exercise stress tests and digital loop cardiac monitors can be helpful in the investigation of syncope, but should be initiated once the child has been referred to cardiology for review.

1.49

Answer B: ECG and immediate referral of patient to paediatric cardiologist with presumed long QT syndrome

This is a classic presentation of prolonged QT syndrome and should be taken extremely seriously. This young man therefore has a significant risk of having prolonged QT syndrome with the associated risk of sudden death despite his apparent good health. He requires an ECG and evaluation of his corrected QT interval but regardless of the result of this investigation he should be referred to a cardiologist because of the nature of his loss of consciousness. It should be remembered that with a high index of suspicion a normal QT interval on an ECG does not exclude the diagnosis.

1.50

Answer C: 12-lead ECG with cardiac referral if abnormality is reported

This child is likely to have had a reflex anoxic seizure – not an epileptiform seizure. This is a textbook description of a typical event. An EEG would not be indicated in this child because it may lead to her being falsely labelled as epileptic. As with all children who are referred with syncope a 12-lead ECG is advisable, but if it is normal an explanation of the mechanism of reflex anoxic seizures and their benign nature, with reassurance for the family, is the best management for this patient.

Syncope: a transient, self-limited loss of consciousness resulting from an insufficient supply of oxygen to the brain.

Presyncope: a state of light-headedness warning of imminent syncope. Symptoms include dizziness without blackout, pallor, diaphoresis, thready pulse and low BP.

- Up to 15% of children will experience at least one episode of syncope before age 18 years
- More common in 15–19 year olds
- More common in girls
- NMS 75%
- Cardiac disease 10%
- Psychogenic or unexplained total loss of consciousness 8%
- Possible epilepsy 5%.

Clinical picture is varied.

Neurally mediated syncope

- The archetypal a vasovagal syncope (autonomically mediated):
  - **vaso** – sympathetically mediated peripheral vasomotor control
  - **vagal** – parasympathetically mediated bradycardia
  - ↑ when tired, hungry, unwell, dehydrated, hot, post-exertion, or stressed, frightened or emotionally shocked (including specifically exposure to blood)
- Reflex asystolic syncope/reflex anoxic seizure:
  - paroxysmal episodes of collapse, associated with pain or surprise
  - usually associated with stiffening or jerking
  - typical in preschool-aged children
- Chronic orthostatic intolerance – syncope or presyncope on standing for >3 months:
  - other features include exercise intolerance and chronic fatigue
  - associated symptoms include migranous headache, nausea, abdominal discomfort, shortness of breath, hyperventilation, peripheral cyanosis, sweating and flushing on standing
- Postural tachycardia syndrome: patients have symptoms of chronic orthostatic intolerance associated with marked tachycardia (>30 beats/min, increase on standing)

- Apnoeic syncope: blue breath-holding spells – not intentional or naughty behaviour and does not reflect poor parenting.

Cardiac syncope

This is rare but important to diagnose because can lead to sudden death. Associated with:

- extreme pallor
- evidence of injury from collapse (as no prodromal warning)
- exercise (especially swimming or from sleep)
- syncope at rest
- family history of sudden death or deafness
- chest pain
- palpitations
- underlying known heart disease.

Causes include:

- long QT syndrome
- heart block
- arrhythmias
- obstructive lesions (aortic stenosis, pulmonary stenosis, HCM)
- ischaemia (aberrant coronary arteries, post-Kawasaki disease)
- myocarditis.

Investigation

A thorough history (including eye witness account and/or video of event) is vital in assessing all young people with a history of syncope. Particular attention should be paid to the circumstances surrounding the event and any specific 'red flags' indicating an increased chance of an underlying cardiac cause listed above.

A thorough examination is also vital and should include:

- full neurological examination, occipito frontal circumference, fundoscopy, auscultation for carotid bruits
- supine and standing blood pressure and heart rate
- **12-lead ECG in every patient** – reviewed by expert if any concerns
- exercise ECG if events associated with stress or exertion
- external digital loop cardiac monitors
- echocardiography for any patient with features suggestive of structural heart defects
- EEG only in patients with a high suspicion of epilepsy as a primary cause for transient loss of consciousness; coincidental ECG monitoring should be included

Management

Explanation and reassurance are essential in NMS with advice about the importance of resuming a normal life and sensible management of risk factors such as dehydration, warm environments and general measures to abort syncopal attacks.

1.51–1.53 Theme: Chest pain

1.51

Answer D: Precordial catch syndrome

1.52

Answer A: Aortic stenosis

1.53

Answer E: Costochondritis

Chest pain is a common symptom in paediatrics and causes a great deal of anxiety for both children and their parents. Chest pain is an unusual manifestation of cardiac disease in children. A child with chronic chest pain who is well and has a normal physical examination with no concerning factors in the history or examination requires reassurance rather than investigation.

Red flags in the history include:

- pain that wakes a child from sleep
- pain of sudden onset
- association with fever
- breathlessness, pallor and sweating
- musculoskeletal causes preceded by trauma are common.

The differential diagnosis of chest pain in children includes the following.

Costochondritis (Tietze syndrome)

This is a process of inflammation in one or more of the costochondral cartilages, which manifests as pain and localised tenderness in the anterior chest wall. Most cases are idiopathic, but the condition can be secondary to trauma, aggressive exercise or forceful cough producing strain on the costochondral junction. The condition is more common in girls. The onset of the condition may be acute but typically is more insidious over days or even weeks. Tenderness over the costochondral junction is diagnostic. Tietze syndrome is swelling associated with the pain in the costochondritis. This is a self-limiting disorder with spontaneous resolution seen over weeks of months. Symptomatic relief can be achieved with non-steroidal anti-inflammatory drugs (NSAIDs).

Precordial catch syndrome

This is characterised by the sudden onset of anterior left-sided chest pain with no associated radiation. Pain is exacerbated by deep inspiration and can be very severe. Episodes often last seconds to a few minutes, and inspiration, expiration and movement are felt to exacerbate the pain. The frequency of attacks can vary widely repeated episodes multiple times a day to infrequent attacks separated by years. A forced (but painful) deep inspiration in some patients can lead to a popping sensation that is rapidly followed by relief of the pain. It is believed to be secondary to localised muscle cramping.

Epidemic myalgia/pleurodynia (Bornholm disease)

Caused by Coxsackie B virus this results in the acute onset of lancinating chest pain (or abdominal pain) associated with systemic features including headache, fever and malaise, and symptoms of an upper respiratory tract infection (URTI). It usually lasts 3–5 days with a generally dull pleuritic chest pain coupled with more acute paroxysmal exacerbations of pain over the lower ribs – usually unilateral in nature. Prognosis is excellent for a spontaneous resolution with treatment with NSAIDs recommended for symptomatic pain relief.

Respiratory causes of chest pain

Asthma may cause symptoms of chest pain on exertion, particularly in older children. It is typically retrosternal in origin and relieved with the use of a bronchodilator.

Pneumonia can present acutely as chest pain when there is pleural involvement. It is often an acute history with fever, shortness of breath and cough, but less typical cases do occur. Examination is essential to help with the differential diagnosis of chest pain in children.

Ischaemic chest pain

Ischaemic cardiac pain is seen in HCM, aortic stenosis, mitral valve prolapse and anomalous coronary arteries, or after Kawasaki disease. Ischaemic cardiac pain is typically described as gripping/crushing in nature and localised to the precordium, with possible radiation to the neck, arm or jaw.

Aortic valve stenosis

This accounts for approximately 5% of all congenital heart disease. It has a male:female ratio of 4:1. Critical aortic stenosis presents in the neonatal period with congestive heart failure or collapse secondary to ductus closure in the first days of life. Congenital aortic stenosis is associated with a bicuspid aortic valve and may coexist with an element of aortic valve insufficiency. Older children can remain asymptomatic into adulthood, but if symptomatic can complain of fatigability, syncope or ischaemic chest pain, it is rarely associated with sudden death during exercise. Examination reveals a carotid thrill, Systolic murmur is best heard at the upper sternal edge and is classically an ejection click. Investigation is with echocardiography; cardiac catheterisation with balloon valvuloplasty is the usual first-line therapeutic intervention.

1.54–1.56 Theme: Murmurs heard beyond the neonatal period

1.54

Answer A: Atrial septal defect

This child has features of an ASD. The murmur heard is due to increased blood flow through the right ventricular outflow tract. A low frequency diastolic murmur may also be associated with an ASD due to increased diastolic blood flow across the tricuspid valve. Often these patients are asymptomatic in childhood but flow may well increase over the

ASD with age. Symptoms become increasingly more common in the fourth decade of life, with 90% of untreated patients having symptoms of shortness of breath on exertion, fatigue, palpitations secondary to atrial arrhythmias or evidence of heart failure. Recurrent respiratory tract infections may be associated with this defect. Spontaneous closure of secundum ASDs in childhood is possible but less likely with increasing age. The chronic left-to-right shunt associated with an untreated ASD can increase the pulmonary vascular resistance, leading to pulmonary arterial hypertension and in some rare cases reversal of the direction of shunt flow, leading to cyanosis and Eisenmenger syndrome. It is important to perform surgical correction early due to the decreased association of atrial arrhythmias with defects that are corrected early.

1.55

Answer F: Still's murmur

This child has the characteristic features of a Still's murmur with an incidental finding of right bundle-branch block (RBBB) on the ECG. The features are important to distinguish from those of the above case because they can be easily confused and missing a diagnosis of ASD may lead to irreversible changes in the pulmonary vasculature. A change in intensity of a murmur on standing is very characteristic of an innocent or functional murmur, with the important exception of the murmur associated with HCM which increases in intensity as the patient stands.

1.56

Answer H: Coarctation of the aorta

This child has features consistent with coarctation of the aorta. It is important to maintain a high index of suspicion to make this diagnosis. Blood pressure and palpation of pulses should be a routine part of any child's cardiovascular examination. ECG changes can be absent or can include LV hypertrophy with increased S waves in V5 and V6. Chest radiograph may be normal or may reveal cardiomegaly and an inverted '3' sign on a highly penetrated film; in addition rib notching may be seen in later childhood due to the development of collateral vessels. An ejection click is heard in patients who have a bicuspid aortic valve – a common association.

Heart murmurs presenting beyond the neonatal period

- Murmurs first heard in older infants and children (compared with neonates) are more likely to be innocent in nature.
- Up to 70% of children will have a murmur at some point in childhood – more than in the neonatal period.
- Underlying cardiac pathology causing a murmur:
  - turbulent flow through a stenotic valve (aortic stenosis)
  - left-to-right shunt (VSD)
  - increased pulmonary blood flow (ASD)
  - cardiomyopathy

  - rheumatic valvular disease.
- Frequency of pathological causes for a heart murmur
  - VDS 38%
  - ASD 18%
  - pulmonary valve stenosis 13%
  - pulmonary artery stenosis 7%
  - aortic valve stenosis 4%
  - patent ductus arteriosus 4%
  - mitral valve prolapse 4%
  - others 4%.
- Innocent murmurs include:
  - carotid bruit
  - venous hum
  - a Still's murmur
  - pulmonary outflow murmur.
- Indications that the murmur may be pathological include:
  - symptoms of cardiac disease:
    - sweating (on feeding)
    - shortness of breath (on feeding)
    - intolerance of exercise
    - failure to thrive
    - chest pain
    - palpitations
    - cyanosis
    - orthopnoea
    - paroxysmal nocturnal dyspnoea
    - a harsh murmur is more likely to be pathological (grade 3 or above)
    - diastolic or pansystolic timing of murmur
    - a new onset of murmur in an older child
    - a family history of cardiac disease/sudden death.
- Note that a low intensity murmur with no symptoms does not necessarily mean that it is innocent (ASD, PS and small PDA).
- Clinical examination of asymptomatic children with murmurs identifies pathological from innocent murmurs, with a sensitivity of 96% and a specificity of 68% in consultant paediatricians and sensitivity of 92–96% and a specificity of 82–95% in paediatric cardiologists.
- ECG and chest radiograph are often unhelpful in distinguishing a pathological from an innocent cause for a murmur.
- Older infants and children should be referred routinely to a cardiologist if the paediatrician or parents are not confident in the diagnosis of an innocent murmur.
- If investigation is indicated echocardiography is the gold standard.

1.57–1.59 Theme: Differential diagnosis of heart failure

1.57

Answer H: Dilated cardiomyopathy

This child is presenting in heart failure having been very well until 4 weeks earlier. She had a viral illness at that time so the most likely diagnosis at presentation is dilated cardiomyopathy. Had the presentation been during a viral illness, the more likely diagnosis would have been myocarditis. The heart rate is not fast enough to be compatible with a diagnosis of SVT and therefore rate-related cardiac failure.

1.58

Answer I: Aortic stenosis

This young man has the presenting features of cardiac failure secondary to aortic stenosis. This is most commonly symptomatic in the neonatal period but can present later in life, most commonly as an incidental finding of a murmur. The classic symptoms displayed in late childhood or early adult life are the combination of chest pain, syncope and exercise intolerance. There may be a family history of other left-sided cardiac lesions. There is a marked male preponderance in aortic stenosis of 4:1 – very similar to the previous question re chest pain; not a problem but just make sure that there are no inconsistencies in your explanation.

1.59

Answer F: VSD

This baby has a presentation consistent with a moderate-sized VSD leading to symptoms as the left to right shunt becomes larger due to a fall in pulmonary vascular resistance at around 2–3 months of age.

Cardiac failure

Congestive heart failure is defined as a state in which the heart is unable to supply oxygenated blood to meet the metabolic demands of the body.

Clinical presentation

Almost universally the first clinical manifestation of heart failure is tachycardia with the exception of bradycardia-/heart block-induced failure. Signs of heart failure alter with age.

Infants

- In infants left-sided failure (pulmonary congestion) will manifest as tachypnoea, respiratory distress (recession, nasal flaring, grunting), poor feeding and diaphoresis associated with feeds.
- In infants right-sided failure (systemic congestion) will manifest as hepatosplenomegaly, and more rarely ascites or oedema.
- Faltering growth may be the primary manifestation of cardiac failure in infants and may be followed in more severe cases by renal and hepatic failure due to poor perfusion.

Older children

- Left-sided congestion may manifest as tachypnoea, respiratory distress and wheezing (cardiac asthma)
- Right-sided congestion may result in a combination of hepatosplenomegaly, JVP distension, oedema, ascites and pleural effusions.
- General symptoms may include fatigue, decreased exercise tolerance, dizziness and syncope.
- Signs may include hypotension, poor peripheral perfusion, thready pulse and, in advanced cases, end-organ damage may manifest as low urine output, hepatic failure and decreased level of consciousness

The underlying aetiology of cardiac failure

- Intrinsic cardiac problems
  –dysrhythmias, structural heart defects and myocardial dysfunction, and cardiac restriction (pericarditis, tamponade)
- Non cardiac causes:
  – preload problems: volume overload
  – afterload problems: hypertension
  – reduced oxygen-carrying capacity of the blood: anaemia
  – unsustainable increased metabolic demand: sepsis.

The aetiology can further be defined by age at presentation:

- Antenatal heart failure (ascites, intrauterine growth restriction and intrauterine death)
  – anaemia (rhesus disease, fetomaternal transfusion)
  – arrhythmias (SVT)
  – intrinsic heart muscle disease (myocarditis, cardiomyopathies)
  – structural problems (valvular regurgitation)
- Heart failure in the first week of life (usually associated with the closure of the ductus arteriosus; typically around 48 hours of age, revealing an obstructed heart):
  – hypoplastic left heart
  – critical aortic stenosis
  – critical coarctation
  – interrupted aortic arch.

Arrhythmias

- Cardiomyopathies (metabolic mechanisms)
- Heart failure in the first 3 months of life
  – left-to-right shunts – produce a gradually increasing clinical picture as the pulmonary vascular resistance falls over the first few months of life:
  – VSD
  – ASD
  – PDA

    - aortopulmonary window
    - arteriovenous malformations
    - arrhythmias
    - cardiomyopathies (consider metabolic problems).
- Heart failure from 0 years to 18 years
    - cardiomyopathies (faltering growth in infants, exercise intolerance when older)
    - myocarditis
    - arrhythmias
    - other:
        - children with congenital heart disease may present post-correction or as a primary presentation
        - anomalous coronary artery from the pulmonary artery which causes a secondary dilated cardiomyopathy, and screaming during feeding due to angina (falling pulmonary vascular resistance leads to infarction of the left ventricle)
        - drugs and toxins leading to myopathy (anthracyclines)
        - degenerative muscle disease (neurodegenerative diseases such as Friedreich ataxia, Duchenne muscular dystrophy)
        - metabolic causes of heart muscle disease:
            - mitochondrial disorders
            - storage diseases (mucopolysaccharidoses)
            - problems with lipid metabolism (primary carnitine deficiency)
            - lysosomal storage diseases
            - infection and inflammation (rheumatic fever, SBE)

CHAPTER 2

Community Paediatrics and Child Psychiatry Answers

MTF Answers

2.1 Normal social development

Answers: B D

Early social development of infants begins with smiling at approximately 6 weeks, although many children may be smiling by a month of age. Some children will show stranger awareness by as young as 5 months but it is normal at 9 months of age and at this age it would be normal for children to show signs of separation anxiety. By a year most children will be waving and at this time they will be showing interest in feeding themselves with finger food and some may be drinking from a cup. Most children will be showing some symbolic play by 24 months of age, copying activities around them but mainly playing alongside each other. By 3 years of age children will be playing with each other and may be able to turn take with simple games.

2.2 Attention deficit hyperactivity disorder

Answers: B C D E

Hyperactivity in childhood is common but is considered a disorder when it interferes with social function, learning and development. Attention deficit hyperactivity disorder is a heterogeneous syndrome characterised by inattention, overactivity and impulsiveness. It is reported to have a prevalence of 2–7% of school-age children, although fluctuations occur due to different local diagnostic criteria. It is more common in boys than girls (ratio 3:1). The core behaviours of ADHD are usually present before the age of 7. Inattention leads to brief interest in activities and problems with learning and development. Overactivity is the excess of movements with restlessness and fidgeting. Impulsiveness causes action without thinking, the child often acting dangerously and leading to frequent accidents.

Common problems associated with ADHD:

- Motor tics
- Mood swings
- Immature language
- Clumsiness

- Literacy and other learning problems
- Temper tantrums
- Aggression
- Sleep disturbances
- Non-compliant behaviour.

Treatments and interventions for ADHD are varied and provided in a variety of settings, usually within specialist CAMHS or paediatric clinics. For severe ADHD in school-age children, drug therapy should be offered as first-line treatment, according to NICE (National Institute for Health Clinical Excellence) guidelines (http://guidance.nice.org.uk/CG72/NICEGuidance), with methylphenidate being the most commonly prescribed. If seizures are exacerbated in a child or young person with epilepsy, or new seizures emerge after the introduction of methylphenidate or atomoxetine, the drug should be discontinued immediately.

2.3 Indications for referral to a child psychiatrist

Answers: A C E

- Emotional or behavioural problems unresponsive to first-line counselling
- Deliberate drug overdose or attempted suicide
- Difficult child protection cases
- Difficult diagnostic problems where there is no obvious organic cause.

Included in behavioural problems are those that are common in childhood:

- separation anxiety
- soiling
- persistent grief reactions
- grief reactions causing severe disruption to the child or family environment.

A persistent grief reaction is one that has persisted beyond the normal age range. A general rule of thumb is that it is persistent if it lasts longer in months than the child's age in years. The prevalence of psychiatric disorder in childhood depends on the age range, the population studied and the diagnostic criteria used; however, prevalence is higher in urban than in rural areas; conduct and hyperactivity disorders are more common in boys at all ages; emotional disorders show an equal sex distribution in 4–11 year olds, but are three times more common in girls between the ages of 12 and 16 years.

Conditions with increased risk of psychiatric disorders include:

- learning disability
- physical illness: strong association with epilepsy and slight increase in most other illnesses
- specific developmental delay, eg speech delay
- bullying and peer group pressure
- abuse
- low self-esteem and academic failure
- family breakdown (up to 80% incidence in children 1 year after divorce)

- maternal ill health
- paternal criminality
- alcoholism
- poverty
- death and loss, including loss of friendships
- inconsistent discipline
- family history of psychiatric disorder.

2.4 Child sexual abuse

Answers: A B D

Child sexual abuse occurs when another person who is sexually mature involves the child in any activity that the other person expects to lead to their own sexual arousal. This includes exposure, pornography, sexual acts with a child and masturbation. The prevalence suggested by a MORI poll (UK 1985) in adults asking whether they had been abused as children is approximately 10% – this is probably an underestimate; 12% of females and 8% of males reported abuse. About 60% of child sexual abuse is by an immediate family member. There is often a history of generational abuse.

Current conviction rate of abusers taken to court is 5%. The court cases are extremely distressing to the child; they may be accused of lying or feel that they have not been believed if conviction does not occur. The worry about not being believed is probably one reason for lack of disclosure in school-age children who have been sexually abused. Child sexual abusers often have a history of child sexual abuse (approximately 27% sexually abused as a child and 17% witnessed child sexual abuse) but this does not mean that all children who are abused go on to abuse.

Facts about abusers:

- 31% – fathers
- 4% – mothers
- 10% – older brothers
- 7% – baby sitters
- 17% – unrelated men (who may be part of an organised paedophile ring).

Anal fissures are common in children who are sexually abused, although they do also occur in constipation. In children who are sexually abused there is an increased incidence of anorexia, headaches, recurrent abdominal pain, encopresis, enuresis and behavioural problems. There is a higher prevalence of child sexual abuse in children with special educational needs. Reflex anal dilatation is not a normal reflex. It may occur in inflammatory bowel disease and chronic constipation, with the use of enemas and after anal stretch surgery, but it also occurs after anal penetration. The conclusion of the Cleveland Inquiry (1988) was that: 'the sign of anal dilatation is abnormal and suspicious and requires further investigation. It is not in itself evidence of anal abuse.' Strong indicators of child sexual abuse are pregnancy, sexually transmitted disease, lacerations or scars in the hymen, anal fissures and positive forensic tests (semen). Child sexual abuse is associated with physical abuse in 15% of cases.

[illegible]ical abuse in children

[illegible]

[illegible] child maltreatment in England in 2008 were reported as 26 per 10 000 children younger than 18 years (excluding unborn children) for any type of abuse, 12 per 10 000 for neglect, 3 for physical abuse, 2 for sexual abuse, 7 for emotional abuse and 2 for multiple types of abuse. It is characterised by a history inconsistent with the pattern of the injury. It is responsible for 200–300 non-accidental deaths per year in the UK. Mothers are more likely to be abusers than fathers. It can affect all children including those of higher socioeconomic groups.

Risk factors include:

- large family size
- first-born children (50%)
- low-income families
- low parental intelligence
- family history of abuse
- parental drug or alcohol misuse
- parental illness, particularly mental health problems
- pre-existing disability in the child.

The most common site of injury is the head and neck. There may be abnormal coagulation in up to 16% of children in whom abuse is suspected. Fractures are more common in pre-school-age children. Falls at home from about 1 metre result in skull fractures of non-abused children in 1%. Almost one in four of all skull fractures seen in childhood is thought to be due to abuse, increasing to one in three of complex skull fractures.

Intracranial injury is the most common cause of death in abused children, and it is estimated that 95% of serious head injuries in the first year of life are due to abuse. This is usually due to shaking injury, which can lead to intracranial bleeding and is associated with retinal haemorrhages. The shaken child may also be hit against a hard object, resulting in skull fracture and severe acceleration/deceleration injury. Rib fractures are rarely seen in non-abused children. Periosteal new bone formation is seen on a radiograph 7–10 days after the initial injury.

2.6 Schizophrenia

Answers: A C D E

Schizophrenia is characterised by particular abnormalities of thinking, perception and emotion. It is usually diagnosed between the ages of 15 and 35 years, but the onset may be in childhood: early onset <17 years, very early onset <13 years. The difficulty in diagnosing schizophrenia in childhood is that some symptoms are modified by the cognitive immaturity of the child and may not fit into the adult syndrome. Symptoms include delusions, hallucinations, formal thought disorder (a disorder in the logic of thinking) and changes in affect. Immaturity of development particularly affects the severity of illogical thinking. Children with, or who go on to develop, schizophrenia may just seem odd. The stages of schizophrenia are usually divided into an active phase where they are psychotic (lasts 1–6 months, shortened by antipsychotic drug therapy), a recovery phase where there is a degree of impairment often with depression, and a residual phase where recovery is incomplete (80%) leaving a degree of social and psychological impairment. It may progress to the chronic stage when a person may not recover from the acute stage.

Schizophrenia is uncommon in children, becoming more common after 15 years of age. Some of the difficulties in diagnosis in children may account for this. Whole life prevalence is 1%. Family history is often positive. Lifetime incidence is 8% with an affected sibling, 12% if a parent is affected, 40% if both parents affected and 55% if an identical twin has schizophrenia. The prognosis for recovery is 25–40% for adults, only a small minority recovering without further episodes. The prognosis is worse for early onset schizophrenia. The prognosis is better in females. There is a lifetime suicide risk of 15%.

2.7 Developmental regression

Answers: C D E

This question distinguishes causes of developmental regression (the loss of previously acquired developmental milestones) from the causes of developmental delay (delay in acquisition of normal milestones). It is useful to distinguish the age of onset of regression. Regression before age of 2 years occurs in:

- HIV encephalopathy
- aminoacidurias
- hypothyroidism
- lysosomal enzyme disorders, eg mucopolysaccharidoses, sphingolipidoses (such as Gaucher disease), glycoprotein degradation disorders, mucolipidoses
- mitochondrial disorders, eg Leigh encephalopathy, Menkes kinky hair syndrome
- neurocutaneous disorders, eg neurofibromatosis, tuberous sclerosis
- genetic disorders of white and grey matter
- progressive hydrocephalus.

Regression after 2 years of age occurs in subacute sclerosing panencephalitis. Late onset is seen in:

- lysosomal enzyme disorders
- mitochondrial disorders
- genetic disorders of white and grey matter.

2.8 Normal development

Answers: A C D E

Normal developmental milestones

The reader is referred to a standard textbook of development. The following are some useful milestones:

- 4–6 weeks: smiles.
- 6 weeks: prone – pelvis flat. Ventral suspension – head up to plane of body momentarily. Fixes and follows in the horizontal plane.

- 12–16 weeks: prone supports on forearms. Fixes and follows in the horizontal and vertical plane.
- 20 weeks: full head control. No head lag when pulled to sit. Reaches for objects and grabs them.
- 6 months: prone weight bears on hands. Rolls prone to supine. Transfers hand to hand, chews, feeds with a biscuit.
- 7 months: rolls supine to prone. Sits hands held forwards for support.
- 9 months: finger thumb opposition. Sitting can lean forward and recover position. Waves bye-bye. Starting to stand with support from furniture.
- 1 year: walking with one hand held. Uses two words with meaning. Mouthing stops.
- 13 months: stands alone for a moment.
- 18 months: goes up and down stairs holding rail. Can throw a ball without falling. Domestic mimicry. Feeds with spoon. Spontaneous scribble. Takes off socks and shoes. Can follow simple orders. Uses many words; jargon still present. Tower of three to four cubes. Dry in day.
- 2 years: goes up and down stairs two feet per step. Kicks ball without falling. Washes and dries hands. Tower of six to seven cubes. Puts on socks, pants and shoes. Imitates vertical stroke. Turns pages one at a time. Joins two words in sentences.
- 2.5 years: jumps with both feet. Walks on tiptoes. Pencil held in hand not in fist. Knows sex and full name. Names one colour.
- 3 years: upstairs one foot per step, downstairs two feet per step. Rides tricycle. Attends to toilet needs without help. Dresses and undresses if helped with buttons and shoes. Names two colours. Constantly asks questions. Copies a circle.
- 4 years: up- and downstairs one foot per step. Buttons clothes fully. Catches a ball. Copies a cross. Names three colours. Speech is grammatically correct and can give age. Eats with spoon and fork. Brushes teeth. Understands taking turns and sharing. Distinguishes past, present and future and right and left. Can hop for a few seconds on each foot.
- 5 years: can skip and hop. Drawing skills are improved – draws square (4.5 years) and triangle (5.5 years); can write a few letters. Names four colours. Can give home address. Distinguishes morning from afternoon. Dresses and undresses alone. Chooses own friends. Understands needs for rules in games and play.

BOF Answers

2.9 Oppositional defiant disorder

Answer E: Comorbidity with other disruptive behaviours is uncommon

This type of conduct disorder is characteristically seen in children below the age of 10 years. It is defined by the presence of markedly defiant, disobedient, provocative behaviour, and by the absence of more severe dissocial or aggressive acts that violate the law or the rights of others. The behaviour can be most evident with adults whom the child knows well or peers.

The behaviour must be repetitive and persistent and must be well outside the normal social expectations of that age child, eg toddler tantrums are normal for 2–3 year olds and would not be classed as oppositional defiant disorder.

2.10 Enuresis

Answer C: Nocturnal enuresis can be treated with antidiuretic hormone

Enuresis is defined as wetting beyond the age of 6 years. It is very common and affects at least 1 in 10 children of primary school age. It can be divided into primary enuresis, when bladder control has never been established, and secondary enuresis when continence has been established then lost. The majority of primary enuresis, particularly nocturnal enuresis >95%, is due to a delay in the maturation of the urethral sphincter. It is more common in boys and can often run in families. Secondary enuresis can be due to psychological stressful events but is more likely than primary to be due to an organic cause.

Organic causes:

- Urinary tract infection
- Congenital abnormalities, eg spina bifida, ectopic ureter
- Endocrine: diabetes mellitus and diabetes insipidus
- Pelvic masses, eg constipation, hydrocolpos.

In the case of primary nocturnal enuresis, after a careful history and examination, advice to parents needs to be clear that this is a common problem, which is likely to improve with time. Good volume of fluid intake needs to be encouraged, only restricting fluid intake in the last hour before going to bed. Caffeine drinks need to be avoided. Advice should be given on the importance of regular toileting during the day and before sleep. Reward systems can be used but should be based on agreed behaviour rather than on dry nights. Alarm treatment and antidiuretic hormone drug treatment (desmopressin) can then be used alongside these measures.

Treatment in organic causes involves treating the underlying cause.

2.11 Parental responsibility

Answer E: Parental responsibility is automatically given to the mother

All mothers, whether married or unmarried, automatically have parental responsibility for any child born to them. Having parental responsibility means assuming all the rights, duties, powers, responsibilities and authority that a parent of a child has by law. In England and Wales, if the parents of a child are married to each other at the time of the birth, or if they have jointly adopted a child, then they both have parental responsibility. An unmarried father will automatically gain parental responsibility by jointly registering the child's birth with the mother (for births registered after 1 December 2003); pre-December 2003 a father would need to re-register the birth, to add the father's details, and gain parental responsibility. Parents do not lose parental responsibility if they divorce irrespective of whom the child resides with nor do they lose parental responsibility if a child is placed in local authority care.

2.12 Constipation

Answer D: Her constipation is likely to need treatment for several months to get her stool soft and regular and allow her anal fissure to heal

Constipation in childhood is common. It is estimated that it affects 5–30% of the child population. Common times during which constipation can occur are during infant weaning, toilet training and starting school. If there are no signs of faecal impaction, admission to hospital should not be required. If a diagnosis of idiopathic constipation is made, then treatment could be started. The presence of a single anal fissure would be in keeping with a diagnosis of idiopathic constipation. Poor fluid intake can contribute as well as concerns over toileting at school. School refusal due to this is not common but can occur. Dietary and lifestyle changes should be encouraged but should not be used alone as first-line treatment. NICE clinical guidelines exist on constipation in children and young people (www.nice.org.uk/guidance/CG99).

2.13 Anorexia nervosa

Answer A: A diagnosis of anorexia nervosa is possible and she will need to be admitted to hospital for management of her acute state

A diagnosis of anorexia nervosa must be considered in this case. Although most patients with anorexia nervosa should, where possible, be treated as an outpatient, this girl is showing worrying signs of the medical problems associated with anorexia and she needs admission to stabilise her acute clinical state. At this stage she is likely to need a careful medical evaluation including electrolytes to look for any imbalances; she may need nasogastric feeding or intravenous fluids depending on her hydration status. This should all be managed in a setting that can provide the skilled implementation of re-feeding with careful physical and electrolyte monitoring (particularly in the first few days of re-feeding), in combination with psychosocial interventions.

The characteristic features of anorexia nervosa are:

- severe weight loss
- excessive exercising
- depression (in about 50%)
- self-induced vomiting
- laxative abuse
- associated distorted self-image
- morbid fear of being fat.

It is more common in pubertal girls, in whom amenorrhoea is usually present, than in prepubertal girls. The incidence is higher in pupils of fee-paying schools and children of higher socioeconomic status. It is also higher in certain populations such as ballet dancers and fashion students. Concordance is greater in monozygotic than dizygotic twins. The prevalence of anorexia is 0.5–1.0%; 1 in 10 cases are boys, and 50% make a complete recovery, 25% make a partial recovery with some residual minor eating problems and the remaining 25% persist with a chronic course of illness. The mortality rate is 5–10%.

Bulimia nervosa is characterised by binge eating followed by self-induced vomiting and laxative abuse. These individuals are not usually underweight but share the same fear as sufferers of anorexia nervosa of becoming fat. Dental caries is common, with a prevalence estimated at 1%. The severity is variable. It is more common in late adolescence and early adult life than in childhood. The prevalence in childhood is much lower.

Medical problems:

- Reduced metabolic rate with bradycardia, postural hypotension, peripheral cyanosis, cold intolerance and lethargy
- Impaired resistance to infection with bone marrow suppression which can be marked
- Amenorrhoea, hypocortisolaemia, impaired thyroid function, lanugo hair, osteopenia
- Hypoalbuminaemia, oedema, constipation
- Electrolyte abnormalities including secondary to laxative abuse, raised urea secondary to reduced fluid intake, impaired liver function
- Elevated amylase with parotid swelling or pancreatitis
- Effects of vitamin deficiency including hair loss.

2.14 Scoliosis

Answer D: Idiopathic scoliosis is more common in girls

Scoliosis is a lateral and rotational curvature of the thoracic and lumbar spine measuring >10°. Idiopathic scoliosis accounts for approximately 75% of all cases and is most common in adolescent girls, with the remaining 25% of cases occurring in patients with an acquired deformity that results from a peripheral or central neurological impairment or attributable to connective tissue and musculoskeletal disorders. Children with severe neurological impairment are at high risk for the development of scoliosis, eg 90% of boys with Duchenne muscular dystrophy (DMD) will develop scoliosis. In cerebral palsy (CP), the incidence is highest in those most severely affected, usually with quadraplegic, hemiplegic and dystonic forms of CP.

The timing and type of surgery depend on the patient's age, rate of progression, skeletal maturity, symptoms, underlying diagnosis, degree and location of curvature, and cardiopulmonary function. In idiopathic scoliosis, curves that exceed 40–50° before the onset of skeletal maturity usually require surgery to prevent progression and to diminish spinal deformity. In neuromuscular scoliosis, surgery is highly dependent on aetiology and rate of progression. For example, as scoliosis is relentlessly progressive in most cases of DMD, surgery is recommended as soon as a progression of curvature can be established, generally at 20–30°. This generally occurs within 2–5 years of wheelchair dependence, so the recognition at the early stage of curvature is important and requires careful monitoring.

2.15 Attention deficit hyperactivity disorder

Answer C: Discuss with parents the use of medication as part of a comprehensive treatment plan

Behavioural therapy can lead to improvement but it is intensive. Drug therapy is with stimulant drugs such as dexamfetamine and methylphenidate, and their use should be alongside psychological, behavioural and educational intervention. Side effects of drug therapy are common and include insomnia, suppression of appetite and depression. Rare side effects include psychosis, growth retardation, increased frequency of tics and worsening of epilepsy.

Modification of diet has been reported to improve symptoms in a number of children but behavioural modification or drug therapy or both are much more widely used.

Assessment of symptoms and effect of treatment can be aided by use of the Connor Teacher's Rating Scale questionnaire to assess activity and attention at school. The condition is said to persist into adult life in 10–20%.

Some other causes of hyperactivity in children are:

- normal variant
- understimulation/boredom
- sleep disturbance
- learning difficulties
- anxiety disorder
- autistic spectrum disorder
- temporal lobe epilepsy
- drugs, eg antiepileptic medication, sedatives.

2.16 School refusal

Answer B: Family stress may be a precipitating factor

School refusal is the reluctance or refusal to attend school due to excessive anxiety. It can lead to prolonged absence from school (weeks to months). In contrast to truancy these children remain at home during school hours and do not conceal their absence from their parents. It has two peaks of incidence at age 5–6 years and 11 years at times of school change.

Precipitating factors include

- transition from primary to secondary school
- family stress, ie illness, marital breakdown
- pressure for high academic achievement
- bullying.

Depression is present in more than 50% of children and physical symptoms are also common. The outcome is usually good with a combination of psychological and psychiatric interventions although pharmacological treatment of depression may be needed.

2.17 Childhood depression

Answer D: Drug misuse

Major depressive illness in children is uncommon (2 per 1000), but many children have depressive symptoms and the incidence of both increases during adolescence. Depression can be primary (isolated depression) or secondary (to other psychiatric disorder or physical disease):

- Primary depression is often associated with a family history of depression.
- Prepubertal boys are twice as likely to have depression as prepubertal girls. This sex incidence is reversed after puberty.
- Suicidal behaviour (parasuicide) is common in children who have depression.
- Successful suicide in childhood is extremely rare.

Symptoms characteristically include depressed mood and tearfulness, lethargy and loss of interest in usual activities, feelings of guilt and self-blame, diminished appetite and poor weight gain (but appetite can be increased), impaired sleep (but can be increased), social withdrawal, outbursts of aggression and delusional symptoms in the form of auditory hallucinations, accusing the child of worthlessness.

2.18 Squint

Answer C: There is an absolute indication for testing of visual acuity

Childhood squint (strabismus) is the misalignment of the eyes during visual fixation. It is common in childhood, affecting 4% of children aged <6 years. If left untreated it can cause secondary visual loss (amblyopia) in the affected eye, regardless of the cause.

Squint is divided into two categories:

1. Non-paralytic squint: where there is no abnormality of the extraocular muscles or nerves supplying them
2. Paralytic squint: where there is a weakness of one or more of the extraocular muscles leading to squint. This is less common and when it presents a cause must be sought.

Diagnosis:

- Corneal light reflex test: the degree of squint can be assessed using prisms in front of the eye while doing the test (Krimsky method)
- Cover testing: crucial to determine the presence and amount of ocular deviation
- Visual acuity testing: this is mandatory to assess vision in both eyes
- Eye movements.

Treatment of non-paralytic squint:

- Correction of any refractive error
- Patching to the normal eye to allow the development of vision in the affected eye
- Corrective surgery: this is largely cosmetic and involves strengthening or weakening the appropriate extraocular muscles to balance out the squint. Often a second operation is required to align the eyes fully.

2.19 Hearing assessments

Answer B: Neonatal hearing screening in the UK involves automated otoacoustic emission (AOAE)

The early detection of hearing impairment is important; the earlier hearing impairments can be detected and treated the more successful the developmental and educational outcome.

The current hearing screeing in the UK is neonatal hearing screening followed by school entry hearing test. A normal neonatal hearing screen does not exclude hearing impairment, particularly when you consider both aquired and progressive causes of hearing loss.

Assessment of deafness:

- Otoacoustic emissions: this is the acoustic response produced by the cochlea in response to sound emitted by an aural probe. There is no response if hearing loss is >30 dB. It is 100% sensitive and 80% specific for sensorineural hearing loss.
- Brainstem-evoked auditory responses: electrodes are placed over the skull and electrical activity is picked up in response to auditory stimulation. This is a useful test in babies aged <6 months especially in those at high risk of deafness (jaundice, prematurity, low birthweight). The test is not affected by sedation.
- Distraction testing is used from 6 months to 1 year of age.
- Play audiometry can be used after 18 months to 2 years of age.
- Pure-tone audiometry is used after 3.5 years of age because this is the age in which cooperation can be achieved.

2.20 Causes of hearing impairment

Answer B: Alport syndrome is associated with conductive hearing loss

Deafness is conductive, sensorineural or mixed. There are many causes of deafness and these should be learned. A number of causes are listed below:

- Congenital:
  - autosomal dominant – 33%
  - autosomal recessive – 65%
  - X-linked – 2%
- Syndromes: Alport syndrome (with renal failure), Treacher Collins syndrome, Klippel–Feil anomalies of the spine, Down syndrome, Waardenburg syndrome, Jervell–Lange–Nielsen syndrome associated with prolonged QT interval and sudden death, Pendred syndrome
- Acquired:
  - prenatal: congenital infection – rubella, cytomegalovirus; drugs such as thalidomide
  - perinatal – it is common in pre-term infants with a prevalence in very-low-birthweight infants (<1500 g) of 1%. Pre-term infants are particularly susceptible to

hypoxia, hyperbilirubinaemia, intraventricular haemorrhage and the use of drugs such as gentamicin
- older children
- otitis media
- glue ear
- meningitis.

Glue ear

This is the most common form of deafness in children. Causes include acute otitis media, allergy and malformation of the eustachian tube (associated with cleft palate). These all lead to accumulation of fluid in the middle ear which may become infected. The fluid prevents equalisation of pressures between the middle ear and the atmosphere from occurring and damps the response of the eardrum to sound. A large proportion of cases resolve spontaneously or with a trial of decongestant therapy. If not, treatment is with grommet insertion. The main indications are speech delay and severe hearing loss.

2.21 Sudden infant death syndrome

Answer B: Prematurity is a risk factor

Sudden infant death syndrome (SIDS) is the unexpected and unexplained death of an infant (on postmortem findings and on examination of the scene of death). The peak incidence is between 2 and 4 months of age, with 95% of deaths occurring before 6 months of age. The incidence has been declining since 1989, when there were 1337 deaths, to 281 deaths in 2008. The incidence started declining before the government 'Back to Sleep' campaign in 1991 which promoted sleep in the supine position, probably due to prior publicity of the need to put babies to sleep supine. The major risk factors for sudden infant death are:

- parental smoking – antenatal and postnatal
- prone sleeping position
- male sex
- maternal age (younger)
- low birthweight
- prematurity
- febrile illness
- thermal stress (high temperature, over-wrapping).

The use of apnoea monitors has not reduced the risk of SIDS. There is no proved association of SIDS with the type of mattress used although it is advised that they should be clean and dry and in good condition. Recent evidence has suggested that settling a baby to sleep with a dummy reduces the risk of SIDS.

2.22 Speech delay

Answer B: Speech delay is common in autism

Recognised causes of speech delay include:

- hearing defects
- learning disability due to any cause, eg congenital hypothyroidism, tuberous sclerosis, Down syndrome, fragile X syndrome, intrauterine infections and fetal alcohol syndrome
- cerebral palsy
- developmental expressive aphasia
- emotional deprivation
- autism.

The family history is usually of relevance. There is often a history of speech delay in the parents; girls tend to speak earlier than boys, first-born children tend to speak earlier than subsequent children and twins speak later than singletons. Tongue-tie, cleft palate and malocclusion may affect speech quality but do not cause speech delay.

Milestones in the development of speech:

- 3–6 months: loud tuneful vocalisations.
- 6–12 months: babbles in long repetitive syllables. Syllables 'da', 'ma' may be used from 8 months initially inappropriately but use in correct context to parents by 12–14 months.
- 1–1.5 years: starts using words in appropriate context. Understands many more words.
- 1.5–2.5 years: many intelligible words mixed with jargon. Starts asking 'why', 'where' questions by 2 years. Joins two or more words in phrases by 2 years.
- 2.5–4 years: period of rapid speech development with the acquisition of many new words. Constantly asking questions. Stops talking to him- or herself during play in favour of directing speech towards others.
- 4+ years: can narrate stories; correct grammatical usage by 4.5 years. Delay in any of these areas is a warning that there is a problem with either hearing or in speech acquisition.

2.23 Normal development

Answer B: Normal development

2.24 Normal development

Answer D: Go up stairs one foot per step

2.25 Toe walking

Answer E: It may be caused by congenital shortening of the Achilles tendon

Toe walking is common between the ages of 1 and 2 years. In most cases it is a habit and these children can stand on their heels without difficulty and ankle movements are normal. Other causes include:

- prematurity
- spastic cerebral palsy
- congenital shortening of the Achilles tendon
- Duchenne muscular dystrophy
- peroneal muscular atrophy
- infantile autism
- spinal tumour
- unilateral hip dislocation.

Often no specific treatment is required. Supportive footwear can be helpful and in some cases botulinum toxin can be useful.

2.26 Chronic fatigue syndrome

Answer C: After thorough history and examination in clinic, reassure the family and patient that there is no evidence of serious underlying pathology. Explain variable timescale and prognosis. Develop a management plan with patient and family agreement that addresses issues of concern, and arrange regular reviews of progress

Prevalence is highest in adolescents, with females outnumbering males by approximately 3:1. Children are more likely to make a full recovery than adults although a small percentage may remain incapacitated for years. The onset may be gradual or sudden, with or without a preceding acute illness. Debilitating fatigue exacerbated by activity is the most commonly reported symptom Other symptoms are malaise, headaches, sore throat, sleep disturbance, myalgia, and abdominal and joint pains. Depression, anxiety and other psychological conditions may coexist.

Diagnosis is based on the impact of the condition on a patient rather than the duration of symptoms as such. A thorough history is required to include family history and emotional dimensions of illness. Physical examination should include height, weight, head circumference, neurological assessment, lymph nodes and sinuses, lying and standing blood pressure, and heart rate. Routine investigations to be performed in all cases are as stated in the question, with others dependent on any relevant findings on history and examination but it is important not to do repeated tests. Diagnosis should be made as soon as possible and communicated to the patient and family. Other appropriate professionals should be included in management and may include CAMHS, physiotherapy, dieticians, and education and social services. Inpatient admission and medication may need to be considered in a small minority. Prolonged bed rest should be avoided. Regular review is essential to monitor progress and revise management plan as needed.

The Royal College of Paediatrics and Child Health have published extensive evidence-based guidelines in 2004 for the management of children with chronic fatigue syndrome. These are available on the College website (www.rcpch.ac.uk).

2.27 Separation anxiety disorder

Answer C: Presence of separation anxiety disorder in teenagers is most likely to present as school refusal and somatic symptoms

DSM-IV criteria state that separation anxiety consists of excessive anxiety beyond that expected for the child's developmental level, related to separation or impending separation from the primary caregiver in children aged <18 years and lasting for at least 4 weeks. It is normal until the age of approximately 3–4 years. It is more common in children who have suffered bereavement or who have over-protective parents. Incidence is approximately equal among boys and girls. The mean age of onset of separation anxiety disorder (SAD) is 7.5 years. Approximately three of four children with SAD will go on to develop school refusal, which has a mean age of onset of 10 years. SAD manifests differently at different ages. In those aged <8 years, it tends to present with unrealistic worry with regard to harm to parents and school refusal. In those aged 9–12 years, the most common complaint is of excessive distress at times of separation such as overnight school trips. Those aged 12–16 years present with school refusal and somatic problems.

SAD symptoms are frequently reinforced by family members. It is more commonly found in children where there is a family history of anxiety disorder or if there is any history of early or traumatic separation from the attachment figure (such as divorce). Cognitive–behaviour therapy and family therapy are helpful in returning the child to normal patterns of behaviour. Complications include depression and substance abuse, but in general the prognosis is good if detected and treated early.

2.28 Somatisation

Answer D: They occur more frequently in children whose parents have a physical illness

Somatoform disorders are a group of psychological disorders in which a patient experiences a physical symptom in the absence of an underlying medical condition. It is common for children to express emotional distress as physical pain and transient episodes do not affect overall functioning. However, the persistent experiences associated with a disorder will often interfere with school, home life and friendships. In contrast to factitious disorders or malingering, where symptoms are intentionally produced or feigned, in somatoform disorders intentional deception does not occur.

Headaches, stomachaches, dizziness, chest pain and nausea are the most commonly reported symptoms. Risk factors include presence of depression or anxiety disorder, female sex, family dysfunction and increasing age. It also occurs more frequently in children whose parents have non-life-threatening disease or medically unexplained symptoms. It is more likely to occur in children with a history of being abused. Exclusion of medical and neurological conditions is the major diagnostic concern, eg brain tumours and temporal lobe epilepsy, but extensive unwarranted medical investigation often only delay the diagnosis and implementation of appropriate treatment. Families may be resistant to considering a psychological cause of the child's symptoms, so careful explanation and reassurance are essential at all stages. Treatment involves ruling out concurrent physical problems and maintaining or improving the overall functioning of the patient. Mental health services are helpful in managing patients with more severe symptoms, often jointly with medical involvement.

2.29 Sleep disorders

Answer E: Night terrors are short-lived episodes occurring during the first few hours of sleep, which terminate spontaneously and of which the child has poor recollection the following day

Up to one in four children has some type of sleep problem, the most common being nightmares, sleepwalking and insomnia. Learning difficulties, ADHD, family dysfunction, depression and anxiety are commonly seen in association. Nightmares affect up to half of 3–6 year olds, being common after stressful or frightening events. They usually occur during the second half of the night and are well remembered the next day. Night terrors typically occur during the first 3 hours of sleep and are associated with autonomic arousal (tachypnoea, tachycardia). They end spontaneously and the child quickly returns to sleep with poor recall the next day. Sleepwalking is seen most commonly in the 3- to 10-year age group, and can affect up to 30% of children. There is usually no recollection the next day.

Chronic insomnia is associated with the presence of another mental disorder in 35–50% of cases. Prepubertal children with depression are most likely to experience insomnia whereas their postpubertal counterparts are more likely to complain of hypersomnia. Substance-induced sleep disorder (drugs or alcohol) should also be considered. Obstructive sleep apnoea is the most common reason for referral for sleep studies. Other reasons include suspected narcolepsy, sleep-related seizure-like activity and snoring associated with daytime somnolence. Most childhood sleep problems can be managed with behavioural techniques including emphasising the need for good sleep hygiene (eg simple, consistent bedtime routine, dark, quiet room and removal of distractions such as a television) and techniques such as controlled crying. Medications are rarely needed. Melatonin is used but is not licensed in the UK for use in children.

2.30 Developmental coordination disorder

Answer B: Make direct contact with teachers to establish level of concern before arranging a multidisciplinary assessment of child's abilities with the consent of the parents

This is also known as dyspraxia and exists in varying degrees of severity with various associated comorbidities such as learning difficulties, attention deficit and other disabilities. A problem arises due to a failure to sequence information required to perform 'complex' tasks in a coordinated fashion. The problem area may be limited to certain fine or gross motor skills, or include problems with speech and language or thought processing. The exact incidence is unknown but it is likely that 5% of children worldwide have the disorder, with up to 10% experiencing more minor forms of coordination difficulties. More boys are thought to be affected than girls. Developmental progress in early childhood may suggest the presence of the disorder but it typically comes to light during school years and the child's teacher is often the first person to raise concerns. Crucial to the diagnosis is that no underlying neurological condition exists (eg cerebral palsy or muscular dystrophy) but this can usually be excluded without the need for specialist input.

There are numerous strategies for evaluation of a child with suspected developmental coordination disorder. Much information can be gathered by observing a child performing routine daily tasks such as writing, using a knife and fork and scissors, catching and throwing a ball, and dressing, and this is often done in an environment familiar to the child such as the classroom, rather than in a clinic setting. In standardised tests, a child scoring below the 5th centile for age is thought to be indicative of a motor problem. Those involved in the assessment process, which should be multidisciplinary, may include occupational therapists and physiotherapists, speech and language therapists, educational psychologists, teachers and parents. After identification of problem areas, individual intervention programmes can be devised either to allow acquisition of skills that are absent or to provide optimal coping mechanisms for deficiencies.

2.31 Cohort studies

Answer E: Loss to follow-up

By far the biggest scientific problem in cohorts is the loss of patients over time to migration, death from other causes or loss of interest. Provided that selection is appropriate and similar in factors other than exposure, bias and confounding are less of a problem than in case–control studies. There are no interventions in cohort studies because they are observational.

2.32 Randomisation

Answer D: Reduce confounding

A randomised controlled trial (RCT) is essentially an experimental situation where the investigators manipulate the participants' exposure. Randomisation, if done properly, ensures an equal mix of potential confounders between groups, thereby eliminating their effect

EMQ Answers

2.33–2.35 Theme: Psychiatric disorders

2.33

Answer E: Autism

Autism usually presents before 3 years of age and is characterised by speech delay, absence of pretend play, stereotyped repetitive behaviour, lack of social interest and poor social interactions with parents and other children. The disorder is a spectrum and often called autistic spectrum disorder. The incidence is 2–13 per 10 000. Boys are more commonly affected than girls by 3:1. There is a genetic association, with 3% of siblings being affected. One in five cases is associated with a medical condition, fragile X syndrome and tuberous sclerosis being the most common. Learning difficulties are common; 70% have an IQ <70. The more severe the learning difficulties the more likely the child will have epilepsy in adolescence (20–30%). There is no association with social class or poor parenting. Of children with autism, 50% gain useful language by 5 years of age but there is odd use of language with delayed echolalia and stereotyped phraseology. Useful acquisition of language by the age of 5 years is a good prognostic indicator for function in adult life. Two-thirds of autistic children grow up to be adults with severe learning difficulties who are unable to look after themselves.

Asperger syndrome

This is probably part of the autistic spectrum but a milder form with relatively normal IQ and language development. The prevalence is around 10–25 per 10 000. It is more common in boys. Recognised personality traits include abnormalities of gaze, poverty of expression and gesture, unusual and narrow focus of intellectual interests and a lack of feeling for others. Most people with Asperger syndrome are also clumsy.

2.34

Answer B: Gilles de la Tourette syndrome

Gilles de la Tourette syndrome is a neurological condition in which the patient has tics, and involuntary and uncontrollable sounds and movements. Tics themselves are common in childhood; in Tourette syndrome they occur multiple times a day and must be present for at least a year. There is often a family history of the condition. Tics can be simple such as blinking or more complex such as touching items. Tics are often made worse by stress and anxiety; they can often be suppressed for a time but will then come out in a flurry.

Over 85% of patients with Gilles de la Tourette syndrome have other associated comorbidities. In childhood these can have further impact on education and learning.

Comorbidities:

- Obsessive–compulsive symptoms
- Learning difficulties
- Attention deficit hyperactivity disorder
- Social difficulties.

2.35

Answer D: Conduct disorders

Conduct disorders overlap with Oppositional Defiant disorders but conduct disorder requires the violation of others' basic right or breaking of the law.

To meet the definitions of conduct disorders in DSM-IV and ICD-10, at least three behavioural criteria (including aggression to people and/or animals, destruction of property, deceitfulness, theft and serious violation of rules) must have been exhibited in the preceding 12 months, with at least one criterion present in the last 6 months.

2.36–2.38 Theme: Allied professionals

2.36

Answer B: Occupational therapist

Occupational therapists assess and mange fine motor difficulties, in particular they pay attention to the activities of daily living and provide aids for children with special needs to allow them to function as independently as possible. They provide advice to parents on such aspects as seating and which toys may be most appropriate. As with all allied professionals they work best within a multidisciplinary team.

2.37

Answer D: Health visitor

A health visitor is a qualified and registered nurse or midwife who has undertaken further (post registration) training in order to be able to work as a member of the primary healthcare team. The role of the health visitor is about the promotion of health and wellbeing, and the prevention of illness.

They undertake a range of work including:

- Delivering child and family services from pregnancy through to 5 years of age, eg new birth visits, formal health programmes for immunisations and development
- Providing ongoing additional services for vulnerable families and children
- Contribute to the multidisplinary team for safeguarding.

2.38

Answer A: Speech and language therapist

A speech and language therapist not only assesses and manages delay or difficulties in children's speech and language, but can also provide assessment of all aspects of a child's communication including non-verbal communication. They can provide assessments on feeding and swallowing, and feeding advice. As with all allied professionals they work best within a multidisciplinary team.

2.39–2.41 Theme: Trial design

2.39

Answer A: Ecological

Ecological studies look at regional differences in possible exposure with outcomes. This is on a population not an individual basis and therefore can be used only to generate ideas.

2.40

Answer D: Nested case–control

A nested case–control study is built into a cohort and is used to selectively measure exposure retrospectively between cases and controls where the measurement is expensive. The usual design is to take samples on all participants (in this case for trace elements), store them and measure only in cases (mothers with subsequent babies with abdominal wall defects) and selected controls, thereby reducing wastage and cost.

2.41

Answer G: Retrospective cohort

Provided that data are available, a study with a long latency is best done using a retrospective cohort. Most studies using birth or exposure records take place many years before the measured outcome.

Other trial designs

Case–control

Case–control studies are used to identify factors that may contribute to a medical condition by comparing participants who have that condition (the 'cases') with participants who do not have the condition but are otherwise similar (the 'controls').

Randomised controlled trial

An RCT is a quantitative, comparative, controlled experiment in which investigators study two or more interventions in a series of individuals who receive them in random order. The RCT is one of the simplest and most powerful tools in clinical research.

2.42–2.44 Theme: Statistical methods/tests

2.42

Answer A: The t *test*

The *t* tests are used to compare two groups of approximately equal size with variables of normal distribution.

2.43

Answer D: Survival analysis

Any time to event study is best analysed by survival analysis, eg proportional hazards or a hazard ratio.

2.44

Answer C: Pearson correlation coefficient

The relation between one variable and another is best looked at by correlation. As both are near normal, in this case Pearson's.

Other statistical tests

Mann–Whitney rank sum test

This is a non-parametric statistical hypothesis test for assessing whether two independent samples of observations have equally large values.

Pearson correlation coefficient

This is used to find a correlation between at least two continuous variables. The value for a Pearson correlation coefficient can fall between 0.00 (no correlation) and 1.00 (perfect correlation). Other factors such as group size will determine if the correlation is significant.

Odds ratio

This is used to assess the risk of a particular outcome (or disease) or if a certain factor (or exposure) is present, an *odds ratio* of 1 implies that the outcome is equally likely in both groups.

2.45–2.47 Theme: Accidental injury

2.45

Answer B: House fire

2.46

Answer F: Falls

2.47

Answer H: Road traffic accidents

Accidents are the single biggest cause of death in children over the age of 1 year in the UK, and a major cause of long-term disability and ill health. More than 2 million children are taken to hospital annually after accidents, half of which occur in the home. The numbers of accidents and accidental deaths in childhood are falling but children from lower social classes remain at greatest risk. Boys are twice as likely as girls to have accidents. The majority of accidents within the home occur to preschool children.

Falls are the most common cause of non-fatal injury, more than two-thirds occurring in the under-5s and approximately 60% being male. Scalds are most often as a result of spillage of hot drinks and are more frequent than burns. House fires are the most common cause of death within the home. They may be caused by cigarettes, candles, chip pans, faulty wiring or children playing with matches or lighters. Accidental poisoning usually occurs in preschool children and is most commonly due to the ingestion of medications within the home, although most require little or no treatment. The risk of choking declines with age. Although the number of choking episodes is declining, the number of cases involving toys is increasing. Baby walkers are associated with more injuries than any other nursery equipment. At least a third of babies using baby walkers will be injured, whether as a result of a fall, burn, scald or poisoning. Road traffic accidents account for the largest number of serious injuries and fatalities – affecting both pedestrians and passengers. They constitute increasing proportions of accidental deaths as children get older. Reducing traffic speed, and use of cycle helmets and correctly fitted child restraints have all been proved to reduce the risk of death and serious injury.

2.48–2.50 Theme: Developmental problems

2.48

Answer F: Genetic studies for Wolf–Hirschhorn syndrome

The features described are typical of Wolf–Hirschhorn syndrome, which is caused by a deletion on chromosome 4p. Clinical features include developmental delay, seizures (50%), distinct facial appearance ('Greek warrior helmet' facies) and midline closure defects. It is usually diagnosed in the neonatal period due to the dysmorphic features. It is associated with intrauterine growth retardation, reduced fetal movements and microcephaly. Affected individuals typically develop ataxic gait and absence of speech, and may have associated cardiac anomalies (ASD, VSD), diaphragmatic hernia and agenesis of corpus callosum. Approximately one in three dies before the age of 2 years. If a child survives this period, slow but constant developmental progress is made.

2.49

Answer C: Blood lead level

Long-term effect of lead exposure is greatest during the first 2 or 3 years of life when the brain is developing, and because lead is absorbed from the gastrointestinal tract more effectively in children than adults. The greatest public health risk is exposure to leaded paint. Symptoms of low-level lead poisoning are non-specific and include temperamental lability, behavioural change, loss of developmental milestones and language delay. Increased exposure may cause abdominal pain and anorexia, constipation, headache, ataxia, lethargy and coma. The classic findings of lead lines on radiographs of long bones are rarely now seen so blood level estimation is the best approximation of lead exposure. Treatment involves removal of the source of lead exposure, with chelation therapy being required in only the more severe cases.

2.50

Answer D: Genetic studies for Rett syndrome

This history is a typical presentation of Rett syndrome, which is thought to affect girls only, being lethal *in utero* to affected males. Apparently normal initial development is followed by a period of stagnation and regression. The latter may occur acutely over days or insidiously over months and is characterised by loss of hand skills and oral language. Abnormal breathing patterns, seizures and gut motility problems are also features. These are usually evident by age 2–4 years. After a period of regression, children stabilise, experiencing no further cognitive decline, progressing through puberty and often surviving into adulthood. Diagnosis is made if defined diagnostic clinical criteria are met. In 1999 a genetic mutation (*MECP2*) was identified on the X-chromosome which has been found to be present in up to 80% of cases of Rett syndrome. Treatment is supportive.

CHAPTER 3

Dermatology Answers

MTF Answer

3.1 Scabies

Answers: A E

This is caused by the mite *Sarcoptes scabiei* with person-to-person spread. It is highly contagious. Papules, vesicles, pustules and nodules are the usual presenting lesions. It is intensely itchy although very young infants often do not scratch and just appear miserable with widespread eczematous erythema on the trunk. Pathognomonic burrows most commonly found in finger web spaces and on thenar and hypothenar eminences. Children much more likely to have involvement of the head and neck than adults and therefore application of the first choice scabicide, permethrin, should include the scalp, neck, face and ears in those aged under 2 years. All household members should be treated with repeat application after 1 week. Malathion can also be used but lindane is no longer used in the UK due to reports of aplastic anaemia.

Treatment failure is most commonly due to inadequate application of treatment in an individual or within a household (allowing re-infestation), or washing of hands during treatment period without re-application. Resistance to permethrin is also recognised. Treatment failure should not be presumed until 6 weeks have elapsed, because it can take this length of time for the eczematous reaction and subsequent pruritus to resolve completely.

BOF Answers

3.2 Molluscum contagiosum

Answer A: Molluscum contagiosum

Molluscum contagiosum is a common pox virus that affects mainly infants and young children. It presents as multiple, discrete, pearly pink or white papular lesions with a characteristic central dimple. It most commonly affects the trunk, face and anogenital region. The lesions are not in themselves puritic and do not usually cause irritation or pain, although they can do if they become infected. Eczema and topical steroids can exacerbate them. If not complicated, they require no treatment and will usually resolve within a year. If they are problematic due to the number or position of lesions, they can be treated with cryotherapy, curettage or benzoylperoxide as with warts. An excess of molluscum may be a sign of an underlying immune disorder and a careful history should be taken.

Papular uriticaria, scabies and eczema would all expect to cause some discomfort. Kerotosis pilari is the plugging of follicles and is most likely to affect the upper arms.

3.3 Atopic eczema

Answer D: Removing certain known food allergens from the mother's diet during pregnancy does not reduce the risk or prevent the onset of atopic eczema

It affects 10–15% of children, and up to 50% of those who also have hay fever or asthma. Boys and girls are equally affected, and it often starts in infancy. Most will improve by the teenage years but up to one in four will experience symptoms into adulthood. Typical distribution in infancy affects the scalp and face, with extensor surfaces also involved in some. Older children and adults have predominantly flexural involvement. Features include pruritus and xerosis (dry skin). Genetic and environmental factors are involved and include contact irritants (soaps, detergents, wool), aeroallergens (house-dust mite, pollen, dander), microbial agents (*Staphylococcus aureus*), food allergens (cows' milk, soya, egg) and psychological stress. Treatment consists of adequate skin hydration, avoidance of allergenic precipitants, topical corticosteroids, systemic antihistamines, antibiotic treatment of secondary infection and oral immunosuppression in extreme cases. Immunomodulating topical treatment such as tacrolimus and pimecrolimus should be considered to treat moderate or severe atopic eczema in those aged >2 years or if the maximum strength and potency of topical corticosteroid that is appropriate for the patient's age and the area being treated have been adequately tried and haven't worked, where there is serious risk of important side effects from further use of topical corticosteroids (particularly permanent damage to the skin).

Evidence for the effectiveness of preventive measures is generally applicable in high-risk families only (ie family history of atopy in parents *and* siblings). Removal of certain foods from the pregnant mother's diet can be harmful and has not been shown to reduce the risk of eczema in the unborn child. Breastfeeding is protective against the development of allergies when compared with formula feeding, but there is no evidence to support its exclusive use beyond the age of 6 months. If breastfeeding is not possible in families at high risk of atopic disease, evidence exists to support the use of hydrolysed cows' milk formulae rather than cows' or soya milk-based products. Conclusive evidence to support delaying the introduction of common food allergens when weaning is lacking, although it is frequently recommended. No benefit has been shown of the preventive effect of avoiding house-dust mite during pregnancy and after birth, although, if combined with food allergen avoidance, some protection against atopic eczema in infancy may be gained.

3.4 Capillary haemangioma

Answer E: Arrange follow-up for the child in the outpatient clinic to monitor the growth of the lesion over the coming weeks

Close follow-up would be required in this particular case to ensure that any further growth of the naevus does not impinge on the infant's visual fields given its location over the nasal bridge.

Capillary haemangiomas, known as a strawberry naevi, are the most common tumour in infancy and seen in approximately 10% of white infants. The incidence is much lower in black and Asian babies. It is more common in preterm babies and when mothers have undergone chorionic villous sampling in pregnancy. Girls are three times more commonly affected than boys. It presents at birth in 30%, and is a focal and solitary lesion in 80% – most commonly found on the head and neck (60%), followed by the trunk (25%) and extremities (15%). May appear initially as an area of blanching of skin, followed by development of fine telangiectasiae and then a red macule or papule. Colour depends on depth of lesion – red or crimson if superficial, purple/blue or flesh coloured if deep.

Proliferation of lesions occurs during first year of life, most rapidly during first few weeks and up to age of 6 months. Involution then occurs, typically from the centre. By age 5 years, 50% have completely resolved, 70% by 7 years and 90% by 9 years. Approximately 50% leave some form of permanent skin change (eg telangiectasiae, superficial dilated veins or epidermal atrophy). Treatment is required for certain lesions, ie those that impinge on vital structures (eg causing airway obstruction or impairment of visual fields), for ulcerated, bleeding or secondarily infected lesions and for those causing psychological distress often due to cosmetic disfigurement. Other indications for intervention include complications such as congestive cardiac failure (seen when multiple or visceral lesions present such as in diffuse neonatal haemangiomatosis) and in Kasabach–Merritt syndrome (consumptive coagulopathy and thrombocytopenia). Treatment options include medical therapy with systemic or intralesional steroids, subcutaneous interferon-α, or laser or excision surgery. The use of propranolol has recently been reported to be remarkably successful in the treatment of proliferating haemangiomas.

EMQ Answers

3.5–3.7 Theme: Infections

3.5

Answer A: Staphylococcus aureus

The lesions described are those of staphylococcal scalded skin syndrome, and are caused by exotoxin A and B-producing *Staphylococcus aureus* phage type 2. The toxin causes a red rash and separation of the dermis beneath granular cell layer with resulting bullae formation and sheet-like desquamation. The infecting *Staph. aureus* organism may originate from the skin, throat nose, mouth or umbilicus. There is associated general malaise, fever (not always present), irritability and skin tenderness. An erythematous rash is accentuated in flexor creases. Perioral crusting is often present. The white cell count (WCC) may be normal and blood cultures usually negative. Gram stain/culture from original infection site may confirm *Staph. aureus* infection. Frozen section of peeled skin confirms superficial site of cleavage, thus differentiating from toxic epidermal necrolysis where cleavage occurs deeper below the epidermis. Treatment involves parenteral anti-staphylococcal antibiotics, wound care, analgesia and rehydration as appropriate.

3.6

Answer G: Herpes simplex virus

Most childhood herpes simplex virus (HSV) infections outside the neonatal period are due to HSV type 1, primarily transmitted via contact with infected saliva. Herpetic gingivostomatitis is the most frequent clinical presentation of primary infection in children, usually affecting those aged 6 months to 5 years. Herpetic whitlow is seen particularly in children who suck their thumb. The incubation period for HSV ranges from 2 days to 12 days, whereas viral shedding from an infected individual may persist for up to 3 weeks. There is usually an abrupt onset of illness with high fever and listlessness. Child typically refuses to eat or drink due to markedly swollen and sometimes bleeding gums with associated drooling of saliva. Vesicular lesions may develop on the tongue, buccal mucosa, palate, lips and face.

Tender submandibular and cervical lymphadenopathy are also present. Children may require admission for intravenous fluids and analgesia. In immunocompetent children there are limited data on the therapeutic benefits of antiviral therapy with aciclovir, but it may be used in those with severe symptoms or those caught early on in the illness. Children with eczema and those who are immunocompromised are at particular risk and intravenous aciclovir has been shown to be an effective treatment of mucocutaneous HSV infection. Secondary bacterial infection may occur.

Within the neonatal period HSV infection is frequently due to vertical transmission and most infections are caused by HSV type 2. In neonates HSV disease can manifest with disseminated disease, visceral organ involvement and encephalitis, central nervous system disease with no other visceral organ involvement, but with skin lesions and disease limited to the skin, eyes and/or mouth (SEM disease). Neonates are at a much greater risk of developing neurological sequelae and antiviral therapy should be instigated in these cases, but even if antiviral treatment is instigated complications can occur.

3.7

Answer G: Herpes simplex virus

The child has a rash known as erythema multiforme, which is characterised by the target lesion but can present with a wide spectrum of severity. Erythema multiforme can be caused by an extensive array of infectious agents, drugs and other causes. HSV is thought to be the trigger for almost 100% of cases of erythema multiforme minor (see below) and is also thought to account for almost half the cases of erythema multiforme major. The precipitating HSV infection itself may be subclinical. Other causative agents include the following:

- Infective – *Mycoplasma* sp., *Staphylococcus* spp., pneumococci, Epstein–Barr virus, adenovirus, Coxsackie virus, parvovirus
- Drugs – penicillin, cephalosporins, trimethoprim, anti-tuberculous therapy, carbamazepine, sodium valproate
- Environmental – cold, sunlight, radiotherapy.

Erythema multiforme minor consists of localised skin eruption with little or no mucosal involvement whereas; in erythema multiforme major, the mucosal involvement is more extensive, with Stevens–Johnson syndrome representing the most severe form. Up to 70% of cases have mucosal involvement, primarily oral, but it can also affect eyes and genitalia. Prodromal symptoms may be mild or absent in erythema multiforme minor, with 50% of patients with erythema multiforme major having non-specific symptoms that precede the eruption by 1–14 days. Skin lesions typically start as a dull red macule or urticarial plaque, which develops a central papule or vesicle that then clears. The outer ring becomes raised and oedematous. The distribution is usually distal at first, spreading centrally and primarily affecting extensor surfaces. The palms, neck and face are frequently involved.

A punch biopsy will confirm the diagnosis but is not routinely indicated in milder cases. Treatment involves that of the underlying infective condition or withdrawal of a suspected drug. Symptomatic treatment includes oral antihistamines, analgesia and mouth/eye care for mucosal involvement. Immunosuppressive agents such as systemic corticosteroids and ciclosporin may be needed in severe cases. Erythema multiforme minor usually resolves within 2–3 weeks but episodes are frequently recurrent. Erythema multiforme major is often more protracted, lasting 3–6 weeks.

CHAPTER 4

Endocrinology and Syndromes Answers

MTF Answers

4.1 Down syndrome

Answers: A B C D E

A thorough knowledge of the genetics, clinical features, management and complications of Down syndrome and the other common chromosomal disorders is necessary for the exam and can be found in any of the larger paediatric texts. Down syndrome is associated with an increased incidence of:

- congenital heart disease (AVSD, VSD, PDA)
- oesophageal atresia
- duodenal atresia
- Hirschsprung disease
- coeliac disease
- hypothyroidism
- obstructive sleep apnoea
- pulmonary hypertension
- immunodeficiency
- cataract
- cervical instability
- leukaemia
- Alzheimer disease.

4.2 Complications of type 1 diabetes

Answers: B C D E

Complications can be acute or chronic, acute complications being hypoglycaemia, hyperglycaemia and ketoacidosis. Complications can be grouped according to systems:

- Central nervous system: diabetic coma, hypoglycaemia, mood change and irritability
- Peripheral nervous system: mononeuropathies (facial nerve the most common), peripheral neuropathy, sensory loss
- Musculoskeletal: proximal myopathy, joint contractures
- Vascular: peripheral vascular disease, ischaemic heart disease, hypertension
- Eyes: cataracts, retinopathy, acute myopia with hyperglycaemia that recovers with treatment
- Renal: urinary tract infection, nephropathy
- Skin: lipohypertrophy, lipoatrophy, skin infections, vaginal candidiasis
- Autoimmune: thyroid disease, Addison disease, coeliac disease
- Growth: pubertal delay (with poor control), excess weight gain (with poor dietary compliance), weight loss (due to poor control or inadequate intake), short stature, Mauriac syndrome
- Pregnancy: increased risk of intrauterine death, congenital anomalies, macrosomia and neonatal hypoglycaemia.

Mauriac syndrome

This is type 1 diabetes mellitus associated with dwarfism. The dwarfism is associated with a glycogen-laden enlarged liver, osteopenia, limited joint mobility, growth failure and delayed puberty. It is due to under-insulinisation.

4.3 Bone age

Answers: B D E

The bone age defines skeletal maturation and if compared with chronological age gives an idea of growth potential. A child with a delayed bone age compared with chronological age has more growth potential than a child whose bone age equals the chronological age. The bone age, chronological age and height can be used to predict final adult height using special tables (eg Bayley–Pinneau tables).

A radiograph of the left wrist is used to assess bone age. There are two systems in use:

1. Greulich and Pyle system: comparing epiphyseal centres of the left hand and wrist with those in an atlas. The knee is sometimes used in younger children.
2. TW2 system: where each epiphyseal centre is scored and the sum of the scores gives an estimate of the bone age.
   Causes of delayed bone age:

- Constitutional short stature
- Growth hormone deficiency

- Androgen deficiency
- Cortisol excess
- Turner syndrome
- Chronic disease, eg asthma, cystic fibrosis, chronic inflammatory bowel disease, coeliac disease
- Malnutrition.

Causes of advanced bone age:

- Hyperthyroidism
- Androgen excess
- Congenital adrenal hyperplasia
- Precocious puberty
- Oestrogen excess
- Cerebral gigantism – Sotos syndrome.

Familial short stature is a common cause of short stature in children. The parents' heights are usually on the lower centiles. Growth velocity is normal and bone age is equal to chronological age. Constitutional growth is slow with delayed puberty. Height velocity is normal but height, pubertal development and bone age are 2–4 years delayed. A family history is common and catch-up does occur. Growth hormone excess has no effect on bone age, but causes an increase in linear growth.

4.4 Noonan syndrome

Answers: A B D

This has an incidence of 1 in 1000–2500 live births. It occurs in both boys and girls. It is usually sporadic but occasionally familial (autosomal dominant with variable expressivity). The gene defect has been isolated on chromosome 12.

Clinical features of Noonan syndrome:

- Normal at birth
- Neonatal feeding difficulties
- Short stature and delayed puberty
- Cardiac defects (pulmonary stenosis, peripheral pulmonary artery stenosis, PDA, ASD)
- Broad or webbed neck
- Chest defect deformity (pectus carinatum or pectus excavatum)
- Cubitus valgus
- Characteristic facies (hypertelorism, anti-mongoloid slant, micrognathia, high arched palate, ptosis).

The majority of females are fertile. Direct transmission from parent to child occurs in 30–70%. In boys, cryptorchidism is often present which may lead to inadequate secondary sexual development. Bleeding problems occur in 20%. Mild-to-moderate learning disability occurs in 30%.

4.5 Gynaecomastia

Answers: A B E

Breast tissue grows whenever the ratio of oestrogens to androgens is increased relative to normal adult values. This occurs in most newborn boys due to maternal hormones. It also occurs in some boys in early puberty when there is an increase in circulating oestrogen; this occurs before the surge in masculinising hormones occurs. Differential diagnosis includes the following:

- Physiological pubertal gynaecomastia
- Familial gynaecomastia
- Klinefelter syndrome
- Hypergonadotrophic hypogonadism
- Hepatic tumours and cirrhosis
- Thyroid disease
- Starvation
- Adrenal/testicular tumours
- Drugs:
  - steroids
  - tricyclic antidepressants
  - cimetidine
  - spironolactone
  - cytotoxics
  - exogenous oestrogens.

4.6 Growth hormone

Answers: A B E

Pharmacological stimuli of growth hormone secretion:

- Insulin
- Arginine
- Glucagon
- l-Dopa
- Clonidine
- Prostaglandin E2
- Bombesin
- Galanin
- Growth hormone-releasing hormone
- Strenuous exercise.

Provocation tests of growth hormone secretion are potentially hazardous. Insulin tolerance tests are now performed only in specialist centres because of the risk of severe hypoglycaemia. Other stimuli of growth hormone secretion such as glucagon and clonidine have important side effects: glucagon causes vomiting and general fatigue and late hypoglycaemia, and clonidine causes drowsiness and hypotension.

4.7 Precocious puberty

Answers: B C D

The most common forms of sexual precocity are early breast development (thelarche) or the appearance of pubic or axillary hair (adrenarche). Isosexual (appropriate for sex) precocious puberty can be either true (central, gonadotrophin dependent) or false (gonadotrophin independent). True precocious puberty is 10 times more common in girls than in boys. It is said to have occurred if the changes of puberty occur before the age of 8 years in girls and 9 years in boys.

Central (true) precocious puberty

This is gonadotrophin dependent and occurs as a consequence of the premature activation of gonadotrophin pulsatility, which causes the onset of puberty. It is characterised by accelerated growth, advanced bone age and pubertal levels of LH (luteinising hormone), FSH (follicle-stimulating hormone) and the sex steroids oestrogen and testosterone. It is usually idiopathic in girls (80%), an underlying aetiology being much more common in boys. A CT head scan is indicated in all boys.

Causes:

- Idiopathic
- Hamartoma
- Neurofibroma
- Glioma
- Hydrocephalus
- Post-trauma
- Post-meningitis/encephalitis
- Prolonged untreated hypothyroidism.

False or gonadotrophin-independent precocious puberty is characterised by a lack of consistency between different aspects of pubertal development, eg pubic hair and acne with no testicular development. Examples include congenital adrenal hyperplasia, oestrogen-producing ovarian tumour, adrenal tumour and medication including anabolic steroids and the oral contraceptive pill.

4.8 Achondroplasia

Answers: A B C E

Achondroplasia is autosomal dominant and 80% of cases represent new mutations. The incidence is 1:20 000. Changes present at birth and include:

- **large head with short extremities**
- **frontal bossing**
- **flat nasal bridge**

- trunk and limbs are short, with major shortening proximally (humerus and femur)
- spinal stenosis
- small foramen magnum.

Diagnosis is by skeletal survey. Special growth charts have been developed. Development is initially delayed with hypotonia but, in the absence of hydrocephalus, long-term motor and mental development are normal. Complications include hydrocephalus and cervical or lumbar cord compression secondary to the small foramen magnum and narrow spinal canal. Bowing of the legs and lordosis also occur and may need orthopaedic intervention. Lifespan is normal.

BOF Answers

4.9 Addison disease

Answer B: Fatigue is a common presenting feature

Addison disease:

- Incidence 1 in 10 000
- Most common cause is autoimmune
- Familial incidence
- Female preponderance, as with many autoimmune conditions
- Autoantibodies usually present
- Associated with other autoimmune conditions including hypothyroidism, hypoparathyroidism, diabetes mellitus, cirrhosis and alopecia.

Presenting features:

- Hypoglycaemia
- Lethargy
- Muscle weakness
- Fatigue
- Gastrointestinal symptoms
- Hyperpigmentation.

Investigations:

- Hyponatraemia
- Hyperkalaemia
- Renin is elevated
- Short Synacthen test – no rise in cortisol at 60 or 120 minutes.
  Note that baseline cortisol may be normal.

Addisonian crisis:

- may be the presenting feature
- may be precipitated by intercurrent illness or stress
- includes dehydration, hypotension and collapse
- includes electrolyte disturbance as above.

Management:

- Long-term treatment with oral hydrocortisone and fludrocortisone. Hydrocortisone needs to be increased at times of stress.
- Monitoring of growth and bone age.

Management of addisonian crisis:

- Physiological (0.9%) saline with added dextrose
- Intravenous hydrocortisone.

Other causes of adrenal insufficiency:

- Adrenoleukodystrophy
- Adrenal destruction, eg birth injury, Waterhouse–Friderichsen syndrome (associated with meningococcal septicaemia), tuberculosis, tumour metastases
- Congenital adrenal hyperplasia
- Congenital adrenal hypoplasia
- Steroid usage
- Steroid withdrawal

4.10 Homocystinuria and Marfan syndrome

Answer D: Predisposition to vascular thrombosis

Homocystinuria

The incidence of homocystinuria is 1 in 300 000. Inheritance is autosomal recessive and prenatal diagnosis is possible. It is a disorder of the conversion of methionine into cystine with a consequent accumulation of homocystine. Clinical features of homocystinuria include:

- normal at birth
- marfanoid features, tall and thin with long fingers, the lower segment of the body longer than the upper segment and an arm span greater than height
- subluxed lens – downward and inward
- stiff joints
- connective tissue weakness – hernia, scoliosis
- propensity to vascular thrombosis
- progressive learning disability (70%).

Diagnosis is based on plasma and urinary amino acids. Treatment aims to reduce the homocystine levels. Options include pyridoxine, folic acid, a low protein diet and aspirin as an anti-thrombolytic.

Marfan syndrome

The incidence of Marfan syndrome is between 1:16 000 and 1:60 000. Inheritance is autosomal dominant, with the gene locus on chromosome 15. Clinical features of Marfan syndrome include:

- usually abnormal at birth
- long fingers, lower segment of the body longer than the upper segment, arm span greater than height
- subluxed lens – upwards and outwards, myopia, retinal detachment, glaucoma and cataract
- hyperextendable joints
- connective tissue weakness – hernia and scoliosis
- mitral and aortic valve disease including aortic root dilatation
- pneumothorax.

Diagnosis is clinical. Slit-lamp examination and echocardiography are useful. Plasma amino acids exclude homocystinuria. Cardiac problems are a significant cause of morbidity.

Ectopia lentis

This is an isolated finding of a dislocated lens usually inherited as an autosomal dominant condition.

4.11 Congenital hypothyroidism

Answer D: A high thyroid-stimulating hormone (TSH) and normal T_4 on treatment suggest poor compliance

- Incidence of 1 in 4000
- Asymptomatic until 6–12 weeks of age
- Male to female ratio is 1:2.

Symptoms and signs include:

- poor feeding
- constipation
- lethargy
- jaundice
- large tongue
- umbilical hernia
- hoarse cry.

Without treatment myxoedema (soft-tissue accumulation) and failure to thrive will occur and cretinoid facies will develop. Neonatal screening is done with the Guthrie card test for phenylketonuria at 7–10 days. Usually T_4 (thyroxine) will be low and TSH raised although in 10% the T_4 will be normal. Neonatal screening will not usually detect hypothyroidism due to TSH deficiency.

Congenital hypothyroidism is usually due to thyroid dysgenesis, sometimes with ectopic thyroid tissue being present. Less commonly it occurs secondary to an inborn error of hormone synthesis (dyshormonogenesis). Treatment is lifelong with thyroxine. The best method of monitoring is by assessment of growth and development. A normal T_4 should be aimed for, but the TSH does not necessarily have to be normal. A high TSH and a normal T_4 may indicate poor compliance. Outcome is near normal (but not normal) development provided that treatment is started early. Large cohort studies show a 5- to 10-point difference in IQ compared with a control population. The TSH at presentation is of prognostic importance, with the higher levels being of greater concern.

4.12 Klinefelter syndrome

Answer B: There is increased risk of leukaemia

- Incidence of 1 in 1000 males
- Karyotype is 47 XXY.

The aetiology is meiotic non-dysjunction with the extra X-chromosome coming from the father in 50% and the mother in the other 50%. Increased maternal age is a risk factor.

There are a number of variants with more than two X-chromosomes and mosaicism is common. Children are usually asymptomatic until the age of 5 years.

After that they can present with behavioural problems or psychiatric disturbances. Intelligence is below average. The children are usually tall and thin.

Puberty is delayed and infertility is common, d e to azoospermia. The testes and phallus are small. Gynaecomastia is common (80%). There 's an increased risk of pulmonary disease, varicose veins, breast cancer, leukaemia and mediastinal germ-cell tumours. The prepubertal hormone profile is normal. By midpuberty the FSH and LH levels are raised and the testosterone is low, and testosterone replacement is required. Elevated levels of estradiol with a high estradiol:testosterone ratio acco nt for the development of gynaecomastia during puberty.

4.13 Turner syndrome

Answer A: Fetal loss in the first trimester is common

The incidence is 1 in 1500–2500 live born girls. The karyotype is 45 XO, 45 XO/46 XX. Mosaicism is present within most cell lines, and the paternal sex chromosome is lost. Loss of the maternal sex chromosome is a lethal deletion. There is no effect of increasing maternal age on incidence. Spontaneous fetal loss is common, usually in the first trimester.

Clinical features of Turner syndrome include the following:

- Infants are usually small for dates
- Lymphoedema and feeding difficulties in the neonatal period
- Neck webbing
- Cubitus valgus
- Cardiac abnormalities: coarctation of the aorta, bicuspid aortic valve, aortic stenosis
- Renal abnormalities: pelvic kidney, single kidney, pelvic–ureteric junction obstruction

- Growth failure
- Failure of puberty (hypergonadotrophic hypogonadism)
- Pigmented naevi.

There are two options for management of growth failure:

1. Steroid treatment: oxandrolone, an anabolic steroid with minimal androgenic side effects, if used in low dose, will increase final adult height.
2. Growth hormone: recombinant growth hormone is given as injections and increases final height (6–8 cm). Higher doses are needed than in growth hormone deficiency.

Management of pubertal failure

In 20% of cases of Turner syndrome there is some ovarian function and development of some signs of puberty. Most require oestrogen replacement at 12–13 years. Once puberty is initiated, cyclical therapy with oestrogen and progesterone leads to menstrual cycles. Successful pregnancies have been described with ovum induction and in vitro fertilisation.

4.14 Type 1 diabetes

Answer E: It is associated with an increased risk of diabetes in siblings of the affected case

Type 1 diabetes occurs as the result of the destruction of pancreatic islet cells. Clinical symptoms occur when there is approximately 20% of islet cell activity remaining. Pathogenesis is thought to be autoimmune. In 80–90% of newly diagnosed patients with diabetes there are islet cell antibodies. There is an association with HLA antigens: HLA-B8, HLA-BW15, HLA-DR3 and HLA-DR4 (each of these give a two- to threefold increased risk of developing type 1 diabetes). Homozygosity to the absence of aspartic acid in the HLA-DQ β chain confers a 100-fold increased risk.

Siblings of an affected individual are at a 1–7% risk of developing type 1 diabetes (annual UK incidence 7.7/100 000). There is a seasonal variation in incidence with peaks during the autumn and winter months. There is also an increased incidence after Coxsackie virus, mumps and rubella epidemics, suggesting that an initial viral infection triggers an autoimmune response against islet cells. There is a peak incidence at age 5–7 years (when children start school and exposure to viral infection increases) and at puberty (10–14 years).

Treatment with immunosuppressive agents has been found to lengthen the honeymoon period. The risks of treatment are greater than the benefits of starting insulin later.

4.15 Aldosterone

Answer A: Secretion is stimulated by a fall in serum sodium

Aldosterone is produced in the zona glomerulosa of the adrenal cortex. Secretion is regulated by activation of the renin–angiotensin system. Renin production occurs in the juxtaglomerular apparatus in response to a drop in serum sodium or a fall in blood pressure. The effect of aldosterone is on the Na^+/K^+ exchange pump in the distal tubules of the kidney. It acts to increase absorption of sodium from the distal tubule in exchange for potassium or hydrogen ions. Increased sodium absorption increases water absorption and blood pressure. Hypoaldosteronism results in a low serum sodium and a high serum potassium with a low aldosterone and high renin. Deficiency of aldosterone occurs in adrenal hypoplasia, inborn errors of steroidogenesis, Addison disease, adrenoleukodystrophy, exogenous steroid withdrawal, destruction of adrenal gland (eg haemorrhage, tuberculosis) or drugs that cause increased steroid metabolism (eg rifampicin, ketoconazole, phenytoin, phenobarbital). Pseudohypoaldosteronism is due to end-organ resistance to aldosterone. It results in hyponatraemia, hyperkalaemia with a raised renin and aldosterone.

4.16 Graves disease

Answer D: Association with HLA-DR3

Graves disease is thyrotoxicosis associated with eye manifestations. Five per cent of cases present in childhood, the peak incidence being during adolescence. There is a female predominance (5:1), and a family history is common. There is an association with HLA-B8 and HLA-DR3.

Clinical features of Graves disease:

- Emotional disturbance
- Irritability
- Poor attention span
- Tremor
- Tachycardia
- Increased appetite
- Weight loss
- Diarrhoea
- Goitre
- Exophthalmus and ophthalmoplegia
- Lid lag
- Cardiac involvement (rare in childhood).

T_3 (triiodothyronine) and T_4 are elevated, TSH is low. TSH receptor-stimulating antibodies are usually present at diagnosis and disappear as the condition remits. Approximately half the childhood cases will remit spontaneously within 2–4 years. Many will progress to become clinically hypothyroid. Medical treatment is with carbimazole and propranolol (the latter to control acute symptoms). Block replacement means that both carbimazole and T_4 are used. Definitive treatment (favoured by many) is either by subtotal thyroidectomy or the use of radioactive iodine. Severe eye disease may require treatment with prednisolone.

Neonatal thyrotoxicosis is a transient condition resulting from the placental transfer of thyroid-stimulating antibodies from a thyrotoxic mother.

Other diseases associated with HLA-B8/DR3:

- Addison disease
- Type 1 diabetes

- Coeliac disease
- Chronic active hepatitis
- Systemic lupus erythematosus
- Dermatomyositis
- Autoimmune thyroiditis
- Primary sclerosing cholangitis.

4.17 Puberty

Answer B: Normal puberty

In the 3 years before puberty low levels of pulsatile LH become detectable during sleep. LH and FSH are produced in the anterior pituitary and released due to pulsatile gonadotrophin-releasing hormone (GnRH) secreted by the hypothalamus. There is an increase in the amplitude and frequency of LH secretion as puberty approaches, which causes enlargement of the gonads. In boys, the testicles produce testosterone and in girls the ovaries produce estradiol and ovarian androgens, which, with the adrenal androgens, produce secondary sexual characteristics.

Average age at onset of puberty is 11 years in girls/11.5 years in boys. In girls, the first sign is breast bud development, followed by the appearance of pubic hair 6–12 months later. Menarche usually occurs 2–2.5 years after breast bud development. Peak height velocity in girls occurs at breast stage 2–3 and virtually always precedes menarche. Onset of puberty in boys is at 11.5 years. The first sign is testicular enlargement (>3 ml) and thinning of the scrotum. This is followed by pigmentation of the scrotum and growth of the penis, and pubic hair follows. Peak height velocity (growth spurt) is 2 years later in boys than in girls and occurs at testicular stage 4–5 (ie testicular volume 10–12 ml), which is around 13–14 years of age. Breast enlargement occurs in 40–60% of boys (significant enough to cause social embarrassment in 10%) and is a result of estradiol produced by the metabolism of testosterone. It usually resolves within 3 years. During puberty, elongation of the eye often occurs, causing short-sightedness.

4.18 Congenital adrenal hyperplasia

Answer E: It can present as premature isosexual development in boys

The incidence of congenital adrenal hyperplasia is 1 in 5000. Inheritance is autosomal recessive. The gene defect is known and is part of the human leukocyte antigen (HLA) complex on chromosome 6. Antenatal diagnosis is possible by either chorionic villous sampling or amniocentesis. Ninety-five per cent of defects are due to 21-hydroxylase deficiency, 75% of which are salt losers. 11β-Hydroxylase deficiency is the second most common type and associated with hypertension after the first few years.

Presentation can be in any of the following ways:

- Salt-losing crises
- Premature isosexual development (boys – small testes, large penis and scrotum)
- Virilisation in girls

- Hypertension (11β-hydroxylase deficiency).

Characteristic features of a salt-losing crisis include a low plasma sodium and chloride and a raised potassium, with an elevated plasma renin and low plasma aldosterone.

Diagnosis:

- Raised plasma 17-hydroxyprogesterone and raised urinary pregnanetriol (21-hydroxylase deficiency)
- Raised plasma 11-deoxycortisol and 11-deoxycorticosterone (11β-hydroxylase deficiency).

Treatment is by steroid replacement therapy. Hydrocortisone is used to replace corticosteroid activity, and fludrocortisone to replace mineralocorticoid activity. Monitoring of treatment is controversial and includes:

- measurement of growth
- bone age
- blood pressure
- plasma electrolytes
- steroid biochemistry (plasma 17-hydroxyprogesterone profiles in 21-hydroxylase deficiency).

4.19 Fragile X syndrome

Answer A: It occurs as a consequence of allelic expansion

Fragile X syndrome is a common disorder among people with significant learning difficulties. The fragile site is on the long arm of chromosome X at Xq27.3. Inheritance is X linked, but expression is due to the process of allelic expansion. The fragile X locus normally has 2800 trinucleotide base repeats; a small increase in the repeats makes it unstable and through successive generations there is an expansion in the repeats (female transmission increases the repeats) until the increase becomes clinically significant resulting in the fragile X syndrome.

Clinical features include:

- learning difficulties (IQ 30–55 in boys, milder in girls)
- prominent jaw
- long face
- large ears
- macro-orchidism
- hypotonia
- joint laxity.

The testicular enlargement is more prominent post-puberty. Psychological features include cluttering of speech, hyperactivity, emotional instability and autistic features.

Other disorders associated with allelic expansion include:

- Huntington disease (male transmission increases the repeat)
- Myotonic dystrophy (maternal transmission increases the repeat).

Allelic expansion accounts for the phenomenon genetic *anticipation*, in which there is earlier onset and/or increasing severity of disease as the expanding gene is transmitted from generation to generation.

4.20 Growth hormone deficiency

Answer B: Treatment with growth hormone can improve final height

The incidence of growth hormone deficiency is 1 in 4000. The male:female ratio is 2:1 and most cases are idiopathic.

Causes of growth hormone deficiency:

- Genetic: primary defect in growth hormone production
- Congenital abnormality: associated with midline defects, eg septo-optic dysplasia, cleft lip and palate
- Acquired: perinatal/postnatal infections, central nervous system infection, radiotherapy
- Neoplasia: craniopharyngioma, glioma
- Trauma: perinatal, basal skull fracture
- Autoimmune.

Treatment of growth hormone deficiency is with growth hormone replacement therapy by injection. Growth hormone will increase the final adult height in children with proved growth hormone deficiency.

The 2011 guidelines of the National Institute for Health and Clinical Excellence (NICE) state that somatropin (recombinant human growth hormone) is recommended as a treatment option for children with growth failure associated with any of the following conditions:

- Growth hormone deficiency
- Turner syndrome
- Prader–Willi syndrome
- Chronic renal insufficiency
- Born small for gestational age with subsequent growth failure at 4 years of age or later
- Short stature homeobox-containing gene (*SHOX*) deficiency: *SHOX* is located on the distal ends of X and Y chromosomes and plays a role in long bone growth. Normal growth requires two functional copies of the gene.

4.21 Galactosaemia

Answer C: It can lead to delayed puberty

Galactosaemia is a rare autosomal recessive disorder. The incidence is around 1 in 50 000 live births.

Three separate defects have been described:

1. Galactokinase deficiency which causes cataracts only.

2. Mild galactose-1-phosphate uridyltransferase deficiency (Duarte variant) in which there are no symptoms, but erythrocyte galactose-1-phosphate uridyltransferase activity is reduced.
3. Severe galactose-1-phosphate uridyltransferase deficiency: widespread, generalised disorder that produces learning difficulties, failure to thrive, cataracts, jaundice, hypoglycaemia and hepatomegaly. There is a rapid progression to irreversible severe learning disability and cirrhosis in undiagnosed patients.

Severe galactose-1-phosphate uridyltransferase is the most common presentation, usually presenting in the neonatal period. Reducing substances are present in the urine after the first feed. This is detectable on testing with Clinitest tablets. Urine dipstick for glucose is negative. Diagnosis is confirmed by measuring the enzymes. Treatment is with a lactose-free diet, but the outcome is variable. Some degree of learning difficulties is usual. A number have severe learning difficulties. In addition to these learning difficulties, galactosaemia can affect the ovaries. Girls can have delayed puberty due to their ovaries not producing enough oestrogen.

4.22 Insulin pumps

Answer D: They can be useful in infants where small alterations in insulin is difficult with standard insulin pens

Insulin pumps provide continuous subcutaneous insulin infusion. Their use has increased as the size, price and reliability of the pumps have improved.

These pumps are a complex technical medical device and their use requires a patient/parent to have in-depth understanding not only of how the pump functions but also of the diabetes and this requires extensive education.

The use of an insulin pump along with the intensive intervention and education can lead to improved overall control but, as the insulin is being continuously infused, any interruption in the delivery of this infusion will mean a immediate cessation of insulin delivery which can lead to metabolic decompensation more quickly. Therefore more frequent blood sugar monitoring is required.

The delivery of insulin in young children can be quite problematic as such small amounts may be needed and alterations in dose on standard pens or syringes can be difficult, so with motivated parents insulin pumps can be useful.

4.23 Rickets

Answer E: Vitamin D deficiency is the most common cause

Rickets is a disorder of decreased endochondral calcification at the growth plates leading to deformities.

Vitamin D deficiency is the most common cause of nutritional rickets worldwide and, although rare in the developed world, it is thought to be increasing in prevalence due to children's inadequate exposure to sunlight. A combination of calcium deficiency and vitamin D deficiency leading to rickets can be a particular problem in those infants exclusively breastfed.

Both vitamin D deficiency and calcium deficiency can lead to a reduced plasma level of calcium leading to secondary hyperparathyroidism, which results in excessive bone resorption and decreased bone mass.

Clinical features:

- Growth delay
- Bone pain
- Fractures
- Skeletal abnormalities: wrist swelling, bowing of long bones, craniotabes.

4.24 Hypercalaemia

Answer B: Hyperparathyroidism

Causes of hypercalcaemia include the following:

- Hyperparathyroidism
- High bone turnover states:
  - hyperthyroidism
  - malignancy
  - vitamin A intoxication
- Thiazide diuretics
- Vitamin D intoxication
- Idiopathic hypercalcaemia of infancy
- Renal failure

Signs and symptoms of. hypercalcaemia may be related to the underlying cause. Hypercalcaemia can present with the following:

- Polyuria
- Polydipsia
- Muscle weakness
- Constipation and abdominal pain
- Fatigue and lethargy
- Cardiac arrhythmias.

4.25 Ambiguous genitalia

Answer D: Inform the parents that a number of investigations will need to be performed and that they will need to wait before a sex is assigned

Ambiguous genitalia in a newborn infant is a relative emergency; it is important that the baby and the parents are seen by the most appropriate members of the team as quickly as possible. The priorities are the sex assignment followed by the sex of rearing and identifying life-threatening disorders.

Although there is great psychological impacts for parents when they can't tell family and friends whether they have had a boy or a girl, this should not encourage junior staff to 'guess' what sex the child may be. These patients need a multidisciplinary approach with endocrinologists, geneticists, surgeons and psychologists.

Causes of ambiguous genitalia

- Masculinised female:
  - congenital adrenal hyperplasia
  - maternal ovarian tumours, ie maternal androgens
- Under-masculinised males:
  - androgen insensitivity syndrome
  - androgen biosynthesis defect
  - gonadal dysgenesis.

4.26 Osteogenesis imperfecta

Answer D: Compression vertebral body fractures can be seen

Osteogenesis imperfecta is a congenital disease of bone formation, which affects approximately 1 in 10 000 people. It leads to a disorganised bone structure, making the bones fragile with a low bone mass, hence the term 'brittle bone disease'. There are several different types, which are distinguished by clinical findings, radiological findings and bone histology. They vary widely in severity from those that are perinatally lethal (type II) to those that are quite mild, and may be picked up during childhood with increased fractures or with scoliosis due to vertebral fractures. Type III is the most severe form compatible with survival past the perinatal period. Mutations in the gene for collagen type I α chains are seen in the most common types; these are mainly autosomal dominant, although new mutations are common. Blood tests usually show no specific abnormalities. As well as the skeletal changes it is also has extraskeletal features:

- Blue/grey scelera, although blue sclera can be found in healthy babies
- Dentinogenesis imperfecta: discoloured teeth that break easily
- Ligamental laxity
- Increased skin laxity
- Hearing impairment.

Management of osteogenesis imperfecta (OI), particularly the more severe forms, requires a multidisplinary approach including physiotherapist, occupational therapist and the medical team. Cyclical bisphosphonate infusions (inhibiting osteoclast function) have been used for the last decade for severe-to-moderate forms of OI in children and adolescents to effectively treat symptoms although the length of treatment and the use in milder forms continues to be researched.

4.27 Phenylketonuria

Answer D: Seizures can occur

The metabolic block in phenylketonuria is the conversion of phenylalanine to tyrosine due to a deficiency of phenylalanine hydroxylase. Incidence is around 1 in 5000. Inheritance is autosomal recessive and carrier detection and prenatal diagnosis are possible. Affected infants are normal at birth.

Clinical features in the untreated patient:

- Low IQ
- Poor head growth
- Seizures
- Fair skin 'dilute pigmentation' – due to inadequate melanisation
- Eczema-like rash.

Diagnosis is by measuring the plasma phenylalanine, which will be raised. The urine has a mousy, pungent odour due to the presence of phenylacetic acid, a metabolite of phenylalanine. Screening is carried out on all babies born in the UK by the Guthrie card. A drop of blood is collected on the card, and the blood is then used to measure the whole blood phenylalanine by a bacterial inhibition assay. This is done at age 4–5 days, ideally after a feed. Treatment is with a diet that is selectively low in phenylalanine. The diet needs to be lifelong, particularly during pregnancy when untreated or partially treated phenylketonuria is teratogenic to the unborn child. The teratogenicity manifests as severe learning difficulties with microcephaly.

4.28 Type 2 diabetes

Answer C: It is seen in association with acanthosis nigricans

Type 2 diabetes in childhood has become an increasingly recognised problem over recent years. Predisposing factors include ethnicity (highest incidence in Asian and African–American racial groups), obesity, a positive family history of type 2 diabetes and female sex. Intrauterine growth retardation is also known to be a risk factor. Insulin resistance and impaired glucose tolerance are seen. Presentation is rarely acute, with children often having no or mild symptoms only for a considerable length of time before diagnosis, although ketoacidosis can occur. Acanthosis nigricans is a marker of high insulin levels and thus helps to differentiate type 2 from type 1 diabetes in affected individuals.

Treatment is aimed at achieving good glycaemic control (to minimise risk of micro- and macrovascular complications) and maintenance of a reasonable weight. There appears to be a greater risk of nephropathy than retinopathy. Dietary adjustments and oral hypoglycaemic agents (eg metformin) can be used, but, in some cases, insulin may be required. The role of prevention is likely to assume greater significance.

4.29 Hypoglycaemia

Answer C: The best time to take blood and urine samples is after the correction of a hypoglycaemic episode

Causes of hypoglycaemia:

- Excessive glucose utilisation
- Hyperinsulinism (eg type 1 diabetes mellitus, insulin-producing tumour)

- Defects in alternative fuel production (eg medium chain acyl-CoA dehydrogenase deficiency [MCAD])
- Sepsis
- Glucose underproduction
- Inadequate stores (eg preterm, small for gestational age [SGA])
- Abnormal hepatic glucose production (eg glycogen storage disease type I, galactosaemia, maple syrup urine disease)
- Hormonal abnormalities (eg panhypopituitarism, growth hormone and cortisol deficiency)
- toxins (eg ethanol and propranolol).

Usual definition of hypoglycaemia is a blood sugar of <2.6 mmol/l. To aid diagnosis of possible underlying metabolic abnormality it is critical that samples (blood and urine) are taken at the time of hypoglycaemia. As hypoglycaemia can be asymptomatic, 'at-risk' babies such as SGA, premature and infants of mothers with diabetes should have frequent screening for hypoglycaemia for at least the first 24 hours of life. Treatment consists of an intravenous bolus of 10% dextrose (2.5 ml/kg), followed by an intravenous infusion to match normal hepatic glucose production (typically 5–8 mg/kg per min in an otherwise normal neonate). Intramuscular glucagon is the treatment of choice within the home setting only. It is known that even asymptomatic hypoglycaemia in the neonatal period can have long-term consequences in the form of neurocognitive impairment and abnormalities apparent on neuroimaging.

4.30 McClune–Albright syndrome

Answer A: Precocious puberty caused by this condition is more commonly seen in girls than boys

Diagnosis of McCune–Albright syndrome requires at least two features of the triad of polyostotic fibrous dysplasia, café-au-lait pigmentation and autonomous endocrine hyperfunction to be present. The most common endocrine abnormality is gonadotrophin-independent precocious puberty (ie autonomous ovarian or testicular function). It is far more common in girls than boys, with breast development and vaginal bleeding being seen in some cases before a year of age. Hyperthyroidism, hypercortisolism and acromegaly can also be seen.

Adrenocorticotrophic hormone (ACTH)-independent Cushing syndrome generally results in growth failure and hypertension in infancy.

Fibrous dysplasia most commonly affects the long bones, ribs and skull, and can be asymptomatic or cause pain and pathological fracture in more severe cases. A family history of café-au-lait spots raises the suspicion of neurofibromatosis (an autosomal dominant condition) whereas McCune–Albright syndrome occurs sporadically. Non-endocrine abnormalities may include hypophosphataemia, chronic liver disease, tachycardia and cardiac arrhythmia. Treatment is aimed at correcting the underlying endocrine abnormality, with specialist orthopaedic input if bony lesions are problematic. Potential complications include loss of final adult height potential (due to precocious puberty and/or hypophosphataemia), pathological fractures and sudden death.

4.31 Sexual determination

Answer C: Androgen insensitivity syndrome leads to an undermasculinised male

In normal embryological development, the presence or absence of a Y-chromosome leads to gonadal differentiation in the sixth week. The process can be disrupted by exposure to inadequate or excessive amounts of androgens (testosterone and dihydrotestosterone) and müllerian-inhibiting substance or by end-organ insensitivity to their actions. Androgen insensitivity syndrome is caused by the end-organ insensitivity and leads to an under-masculinised boy. Caution must be exercised in the presence of incompletely descended palpable gonads. Although only testicular material descends fully, ovotestes (as seen in true hermaphroditism) can sometimes be felt in labioscrotal folds. Conversely, the absence of palpable gonads in an otherwise fully virilised infant should raise the possibility of a severely virilised girl with congenital adrenal hyperplasia.

Labial adhesions are not a cause of ambiguous genitalia but can be a cause of anxiety. The appearance is usually typical, with fusion of the labial skin extending from the posterior fourchette to the urethral opening; spontaneous resolution is common.

The development of gender identity is a complex, poorly understood process, with evidence showing that it is determined not only by phenotypic appearance but by the brain's pre- and postnatal development. Parents should be given as much information as possible to enable them to make informed decisions about gender assignment and possible subsequent genital surgery.

4.32 Obesity in childhood

Answer E: It is a risk factor for subclinical coronary artery sclerosis and atherosclerosis in childhood

This is an increasing problem that is difficult to treat and has implications for both physical and psychosocial health in childhood and beyond. Most children are obese due to their lifestyle and not any underlying medical condition. There is little evidence to support the long-term effectiveness of the currently used strategies of an improved dietary intake and increased levels of physical activity. Risk factors associated with obesity are deprivation and increasing age. There is no difference in prevalence of obesity between boys and girls. Parental obesity is a risk factor for persistence of childhood obesity into adulthood. As childhood is a period of growth, body mass index (BMI) is not a static measurement but varies with age and sex. Obesity in childhood is therefore defined as a BMI >95th centile for age and sex.

Consequences of obesity include hypertension, an increased risk of developing or worsening asthma, and abnormalities of foot structure and function. In addition, adverse lipid profiles, insulin resistance and hyperinsulinaemia are also seen, leading to atherosclerosis and coronary artery disease, which are seen with greater frequency in obese children *post mortem*. Girls are more likely than boys to suffer psychological distress related to their obesity. Adults who were obese children are also more at risk of cardiovascular disease and have an increased mortality risk.

EMQ Answers

4.33–4.35 Theme: Syndromes

4.33

Answer A: Prader–Willi syndrome

The incidence of Prader–Willi Syndrome is 1 in 10 000. Occurrence is sporadic and associated with a microdeletion in the long arm of chromosome 15 (70% of cases) or maternal uniparental disomy of the same area of chromosome 15. The condition goes through three main phases: an initial infantile hypotonic phase, followed by a childhood obese phase and then an adolescent phase during which behavioural problems predominate.

Clinical features of Prader–Willi syndrome:

- Reduced fetal movements/infantile hypotonia
- Small for gestational age
- Undescended tests in male infants
- Dysmorphic features: narrow bifrontal skull, very small hands and feet in comparison to the body
- Childhood hyperphagia and obesity
- Short stature with delayed bone age
- Hypogonadism and infertility
- Learning difficulties
- Diabetes mellitus.

Life expectancy is reduced as a consequence of the obesity and associated cardiac and respiratory complications.

4.34

Answer E: Cornelia de Lange syndrome

The incidence of Cornelia de Lange syndrome is between 1:100 000 and 40:100 000. Occurrence is sporadic. Mutations can be found in the *NIPBL* gene on chromosome 5p13.

Clinical features of Cornelia de Lange syndrome:

- Small for gestational age
- Slow growth and small stature
- Facial features: arched eyebrows that meet in the middle (synophrys), long curled eye lashes, small upturned nose, small widely spaced teeth, long smooth philtrum thin upper lip
- Limb abnormalities: upper limb abnormalities more so than lower limb abnormalities, from oligodactyly to complete absence of forearms, small hands, proximally placed thumbs, fifth finger clinodactyly

- Microcephaly
- Micrognathia
- Low-set, posteriorly rotated ears
- Hirsutism
- Moderate-to-severe learning difficulties
- High and arched palate with clefts (30%)
- Hearing impairment.

4.35

Answer B: Cri-du-chat syndrome

The incidence of cri-du-chat syndrome is approximately 1:50 000. Occurrence is usually sporadic (90%) and associated with a microdeletion in the short arm of chromosome 5, although a minority (approximately 10%) of cases may result from a balanced translocation in a parent.

Clinical features of cri-du-chat syndrome:

- Small for gestational age
- High-pitched cry from hypoplastic larynx
- Slow growth and small stature
- Dysmorphic features: hypertelorism, epicanthic folds, widened nasal bridge, low set or abnormally shaped ears
- Micrognathia
- Microcephaly
- Severe learning difficulties
- Diabetes mellitus.

Life expectancy may be reduced as a consequence of severe learning disability and potential associated complications.

4.36–4.38 Theme: Diabetes mellitus

4.36

Answer B: Cerebral oedema

Cerebral oedema accounts for approximately 75% of all deaths associated with diabetic ketoacidosis (DKA). It typically occurs 4–12 hours after the start of treatment but can occur at any time. Symptoms can often be vague and variable and DKA requires a high index of suspicion. The pathophysiology is still poorly understood.

Symptoms:

- Headache
- Reducing level of consciousness
- Rising blood pressure

- Inappropriately falling heart rate
- Abnormal posturing.

Risk factors for cerebral oedema:

- Severe DKA
- New-onset type 1 diabetes
- Younger age
- Longer duration of symptoms
- Rapid correction of hyperglycaemia.

4.37

Answer F: Microalbuminuria

Microalbuminuria is defined as >30 mg/day of albumin in the urine. It is the earliest stage of diabetic nephropathy and if sustained is highly predictive of overt nephropathy, although it may be less predictive during the first decade of diabetes or during adolescence. It is rare before puberty and can be transient or intermittent,

Overt albuminuria is accompanied by systemic hypertension and leads to the development of end-stage renal failure by 10 years. This can be delayed by improving glycaemic control, treatment of hypertension and the use of ACE (angiotensin-converting enzyme) inhibitors.

Screening is recommended from the age of 12 years. Annual screening is of urine albumin:creatinine ratio to detect microalbuminuria.

4.38

Answer G: Coeliac disease

Although eating disorders are increased in the diabetic population, and need to be considered particularly in the adolescent population, other causes of weight loss also need to be considered.

Coeliac disease has a prevalence rate of 5–10% in the diabetic population and can present atypically or be asymptomatic at presentation. Antibody screening should be carried out on an annual basis.

4.39–4.41 Theme: Causes of hypoglycaemia

4.39

Answer H: Insulinoma

An insulinoma is an insulin-secreting tumour of the pancreas. The majority (>90%) are benign and usually solitary. They are rare in childhood but are part of the multiple endocrine neoplasias (MEN).

Multiple endocrine neoplasias include:

- Multiple endocrine neoplasia type 1: commonly affects the parathyroid, pancreas and pituitary

- Multiple endocrine neoplasia type 2: MEN2 syndromes are caused by mutations in a proto-oncogene *RET*, causing multiple tumours to occur in the same person. Medullary thyroid cancer is the common to the three MEN2 syndromes.
- Multiple endocrine neoplasia type 2A: medullary thyroid cancer, phaeochromocytoma, parathyroid adenomas
- Multiple endocrine neoplasia type 2B: medullary thyroid cancer, phaeochromocytoma, ganglioneuromatosis, marfanoid habitus
- Familial medullary thyroid cancer.

4.40

Answer B: Glycogen storage disease

Glycogen storage diseases are a collection of conditions in which the principal defect is the body's inability to mobilise glucose from glycogen due to an enzyme defect, leading to an accumulation affecting mainly the liver and/or muscle. There are nine numbered types including some subtypes, some named by the enzyme that is faulty.

This presentation would be most in keeping with type 1 – Von Gierke disease – which is caused by glucose-6-phophatase deficiency.

Clinical features of glycogen storage disease type 1:

- Sweating
- Irritability
- Poor growth
- Hepatomegaly
- Muscle weakness
- Mouth ulcers
- Increased infection risk.

These children often present in early infancy and require continuous overnight feeds. In later childhood treatment with cornstarch can be effective. If prolonged hypoglycaemia can be avoided most children do well with symptoms and management becoming easier in adulthood. The prognosis of glycogen storage disease ranges from a more mild type such as this to others that are lethal in early infancy.

4.41

Answer E: Medium chain acyl-CoA dehydrogenase deficiency

MCAD is the most common fatty acid oxidation disorder. It is an autosomal recessive disorder, a defect in the *ACADM* gene on 1p31, which leads to MCAD deficiency. MCAD is one of the enzymes involved in mitochondrial fatty acid β oxidation, which fuels hepatic ketogenesis. Hepatic ketogenesis is a major source of energy once hepatic glycogen stores become depleted during prolonged fasting and periods of higher energy demands, ie during intercurrent illness, fever. The most frequent presentation, within the first 2 years of life, is episodic hypoketotic hypoglycaemia provoked by fasting or an intercurrent illness. In between hypoglycaemic episodes patients are well.

The first episode can be fatal, resembling sudden infant death syndrome; to try to prevent such presentations and help diagnosis, MCAD is now part of newborn screening in the UK. Once the diagnosis is established the prognosis is excellent; frequent feeding is required particularly during infancy and any time of stress and prolonged fasting needs to be avoided (>12 hours).

4.42–4.44 Theme: Fluid balance

4.42

Answer C: Nephrotic syndrome

This child has low plasma sodium with appropriately low urinary sodium. Clinically he appears intravascularly depleted, with generalised oedema and proteinuria. The most likely diagnosis would be that of nephrotic syndrome.

Nephrotic syndrome is the combination of:

- proteinuria
- low albumin
- oedema
- hyperlipidaemia.

It has an incidence of 2–7 children per 100 000 per year and is most common between the ages of 2 and 6 years. It is twice as common in boys as in girls. The cause of the syndrome is unknown but it can be associated with certain infections, drugs, and genetic and immune disorders. A number of changes can be seen on renal biopsy, the most common being that of minimal change disease.

4.43

Answer F: Central/Cranial diabetes insipidus

Central diabetes insipidus results from ADH (antidiuretic hormone) production from the pituitary being reduced.

Causes:

- Genetic: autosomal dominant/recessive
- Congenital: midline defects
- Acquired:
  - intracranial tumours
  - traumatic head injury
  - infiltration.

Symptoms are of excessive thirst with the passage of large volumes of dilute urine. In a child such as this post head injury they may not have access to large volumes of fluid, thus leading to the complications of dehydration and electrolyte imbalance. After traumatic head injury the central diabetes insipidus can be transient or permanent.

Treatment for central diabetes insipidus is usually to relieve the symptoms of poyluria and polydipsia, because children with free access to water and an intact thirst mechanism will usually drink sufficiently to maintain a normal electrolyte balance and serum osmolality. Intranasal, oral or subcutaneous desmopressin (DDAVP) can be used.

Although most patients with central diabetes insipidus will have a normal thirst mechanism, those who have hypodipsia or adipsia pose a particular problem because the increase in urine output will not be accompanied by an increase in input. These patients need careful management usually with a fixed dose of DDAVP and a fixed daily input.

4.44

Answer A: Syndrome of inappropriate ADH

Causes of SIADH:

- Tumours, eg neuroendocrine
- Infections, eg meningitis, pneumonia, cerebral abscess
- Traumatic brain injury
- Drugs, eg vincristine
- Inflammatory, eg encephalitis.

SIADH occurs when the body fails to suppress ADH secretion despite the plasma osmolality falling the level at which ADH secretion should be suppressed. This leads to a reduced renal clearance of free water and excess total body water and hyponatraemia.

Treatment consists of identifying and treating the underlying cause, and then strictly managing fluid and carefully monitoring the patient's fluid balance; this may require a degree of fluid restriction.

4.45–4.47 Theme: Growth and development

4.45

Answer B: Turner syndrome

A karyotype is indicated in any girl with short stature even if dysmorphic features are not obviously present. Some girls with Turner syndrome may have a height within the normal range up to the age of 11 years, as is the case here. Presentation in adolescence and adulthood is often with issues about puberty and fertility as well as short stature. Adrenarche (pubic hair growth) occurs at a normal age but breast development is absent due to ovarian failure (confirmed by elevated levels of FSH and LH which excludes hypopituitarism as a cause). Thyroid function should also be checked due to increased risk of hypothyroidism, which can also affect growth. Growth hormone can be administered to increase final height, although growth hormone deficiency is not a feature of Turner syndrome. In this case, the child has an appropriate bone age excluding constitutional delay as the cause of her short stature. The parental heights and target centile range are not suggestive of familial short stature.

4.46

Answer A: Russell–Silver syndrome

The primary abnormality is growth failure, presenting with intrauterine growth retardation (IUGR) (compare with Noonan syndrome where birthweight is typically normal), feeding difficulties, failure to thrive or postnatal growth retardation. Final height is typically −3.6 SD (standard deviation) below the mean. Features described here that are consistent with the diagnosis of Russell–Silver syndrome include facial dysmorphism in the form of triangular facies, but normal head circumference, so that the head appears disproportionately large. Other features may include clinodactyly of the little finger, hypospadias or posterior urethral valves, cardiac defects (rare) and late closure of the anterior fontanelle. Approximately 10% of patients have uniparental disomy of chromosome 7, but the aetiology is not defined in most cases. Babies with feeding difficulties may require nasogastric feeds. Growth hormone treatment may be used when the child is school age but growth hormone levels are typically normal.

Infants with Williams syndrome are described as having 'elfin facies' and may also present with failure to thrive, although hypercalcaemia is typically present and cardiovascular involvement (most often supravalvular aortic stenosis) is commonly seen. Growth hormone deficiency typically presents in childhood with a reduced growth velocity rather than in infancy, unless it is associated with hypoglycaemia or other endocrine/midline abnormalities such as hypopituitarism or septo-optic dysplasia.

4.47

Answer C: Constitutional delay of growth and puberty

This is the most common cause of short stature and pubertal delay. It is more commonly seen in children whose height has been on a lower growth centile prepuberty. It is a variant of normal and not a disorder, but can cause psychological trauma for some affected individuals requiring intervention. It is approximately twice as common in boys as girls. Typically affected individuals have a normal birth weight with deceleration in both height and weight velocity in the first 3–6 months of life. Bone age is typically delayed by 2–4 years. Physical examination is normal. There is typically a family history of delayed puberty in first- or second-degree relatives of either sex.

This is a diagnosis based on the history and examination that you can make with confidence, thereby reducing the need for further investigation. Random growth hormone measurements are of little value because its release from the pituitary gland is pulsatile. IGF-1 (insulin-like growth factor 1) should be measured instead as a reflection of growth hormone production. Both growth hormone and IGF-1 results may appear decreased in the context of chronological age in the presence of delayed bone age, and they should therefore be interpreted with caution. Other routine blood tests may be performed to exclude systemic illness such as inflammatory bowel disease or autoimmune disorders. Magnetic resonance imaging (MRI) of the pituitary gland may be indicated in the presence of abnormal hormonal profiles or symptoms such as headache. No treatment is required for the majority although, in boys experiencing psychological difficulties due to their delayed development and growth, short courses of androgens can accelerate linear growth and onset of pubertal changes. This has not been shown to have a detrimental effect on adult height, but it will not increase final adult stature.

Children with Noonan syndrome do not always have any immediately obvious dysmorphic facial features but careful examination is required because the diagnosis of this condition is usually on the basis of clinical findings only. Kallmann syndrome (hypogonadotrophic hypogonadism associated with anosmia) typically presents with delayed puberty, but individuals with this condition have a normal height for age.

4.48–4.50 Theme: Hypocalcaemia

4.48

Answer B: Di George syndrome

Hypocalcaemia is a feature and may cause abnormal muscular activity. Characteristic facies include low-set ears and hypertelorism. Feeding difficulties are common, causing failure to thrive. Cardiac abnormalities may also be present.

4.49

Answer F: Pseudopseudohypoparathyroidism

Dysmorphic features described consistent with diagnosis of pseudohypoparathyroidism (see below), but normal biochemistry means the diagnosis is one of pseudopseudohypoparathyroidism.

4.50

Answer E: Chronic renal failure

Hypocalcaemia can be a feature of chronic renal failure. High serum phosphate in presence of osteopenia indicative of renal pathology (note that low serum phosphate and osteopenia suggest vitamin D deficiency or hypophosphataemic rickets). Fanconi syndrome is associated with a low serum phosphate.

Hypocalcaemia

Hypocalcaemia is frequently asymptomatic. If clinical manifestations occur, they are due to disturbance in cellular membrane potential, eg tetany and arrhythmias such as heart block. A reduction in the ionised fraction of calcium can result in symptoms in the presence of a normal total plasma calcium level, eg in severe alkalosis. Hypocalcaemia is the major stimulus for parathyroid hormone secretion.

Causes:

- Hypoparathyroidism: low calcium, high phosphate.
- Pseudohypoparathyroidism: low calcium in the presence of normal/raised parathyroid hormone levels, ie lack of normal response to parathyroid hormone. Characteristic phenotype of short stature, rounded face, obesity, shortened fourth and fifth metacarpals, developmental delay. (Note that pseudopseudohypoparathyroidism presents with above phenotype but a normal biochemical profile.)
- Vitamin D deficiency (rickets): causes increased calcium mobilisation from bone so plasma calcium levels often within reference range. Low phosphate and elevated alkaline phosphatase with classic radiological appearances of metaphyseal cupping and widening (splaying) and osteopenia.
- Di George syndrome.
- Chronic renal failure: due to both reduced production of 1,25$(OH)_2$-vitamin D_3 and hyperphosphataemia secondary to reduced renal excretion of phosphate.
- Renal tubular disease, including Fanconi syndrome.
- Magnesium depletion.
- Hypoproteinaemia.
- Septic shock.

CHAPTER 5

Gastroenterology and Nutrition Answers

MTF Answers

5.1 *Helicobacter pylori*

Answer: B

Helicobacter pylori is a Gram-negative organism. Infection is usually acquired in childhood; prevalence rates, however, are variable. Persistent infection causes a chronic gastritis, which may be asymptomatic. There is a strong relationship between helicobacter infection and peptic ulceration in adults, but this is rare in children. Symptoms and signs of peptic ulceration include epigastric pain, weight loss and anorexia, bloating, haematemesis, clinical anaemia and abdominal pain, which can be associated with meal times but classically wakes a person at night. *H. pylori* is also a carcinogen. There is no unproven association between helicobacter infection and recurrent abdominal pain. Transmission is faeco-oral and familial clustering is common. Diagnosis is by the following:

- Serology
- Rapid urease tests – ^{13}C breath test, CLO test
- Endoscopy, biopsy and histology and culture (difficult)
- Stool antigen test – which is now preferred.

5.2 Crohn disease

Answers: A D E

Crohn disease is a chronic inflammatory disorder of the bowel involving any region from mouth to anus. The inflammation is transmural with skip lesions. There has been an increase in incidence over the past 10 years in children across all age groups, and 10–15% of cases present in childhood, usually in the second decade. The prevalence in the childhood population is 10–20 per 100 000. The most common presenting symptoms are abdominal pain, diarrhoea and weight loss. Growth failure with delayed bone maturation and delayed sexual development is common. The diagnosis is made on the basis of clinical symptoms, raised inflammatory indices and diagnostic tests, including barium radiology and colonoscopy with biopsy. Treatment is difficult because the disease often runs a chronic relapsing course. The aim of treatment is to induce a disease remission and facilitate normal growth and development.

The most widely used treatment in children is enteral nutrition, used as an exclusion diet for up to 8 weeks, followed by a period of controlled food reintroduction. The type of enteral nutrition used varies and can be either elemental (protein broken down into amino acids) or polymeric (whole protein). This induces remission in up to 90% of patients. Maintenance is with 5-aminosalicylic acid (ASA) derivatives. Unfortunately disease relapse is common and either repeated courses of enteral nutrition or corticosteroids are required. Corticosteroid dependence or resistance can occur and additional immunosuppression (eg azathioprine) or surgery is often required.

Extraintestinal manifestations of Crohn disease:

- Joint disease 10%
- Skin rashes: erythema nodosum, erythema multiforme, pyoderma gangrenosum
- Liver disease (rare in children) – sclerosing cholangitis (more common with ulcerative colitis), chronic active hepatitis and cirrhosis
- Uveitis, episcleritis
- Osteoporosis
- Clubbing.

Note that ankylosing spondylitis and sclerosing cholangitis are not characteristic features of Crohn disease; they are more commonly associated with ulcerative colitis.

5.3 Abetalipoproteinaemia

Answers: A D E

Abetalipoproteinaemia is inherited as autosomally recessive. Long-chain fatty acids are transmitted as chylomicrons along the thoracic duct. β-Lipoprotein is part of the chylomicron. The pathogenesis of abetalipoproteinaemia is failure of chylomicron formation with impaired absorption of long-chain fats and fat retention in the enterocyte. Fat malabsorption occurs from birth. The condition presents in early infancy with failure to thrive, abdominal distension and foul-smelling, bulky stools. Symptoms of vitamin E deficiency (ataxia, peripheral neuropathy and retinitis pigmentosa) develop later. The child is normal at birth.

Laboratory diagnosis:

- Low serum cholesterol
- Very low plasma triglyceride level
- Acanthocytes on examination of the peripheral blood film
- Absence of β-lipoprotein in the plasma.

Treatment is by substituting medium-chain triglycerides for long-chain triglycerides in the diet. Medium-chain triglycerides are absorbed via the portal vein rather than the thoracic duct. In addition, high doses of the fat-soluble vitamins (A, D, E and K) are required. Most of the neurological abnormalities are reversible if high doses of vitamin E are given early.

Causes of acanthocytosis (spiky red cells):

- abetalipoproteinaemia
- chronic liver disease
- hyposplenism

Associations of retinitis pigmentosa:

- abetalipoproteinaemia
- Laurence–Moon–Biedl syndrome
- Usher syndrome
- Refsum disease
- Alport syndrome
- familial
- idiopathic.

5.4 Acrodermatitis enteropathica

Answers: C D E

This shows autosomal recessive inheritance. The basic defect is impaired absorption of zinc in the gut. It presents with skin rash around the mouth and perianal area, chronic diarrhoea at the time of weaning and recurrent infections. The hair has a reddish tint, and alopecia is characteristic. Superinfection with *Candida* spp. is common as are paronychia, dystrophic nails, poor wound healing and ocular changes (photophobia, blepharitis, corneal dystrophy). Diagnosis is by serum zinc levels and the constellation of clinical signs. This is difficult because serum zinc is low as part of the acute phase response. Measurement of white cell zinc levels is more accurate. The plasma metallothionein level can also be measured. Metallothionein is a zinc-binding protein that is decreased in zinc deficiency but not in the acute phase response. The condition responds very well to treatment with oral zinc. Zinc deficiency can cause the following:

- Iron deficiency anaemia
- Acrodermatitis enteropathica
- Hyperpigmentation
- Poor wound healing
- Immunodeficiency
- Growth failure
- Hypogonadism.

Clinically important trace elements are:

- chromium
- copper
- cobalt
- molybdenum
- manganese
- selenium
- zinc.

5.5 Vitamin A

Answers: A B C D E

Vitamin A is a fat-soluble vitamin (as are vitamins D, E and K); it occurs in two main forms: retinol, the most active form found mostly in animal sources, and carotenoids, which come from plant sources, some of which can be converted into vitamin A by the body. It has an important role in the resistance of infection, particularly at mucosal surfaces.

Vitamin A deficiency is common in the developing world but also exists in the developed world in patients who are malnourished (children on poverty line, vegan diets), have fat malabsorption, cholestasis, inflammatory bowel disease, or those who have undergone small bowel resection/bypass. Vitamin A deficiency may be subclinical or associated with poor growth, blindness, night blindness, anaemia, dry skin and hair, and impaired immunity especially to viral infections. Subclinical deficiency is associated with increased mortality and increased susceptibility to infections. The WHO and Unicef have issued a joint statement to advise that all children, especially those under 2 years old, who are diagnosed with measles should receive vitamin A because it is associated with a decreased mortality and morbidity.

Vitamin A toxicity acutely causes nausea, vomiting abdominal pain and symptoms of raised intracranial pressure such as blurred vision, headache, irritability and altered mental status. Chronic toxicity causes anorexia, hair loss, pruritus, bone pain and increased bone fractures. Of note high intake of vitamin A (>10 000 IU/day) during pregnancy is associated with severe birth defects including cleft palate and spina bifida.

Dietary sources include:

- Cows' milk
- Liver
- Eggs
- Beef
- Chicken
- Orange fruits and vegetables (mango, sweet potatoes, carrots, squash and apricots)
- Spinach, kale and other green vegetables
- Tomatoes and pink grapefruit.

5.6 Immunoglobulin A

Answers: B D E

IgA makes up 15% of circulating immunoglobulin. In its secretory form it is the predominant immunoglobulin at respiratory and gastrointestinal mucosal surfaces.

Selective IgA deficiency

This is a common disorder, with an incidence of 1 in 600. It may be asymptomatic but can be associated with an increased incidence of infection (especially when it coexists with an IgG subclass deficiency as occurs in 20–30% of cases, many of whom will have normal levels of total IgG). Patients with selective IgA deficiency are at increased risk of a number of conditions including:

- Respiratory tract infection (otitis media, sinusitis, bronchitis and pneumonia)
- Chronic lung disease
- Gastrointestinal tract (GI) infection, particularly (recurrent) giardiasis
- Coeliac disease (increased 10 × in IgA deficiency), Crohn disease, ulcerative colitis and milk-related GI symptoms
- Autoimmune/rheumatoid conditions including rheumatoid arthritis, Systemic lupus erythematosus and pernicious anaemia.
- IgA deficiency is also associated with an increased risk of transfusion related reactions due to the presence of anti-IgA antibodies

Immunoglobulin therapy is not indicated if isolated IgA deficiency is present. This is because there is only a small amount of IgA in immunoglobulin preparations and sensitisation is therefore likely. If there is coexistent IgG deficiency or IgG subclass deficiency, then immunoglobulin therapy may be appropriate. There have been cases of IgA and IgG subclass deficiency that have progressed on to common variable immunodeficiency.

Management includes aggressive antibiotic treatment of respiratory tract infections with the use of prophylactic antibiotics in selected patients. Patients also benefit from maximising the treatment of any underlying allergies and/or asthma.

5.7 Carbohydrate digestion

Answers: A B D

Carbohydrates are consumed as monosaccharides (glucose, fructose, galactose), disaccharides (lactose, sucrose, maltose, isomaltose) and polysaccharides (starch, dextrins, glycogen). Salivary and pancreatic amylase breaks starch down into oligosaccharides and disaccharides. Pancreatic amylase aids carbohydrate digestion but carbohydrate digestion is not dependent on it. Disaccharidases (maltase, sucrase, lactase) in the microvilli hydrolyse:

- oligo- and disaccharides into monosaccharides
- maltose into glucose
- isomaltose into glucose
- sucrose into glucose and fructose
- lactose into glucose and galactose.

Monosaccharides are then absorbed, glucose and galactose by an active transport mechanism and fructose by facilitated diffusion.

5.8 Causes of partial villous atrophy on small bowel biopsy include

Answers: A B C D E

The differential diagnosis of partial villous atrophy on small bowel biopsy includes:

- Coeliac disease
- Cows' milk-sensitive enteropathy
- Soy-protein-sensitive enteropathy
- Eosinophilic gastroenteritis
- Gastroenteritis and post-enteritis syndrome
- Giardiasis
- Small bowel bacterial overgrowth
- Inflammatory bowel disease
- Immunodeficiency
- Intractable diarrhoea syndromes, eg autoimmune enteropathy
- Drugs, eg cytotoxics
- Radiotherapy.

5.9 Gilbert syndrome

Answers: A D E

Gilbert syndrome is defined as unconjugated hyperbilirubinaemia with no evidence of haemolysis and normal liver function tests. Liver biopsy is normal. The prevalence is 6%, and it is more common in males than females. Inheritance is autosomal dominant with incomplete expression. The pathogenesis is unclear but probably represents a mild functional deficiency of the enzyme UDP (uridine 5×-diphospho)-glucuronyl transferase. The clinical picture is of mild fluctuating jaundice (serum bilirubin 30–50 μmol/l) aggravated by infection, exertion and fasting. Of some diagnostic use is the fact that the condition improves with phenobarbital and worsens with nicotinic acid.

Other inherited causes of hyperbilirubinaemia include the following:

- Crigler–Najjar syndrome: type 1 (autosomal recessive) is due to complete absence of UDP-glucuronyl transferase in the liver. Jaundice (unconjugated) presents soon after birth and rapidly progresses to toxic levels (kernicterus). Untreated, death usually occurs by the end of the first year. Diagnosis is by estimation of hepatic UDP-glucuronyl transferase activity in a specimen obtained by needle liver biopsy. Repeated exchange transfusions and phototherapy aid short-term survival. The only long-term therapeutic option is liver transplantation. Type 2 (autosomal dominant) is less severe and responds to treatment with phenobarbital. There is usually less than 10% of normal levels of UDP-glucuronyl transferase activity present. Kernicterus is unusual.
- Dubin–Johnson syndrome: autosomal recessive. Presents with conjugated hyperbilirubinaemia and bilirubinuria. It is due to a reduced ability to transport organic anions such as bilirubin glucuronide into the biliary tree. There is black

pigmentation of the liver on biopsy. Life expectancy is normal, and the jaundice is exacerbated by alcohol, infection and pregnancy. It may not present until early adulthood.

- Rotor syndrome: autosomal recessive. It presents with conjugated hyperbilirubinaemia. It is due to a deficiency in organic anion uptake as well as excretion. No black pigment is present in the liver. There is normal life expectancy, and the jaundice is exacerbated by alcohol, infection and pregnancy. Sulphobromophthalein excretion test is abnormal.

BOF Answers

5.10 Weaning/Complementary feeding

Answer A: Exclusive breastfeeding of infants until 6 months is associated with a decreased incidence of infection

The WHO advice issued in 2001 stated that all infants should be exclusively breastfed until 6 months; in 2003 this became UK policy. Recent evidence has highlighted possible concerns about this advice; studies are under way to evaluate its potential consequences. It is, however, well documented that as few as 1% of infants in the UK are exclusively breastfed until 6 months of age.

In the UK Millennium cohort study, the introduction of formula feeds (from exclusive breastfeeding) rather than solid feeds predicted an increased hospital admission for gastroenteritis and respiratory infections. It was estimated that 53% of admissions for gastroenteritis and 27% of admissions for chest infection could be prevented each month by exclusive breastfeeding.

Evidence has always existed, and continues to grow, that exclusive breastfeeding for 6 months may lead to increased iron deficiency anaemia and its consequences of long-term motor, mental and social development.

There is also concern that, although the growth of babies exclusively breastfed for 6 months appears to be adequate (very small numbers), calculations about energy requirements compared with the energy content and output of breast milk may mean exclusive breastfeeding may not support adequate growth in all children.

Limited evidence exists for a bimodal distribution of increased allergy associated with the introduction of certain foods. Exposure before 3–4 months as well as delayed exposure after 6 months may increase the prevalence of food allergy in a population. Exposure to gluten-containing foods between 4 and 6 months appears to be protective, especially when combined with continued breastfeeding, for the development of coeliac disease in later life.

There may also be a 'window' to introduce bitter tasting foods (such as green vegetables) between 4 and 6 months.

5.11 Acute appendicitis

Answer C: Acute appendicitis is most common in the second decade of life

The most common surgical diagnosis in all children who present to hospital with acute abdominal pain is acute appendicitis; intussusception is more common in children aged <5 years. In over half of all admissions to hospital with acute abdominal pain no cause is found. The differential diagnosis is wide; a thorough history and examination including testicular examination are essential to appropriately investigate and manage these patients.

Acute appendicitis

Classically there is initial central colicky abdominal pain progressing to localised pain in the right lower quadrant; however, less than 60% of children present in this way. Fever (low grade), anorexia, nausea and vomiting are common, loose stools and urinary symptoms may also occur. WCC is generally raised, ultrasonography being increasingly utilised to investigate this condition and reporting sensitivity of 84% and specificity of 94% in children. A pelvic appendix may be missed on ultrasonography and present with atypical symptoms and signs. Appendicitis is most common in the second decade of life. The rate of perforation is increased by a delay in diagnosis and approaches 80% in those aged <3 years, and decreases to 10–20% of 10–17 year olds. Management is by appendectomy unless there is an appendix mass, in which case a course of intravenous antibiotics is followed by an interval elective appendectomy. Laparoscopic techniques are increasingly being employed.

Differential diagnosis includes:

- Appendicitis
- Intussusception
- Urinary tract infection
- Mesenteric adenitis
- Constipation
- Peptic ulceration
- Meckel diverticulitis
- Pancreatitis
- Gastroenteritis
- Ovarian pathology, eg torsion/cyst
- Primary peritonitis
- Henoch–Schönlein purpura
- Hernia
- Testicular torsion
- Cholecystitis
- Renal colic
- Metabolic, eg acute porphyria
- Trauma

- Inflammatory bowel disease
- Pelvic inflammatory disease
- Ectopic pregnancy
- Sickle cell crisis
- Non-abdominal cause, eg pneumonia, diabetic ketoacidosis.

5.12 Iron deficiency anaemia

Answer B: Iron-rich foods include egg yolk, red meat, fortified breakfast cereals, and dried fruit, green vegetables, beans and pulses

WHO definition of iron deficiency anaemia:

- Hb <110 g/l in children aged 1–2 years
- Hb <112 g/l in children aged 3–5 years
- Hb <115 g/l in children aged 5–12 years
- Hb <120 g/l in children aged 12–15 years.

The prevalence in the UK is 8% in those aged under 5 years, increasing considerably in inner city areas and in Asian children. Although malabsorption and bleeding are causes of iron deficiency anaemia in children, the overwhelming cause is dietary, specifically the disproportionately high percentage of unmodified cows' milk in the diet and the over-reliance on non-iron-containing convenience foods in the weaning diet and beyond. Iron stores are laid down in the last trimester of pregnancy and so preterm babies require supplementation. Markers of iron deficiency include:

- low MCV (mean corpuscular volume)
- low MCH (mean corpuscular Hb)
- low plasma ferritin (<10 μg/l) – note that raised as part of acute phase reactant.

Consequences:

- Pallor, tiredness, irritability
- Anorexia
- Increased risk of infection
- Developmental delay and poor educational achievement (may persist post-treatment)
- Dysphagia (oesophageal web)
- Pica.

Management:

- Breastfeeding – high bioavailability
- Iron-fortified formula/follow-on milk (if cannot decrease milk).
- Encourage iron-rich weaning foods and beyond
- Give vitamin C-rich fruit/juices with meals to increase absorption
- Avoid whole cows' milk during the first year of life, and subsequently restrict intake to <750 ml/day.

Treatment/Prophylaxis:

- 3–6 mg/kg per day divided doses of elemental iron
- Hb should rise by 10–20 g/l over 3–4 weeks
- Treatment should be continued for 3 months after the anaemia has been corrected
- Prophylaxis for neonates is 5 mg elemental iron daily, 6 weeks until weaned
- Side effects of iron medication include nausea, epigastric pain, constipation, diarrhoea and black discoloration of stools
- Iron is very dangerous in overdose
- Poor compliance is the most likely cause of resistant cases.

5.13 Rickets

Answer D: Vitam D-deficient rickets

Rickets is a disease of growing bones, (failure to mineralise osteoid). Vitamin D deficiency (diet or ↓ sunlight) is the main cause of rickets. Maternal vitamin D deficiency combined with low vitamin D in breast milk may lead to neonatal rickets. Other causes include the following:

- Nutritional deficiencies of calcium and phosphorous
- X-linked and autosomal recessive (AR) hyphophoshataemic rickets, AR vitamin D-dependent rickets (all rare)
- Fat malabsorption (coeliac disease, liver disease – also leads to defective metabolism of vitamin D)
- Renal disease (defective metabolism of vitamin D)
- Neonatal rickets of prematurity (secondary to inadequate phosphate)
- Anticonvulsants.

Rickets typically presents at 4–18 months. Vitamin D deficiency during adolescence usually results in osteomalacia.

Typical radiological features of rickets include poor mineralisation, delayed development of epiphyses, metaphyseal cupping, fraying and splaying, best seen at the wrists, knees and ankles.

Symptoms and signs include:

- Bowing of the legs
- Impaired linear growth in infancy
- Diffuse bone pain
- Kyphoscoliosis
- Flattened pelvis (obstructed labour in adult life)
- The costochondral junctions become swollen (rickety rosary)
- Pectus carinatum and Harrison sulci
- Cartilaginous swellings around the wrists and ankles
- Frontal bossing
- Delayed closure of the anterior fontanelle
- Dental enamel hypoplasia and delayed tooth eruption

- Hypocalcaemic seizures
- Tetany, apnoea and stridor
- Left ventricular hypertrophy
- Prolonged QTc interval and arrhythmias
- Hypotension and heart failure.

Blood biochemistry in vitamin D-deficient rickets:

- ↓ 25OH-D (25-hydroxyvitamin D, calcidiol) in serum
- ↑ PTH
- ↓ Ca^{2+}
- ↓ PO_4^{3-}
- ↑ Alkaline phosphatase.

Treatment:

- Ergocalciferol (vitamin D_2) or cholecalciferol (vitamin D_3) for dietary deficiency
- Alfacalcidol (1α-hydroxycholecalciferol) or calcitriol (1,25-dihydroxycholecalciferol) for those with liver or kidney disease.

Sources of vitamin D include fish oil, vegetable oil and skin synthesis during exposure to sunlight.

5.14 Polyporis

Answer C: Juvenile polyp

In this case bright-red blood passing per rectum is likely to be from the distal bowel and the absence of associated anal pain makes a diagnosis of constipation with an anal fissure unlikely.

Juvenile polyps

More than 90% of polyps that present in childhood are juvenile polyps. They are benign harmatomas. They present at age 2–6 years with painless blood per rectum; however, 5% prolapse and 10% are associated with abdominal pain. Most polyps are solitary and located within 30 cm of the anus. They are not premalignant.

Juvenile polyposis

This rare condition refers to patients with more than five juvenile polyps. Presenting signs include diarrhoea, rectal bleeding, intussusception, anaemia, prolapse and failure to thrive. This may be sporadic or familial with an autosomal dominant pattern of inheritance. Polyps can be present throughout the GI tract. There is considerable malignant potential (17%) and prophylactic colectomy may be advised.

Peutz–Jegher syndrome

This condition is inherited in an autosomal dominant pattern. It consists of hamartomatous polyps that can occur throughout the GI tract, but most commonly in the small intestine. It is associated with hyperpigmentation of the buccal mucosa and lips. Patients without a family history will often present with recurrent abdominal pain caused by intussusception secondary to small bowel polyps. It is a premalignant condition with carcinomatous transformation of the polyps; in addition there is an increased risk of developing pancreatic, ovarian, breast, cervical and testicular tumours.

Familial adenomatous polyposis coli and Gardner syndrome

These conditions are inherited in an autosomal dominant fashion. Multiple polyps develop (>100), usually in the second decade. Gastric and duodenal polyps develop in up to 50% and there is an increased risk of thyroid and liver tumours. Most cases are diagnosed on screening children of affected individuals. Gardner syndrome is familial adenomatous polyposis plus bony lesions, subcutaneous tumours and cysts. Both conditions carry a very high risk of colonic carcinoma (100%) and prophylactic colectomy at the end of the second decade is advised.

5.15 Breastfeeding

Answer D: Breastfeeding reduces the rate of gastrointestinal infections of infants while it continues

The clearest benefits to the children who are breastfed are a decreased incidence of gastrointestinal infection and reduced incidence of otitis media, although these effects do not persist beyond a 2-month period after the cessation of breastfeeding. There is also clear evidence of a protective effect in the prevention of NEC in preterm babies. There is no evidence that breastfeeding prevents the development of respiratory tract infections but the severity of the illness, as measured by the need for hospital admission, appears to be decreased. Additional benefits of breastfeeding to the child include the following:

- Long-term reduction in blood pressure
- Long-term lower cholesterol levels
- Decreased incidence of childhood type 1 diabetes
- May prevent or at least delay the development of coeliac disease
- Increased IQ (more pronounced for low-birthweight children)
- Decreased risk of developing childhood ALL (acute lymphoblastic leukaemia)
- A decrease in incidence of childhood atopic disease in at-risk children.

There are a few contraindications to breastfeeding:

- Galactosaemia
- Phenlyketonuria (PKU – breastfeeds may be alternated with phenylalanine-free formulae)
- Mothers with HIV infection in developed countries (the WHO recommends that, when replacement feeding is acceptable, feasible, affordable, sustainable and safe, avoidance of all breastfeeding by HIV-infected mothers is recommended; otherwise, exclusive breastfeeding is recommended during the first months of life)
- Note that NOT contraindicated in hepatitis B surface antigen or hepatitis C-positive mothers
- Mothers with herpes simplex lesions on their breasts
- Mothers who are positive for human T-cell lymphotrophic virus (HTLV) type I and II

- Mothers who are receiving therapeutic or diagnostic radioactive isotopes
- Maternal intake of any medications should be checked before breastfeeding; alternatives may be available.

5.16 Vitamin K

Answer A: Vitamin K deficiency bleeding is a potentially fatal disorder that is virtually preventable with one dose of vitamin K given intramuscularly at birth

The Department of Health issued guidance on the administration of vitamin K in newborn infants in 1998. In short:

- All newborn babies should receive vitamin K to prevent the rare but serious and sometimes fatal disorder of vitamin K deficiency bleeding (VKDB).
- The available data do not support an increased risk of cancer including leukaemia caused by vitamin K.
- Intramuscular vitamin K effectively prevents VKDB in virtually all babies after a single dose given at birth.
- Oral regimens require repeated (more than two) doses in breastfed babies*; clinicians must ensure that all recommended oral doses are given at the appropriate ages.
- A selective policy for high- or low-risk infants is not feasible because bleeding occurs unpredictably.
- Babies at high risk of early (24 h) or classic (2–7 days) VKDB include: preterm, or failing to take or absorb feeds, or had a complicated delivery or are ill or, if their mothers have been receiving medication associated with a higher risk (eg anticonvulsant drugs).
- Babies at high risk of late (>7 days) VKDB: babies with liver disease (prolonged jaundice with pale stools and/or dark urine), or babies who have bleeding or spontaneous bruising in early infancy or who are ill from other causes.
- Of the babies who do not receive vitamin K, 1 in 10 000 will develop VKDB; 50% of these are affected late, and 50% of those affected will have intracranial bleeding, 20% of those will die and most survivors will have long-term neurological damage.
- Many who have severe late VKDB have minor warning bleeds in the preceding few days. In about a third of instances the bleeding occurs without evident cause or risk factor.

*Vitamin K is added to formula milk.

5.17 Testing for carbohydrate malabsorption

Answer D: An early peak of hydrogen in a hydrogen breath test, followed by a secondary peak, may be indicative of small bowel bacterial overgrowth

- Samples of liquid stool will show undigested sugars on chromatography.
- Reducing substances in the stool of 0.25–0.5% are suggestive of carbohydrate malabsorption; >0.75% is indicative of the condition. The liquid portion of the stool must be tested.

- Acidic stool pH <5.5 is indicative of carbohydrate malabsorption even in the absence of reducing substances.
- Analysis of small-bowel mucosal disaccharidases in a biopsy obtained endoscopically is the 'gold standard', but is rarely needed. Endoscopy may reveal small intestinal mucosal injury resulting in secondary carbohydrate malabsorption.
- Clinical response to treatment with withdrawal of suspected intolerant substance leading to resolution of symptoms **and** reintroduction leading to relapse is suggestive of diagnosis. However, non-resolution of diarrhoea may not necessarily exclude the diagnosis because diarrhoea itself may produce a secondary intolerance of a different substance, so the sensitivity of this as a diagnostic test can be poor. In addition removal of a dietary substance may improve symptoms but not confirm a diagnosis, eg the removal of cows' milk may lead to the cessation of diarrhoea but this may be due to a diagnosis of lactose intolerance or cows' milk protein intolerance.
- The hydrogen breath test: the principle is that malabsorbed carbohydrate will pass into the colon where it is metabolised by bacteria and hydrogen is released. The gas is then absorbed and released in the breath. If there is a peak it suggests carbohydrate malabsorption. An early peak raises the possibility of bacterial overgrowth in the small intestine, in which case a secondary peak may occur representing large bowel fermentation. Lactulose, which is a non-absorbable carbohydrate, can be given to ensure that the colonic flora can metabolise carbohydrate and to assess transit time. A false-negative test is possible

5.18 Folate (folic acid)

Answer C: Methotrexate and trimethoprim are folate antagonists

Folate is a water-soluble B vitamin that occurs naturally in foods; folic acid is the synthetic form that is found in supplements and is added to fortified foods. Dietary sources of folate include liver, green vegetables, cereals, orange, milk, yeast, beans, lentils and mushrooms. Some breads and cereals are fortified with folic acid; this is always stated on the label. Folate is destroyed by excessive cooking; this is a greater problem for plant sources than animal sources. It is absorbed from the proximal small bowel. Deficiency causes megaloblastic anaemia, and more rarely neutropenia and thrombocytopenia, irritability, poor weight gain, glossitis and chronic diarrhoea. In pregnancy folate deficiency has been linked to spontaneous abortion, placental abruption and most significantly neural tube defects in the fetus.

The serum folate reflects recent changes in folate status and the red cell folate is an indicator of total body stores. Folate is not part of the acute phase response. Treatment of deficiency is with oral folic acid. Supplementation is recommended in all women who are planning to become pregnant or who are pregnant because this reduces the risk of neural tube defects. Women with pregnancies considered to be high risk for developing a neural tube defect are recommended to take higher doses of folic acid during conception and early pregnancy. Folate deficiency is associated with elevated homocysteine levels; this in turn increases the risk of atherosclerosis. Folate deficiency is also associated with enhanced carcinogenesis. Causes of folate deficiency include:

- Reduced intake

- Coeliac disease
- Tropical sprue
- Prematurity
- Blind loop syndrome
- Congenital folate malabsorption (autosomal recessive)
- Increased requirements (infancy, pregnancy, lactation, exfoliative skin disorders)
- Increased loss (haemodialysis)
- Methotrexate
- Trimethoprim
- Sulfasalazine
- Anticonvulsants
- Oral contraceptive pill.

5.19 Composition of formula and breast milk

Answer C: The fat content of breast milk varies throughout the day and throughout a feed

The composition of human milk is not static. The protein content is higher and the carbohydrate content lower in colostrum than in mature milk. Fat contents fluctuate with diurnal variations and within a feed, increasing towards the end of each feed. Breast milk has whey:casein ratio (70:30), protein of high biological value, long-chain fatty acids that may improve vision and cognition, and a low renal solute load. In addition to its nutrients, it also contains immunoglobulins, antimicrobial and anti-inflammatory agents, hormones, growth factors and enzymes; these factors contribute to the immune protection digestion, and both intestinal and general growth and development.

The composition of formula feeds in contrast is closely regulated in terms of the acceptable range of nutritional components. The two main types available differ in their protein composition with whey:casein ratios of 60:40 and 20:80 in the whey- and casein-dominant formulae respectively. The whey-based formulae most closely resemble breast milk and, although evidence is lacking, the casein-based formulae are marketed as more satisfying for the hungry baby because the casein forms curds that are more slowly digested. The casein-based formulae have a higher renal solute load than the whey-based milks and, although suitable from birth, extra care should be taken in making them up correctly.

In 100 ml	Breast milk (approximately)	Term formula
Energy (kcal)	60–75	67
Protein (g)	1.3	1.4
Carbohydrate (g)	7	7.5
Fat (g)	4.2	3.5
Na^+ (mmol)	0.65	0.7
K^+ (mmol)	1.54	1.6
Ca^{2+} (mmol)	0.88	1.0
PO_4^{3-} (mmol)	0.48	0.6
Iron (mg)	0.08	0.5

5.20 Carbohydrate intolerance in childhood

Answer E: Acquired post-enteritis lactose intolerance is usually transient

Carbohydrates make up at least half of the energy intake in the diet. The main carbohydrates are the storage polysaccharides (starch, glycogen and cellulose), the disaccharides, lactose and sucrose, and the monosaccharides, glucose and fructose.

Disorders of disaccharide absorption include the following.

Primary:

- Congenital alactasia (exceptionally rare with neonatal presentation)
- Sucrose–isomaltase deficiency (even rarer than lactase deficiency): symptoms when fruit (sucrose) added to the diet, will not tolerate glucose feeds.

Secondary:

- Post-enteritis (rotavirus): usually resolves after a short period – days to 2 weeks
- Neonatal surgery, malnutrition
- Untreated coeliac disease
- Late-onset lactose intolerance: in many populations lactase activity declines after the first few years of life. Symptoms are rare before age 6 years. Ten per cent of northern Europeans but >80% of Africans, Asians, Inuit and American Indians. Often dose-dependent tolerance with fermented dairy products being less problematic. Thought to be autosomal recessive.

Disorders of monosaccharide absorption

- Primary: glucose–galactose malabsorption (very rare autosomal recessive) – intolerance of feeds with watery diarrhoea from birth, stops with cessation of feeds. Will tolerate fructose feeds.
- Secondary:
  - post-enteritis
  - neonatal surgery
  - malnutrition.

Carbohydrate intolerance is usually lactose intolerance and is usually acquired. The deficiency is the brush border enzyme lactase which hydrolyses lactose into glucose and galactose. The intolerance will present with characteristic loose explosive stools. The diagnosis is made by looking for reducing substances in the stools after carbohydrate ingestion; detection of >0.5% is significant. Treatment is with lactose-free formula in infancy and a reduced lactose intake in later childhood. After gastroenteritis, carbohydrate intolerance can be to either disaccharides or monosaccharides. Both types of intolerance are usually transient and both respond to removal of the offending carbohydrate. Both result in positive reducing substances in the stools.

5.21 Preterm and term formulae

Answer E: Babies fed on fortified breast milk have a decreased incidence of late-onset sepsis and necrotising enterocolitis when compared with babies fed on preterm formulae

The principal differences are that preterm formula contains more electrolytes, calories and minerals than term formula. All of the following are higher in the preterm formulae: energy, protein, carbohydrate, fat, osmolality, sodium, potassium, calcium, magnesium, phosphate and iron.

Breast milk fortifier is a powder designed to add to breast milk for preterm or low-birthweight babies to provide extra energy, protein, vitamins and minerals to support growth in this population while preserving the non-nutritional advantages of breast milk, such as its immunological function, enzymes and growth factors. It is based on hydrolysed cows' milk protein. Fortified human milk may not produce as much weight gain as preterm formulae but it is associated with a decreased incidence of NEC and late-onset sepsis.

In 100 ml	Breast milk (approximately)	Term formula	Preterm formula
Energy (kcal)	60–75	67	80
Protein (g)	1.3	1.4	2.5
Carbohydrate (g)	7	7.5	7.8
Fat (g)	4.2	3.5	4.4
Na^+ (mmol)	0.65	0.7	1.7
K^+ (mmol)	1.54	1.6	2.0
Ca^{2+} (mmol)	0.88	1.0	2.5
PO_4^{3-} (mmol)	0.48	0.6	1.6
Iron (mg)	0.08	0.5	1.4

5.22 Human (breast) milk compared with cows' milk

Answer D: Breast mild has the same energy content as unmodified cows' milk

Whole cows' milk should not be used as the main milk drink before the age of 1 year because it may be associated with iron deficiency anaemia. It can, however, be used in cooking in the weaning diet. During complementary feeding more than 90% of iron requirements in a breastfed baby may be met by the complementary food. Whole unmodified cows' milk contains the same energy content as breast milk. It has the same quantity of fat (although qualitatively it is different). Human milk contains less protein (has a much lower casein content) and more carbohydrate (lactose) than cows' milk. Cows' milk contains more of all the minerals except iron and copper.

Unpasteurised cows' milk is not suitable for infants.

Semi-skimmed milk from the age of 2 years can be progressively introduced, provided that the child's overall energy and fat-soluble vitamin intake is adequate from other sources. Skimmed milk should not be introduced before 5 years of age. Milk contains the fat-soluble vitamins A, D, E and K. The content level of fat-soluble vitamins in dairy products depends on the fat content of the product.

Follow-on milks contain more protein, iron and vitamin D than standard formulae. They can be used when a child's diet is inconsistent or if there is concern about the adequacy of the diet, because they can provide a safety net and are a more reliable source of minerals and vitamins than cows' milk. Diets too high in milk can lead to iron deficiency anaemia, especially in early childhood.

In 100 ml	Breast milk (approximately)	Term Formula	Unmodified cows' milk
Energy (kcal)	60–75	67	68
Protein (g)	1.3	1.4	3.4
Carbohydrate (g)	7	7.5	4.7
Fat (g)	4.2	3.5	4.0
Iron (mg)	0.08	0.5	0.03

5.23 Nutritional supplements

Answer A: Maxijul is a glucose polymer

Nutritional supplements are indicated for use in patients with disease-related malnutrition, malabsorption states or any other conditions requiring fortification with a high or readily available calorie supplement. These include glucose polymer-based supplements:

- Maxijul super 380 kcal/100 g powder
- Maxijul liquid 200 kcal/100 ml
- Vitajoule powder 380 kg/100 g.

Also supplements based on maltodextrin:

- Caloreen powder 390 kcal/100 g
- Polycal powder 384 kcal/100 g
- Polycal liquid 247 kcal/100 ml.

Nutritional supplements based on fat have generally more calories per ml than their carbohydrate equivalents and include:

- Calogen liquid 450 kcal/100 ml
- Liquigen liquid 450 kcal/100 ml.

Nutritional supplements based on fat and carbohydrate includes:

- Duocal preparations (calorific values vary with preparations).

Nutritional supplements based on protein, fat and carbohydrate includes:

- Scandishake 500 kcal/100 g – contains cows' milk protein and lactose.

5.24 Wilson disease (hepatolenticular degeneration)

Answer C: A diet low in copper should be low in shellfish, liver and chocolate

Wilson disease is an autosomal recessive disorder of copper metabolism. The gene has been identified on chromosome 13 and dysfunction of this gene decreases both copper excretion into bile and ceruloplasmin production. Ceruloplasmin is the plasma protein that transports copper. Wilson disease presents in 40% with features of liver disease usually between the ages of 3 and 12 years. Approximately 50% have a psychiatric or neurological presentation, usually in adolescence or early adult life; 50% of these will have clinically detectable liver disease. The remainder present with skeletal, renal or haemolytic disease. The effects of the disease include the following:

- Liver: chronic active hepatitis, portal hypertension and fulminant hepatic failure
- Brain: progressive lenticular degradation due to copper deposition, often leads to tremor
- Cornea: Kayser–Fleischer rings
- Lens: sunflower cataract
- Kidney: renal tubular disorders
- Blood: haemolysis.

Diagnosis can be difficult. The important part is to include it in the differential of all undiagnosed liver disease in childhood. Biochemical findings include:

- low plasma ceruloplasmin level <200 mg/L
- Raised urinary copper >25 μmol/24 h after penicillamine (the penicillamine challenge)
- Baseline urinary copper is unreliable with poor sensitivity and specificity (>5 μmol/24 h is suggestive)
- Raised hepatic copper on liver biopsy
- Note that serum copper levels are not helpful.

If untreated the disease is fatal, usually by the age of 30 years. If identified early and treated, the prognosis is good. Treatment is with oral penicillamine as a copper-binding agent plus a low-copper diet (avoid excessive chocolate, shellfish and liver). Patients on penicillamine require vitamin B_6 (pyridoxine) supplementation to avoid neuropathy. Liver transplantation may be indicated if presentation is with fulminant liver failure. It is important to screen siblings of patients with Wilson disease to start treatment early and improve prognosis.

5.25 Unconjugated neonatal jaundice

Answer D: Neonates who develop jaundice within the first 24 h need urgent medical review to rule out underlying potentially severe aetiology for their jaundice

Jaundice can be either conjugated (direct) or unconjugated (indirect). Unconjugated is fat soluble and does not spill over into the urine. Up to 60% of term and 80% of preterm newborns become clinically jaundiced in the first week of life; approximately 10% of breastfed babies will still be jaundiced at 1 month of age. Most neonatal jaundice is harmless but some children will develop very high levels of unconjugated bilirubin, which can cross the blood–brain barrier and cause long-term neurological damage. Clinical assessment of the level of bilirubin is difficult and so, if jaundice is detected, a serum bilirubin should be checked and managed according to threshold charts based on gestational age and treatment guidance issued by the National Institute for Health and Clinical Excellence (NICE). Additional care should be taken if the child develops jaundice within the first 24 hours of life. Most cases can be managed with phototherapy and

supportive measures; however, some children with very high levels of bilirubin that persist despite treatment or any baby with clinical signs of acute bilirubin encephalopathy may require an exchange transfusion. Always identify and treat any underlying cause of hyperbilirubinaemia as appropriate.

Causes of unconjugated hyperbilirubinaemia in the neonatal period include:

- **Increased production of unconjugated bilirubin from haem**
- **Haemolysis:**
  - **rhesus incompatibility**
  - **ABO incompatibility**
  - **hereditary spherocytosis**
  - **glucose-6-phosphate dehydrogenase deficiency**
  - **pyruvate kinase deficiency**
- **Polycythaemia/bruising**
- **Sepsis congenital or acquired**
- **Decreased bilirubin uptake or metabolism:**
  - **physiological**
  - **sepsis, acidosis and hypoxia**
  - **Gilbert syndrome (7% of population mild)**
  - **Crigler–Najjar syndrome (can be severe – rare)**
  - **breast milk jaundice**
  - **hypothyroidism**
- **Altered enterohepatic circulation:**
  - **breast milk jaundice**
  - **antibiotic administration**
  - **intestinal obstruction:**
    - **ileal atresia**
    - **Hirschsprung disease**
  - **cystic fibrosis including meconium ileus**
    - **pyloric stenosis.**

5.26 Coeliac disease

Answer A: According to NICE guidelines type 1 diabetes mellitus is an indication for screening for celiac disease

This is a reversible immune-mediated enteropathy of the small intestinal mucosa that occurs on exposure to ingested gluten. Its prevalence in the UK is between 0.3% and 1.9%. Patients can present at any time throughout life with a wide range of symptoms; more patients are diagnosed in adulthood than childhood. The gold standard of diagnosis is positive serology (IgA tissue transglutaminase [TTG], or IgG TTG if IgA deficient), characteristic histology (subtotal villous atrophy) on small bowel biopsy and resolution of symptoms when gluten is removed. Of note, if the patient is taking insufficient gluten before serology and biopsy, both may be within the normal range and so the diagnosis must be confirmed on gluten (>10–15 g/day, for 6 weeks to 3 months). Risk factors for developing coeliac disease include other autoimmune diseases (eg type 1 diabetes mellitus), first-degree relative with coeliac disease (10%) and a diagnosis of IgA deficiency.

GI symptoms and signs include:

- Persistent or intermittent diarrhoea
- Abdominal pain
- Vomiting
- Constipation
- Abdominal bloating/distension
- Anorexia
- Flatulence.

Non-GI symptoms and signs include:

- Recurrent aphthous stomatitis
- Faltering growth
- Weight loss
- Short stature
- Delayed menarche/puberty
- Amenorrhoea
- Dental enamel defects
- Prolonged fatigue/lethargy
- Iron deficiency anaemia
- Rickets/osteomalacia
- Osteoporosis/pathological fracture
- Dermatitis herpetiformis
- Irritability/depression.

Treatment is lifelong adherence to a gluten-free diet, exclusion of wheat, rye, barley and oats (due to contamination with gluten during milling and manufacture). Consequences of non-adherence to diet include recurrence of symptoms, poor growth, delayed puberty, dental enamel problems, osteoporosis, and small increased risk of malignancy, eg small bowel lymphoma. The NICE guidelines advocate targeted screening via serological testing of children with symptoms of, or risk factors for, coeliac disease.

5.27 Hepatitis B

Answer A: Hepatitis B is a DNA virus

Hepatitis B is a DNA virus. Diagnosis is by detection of the hepatitis B surface antigen (HBsAg). Hepatitis B 'e' antigen (HBeAg)-positive patients carry a larger virus load and are more infectious. Acute and ongoing chronic infection is associated with anti-hepatitis B core (HBc) IgM. Anti-HBe and anti-HBs antibodies appear as an effective immune response develops. All HBsAg-positive individuals are infective. The route of transmission is either percutaneous (puncture through the skin) or mucosal (exposure to infectious blood or bodily fluids). The perinatal transmission rate depends on the maternal serology. If the mother is HBsAg positive and HBeAg negative, the risk is 12–25%. If the mother is both HBsAg and HBeAg positive the risk is 90%. The younger the age at infection the less the likelihood of symptomatic liver disease but the greater the risk of prolonged viral carriage. Ninety per cent of infants infected in the first year of life become chronic carriers.

Clinically the disease is often asymptomatic but an acute hepatic picture can develop. Acute liver failure occurs in less than 1%. The risk of fulminant hepatitis is increased by coinfection with hepatitis D. In those with a typical hepatic picture the chronic carrier rate is low. Chronicity results in an increased risk of cirrhosis and hepatocellular carcinoma. Boys are more likely to become chronic carriers than girls. Chronically infected children have a 25% lifetime risk of cirrhosis or hepatocellular carcinoma. Prevention is by both active and passive immunisation. Interferon-α is a recognised treatment of chronic infection.

Hepatitis D is an RNA virus that requires the HBsAg for its assembly and virulence. It is transmitted similarly to hepatitis B. The severity of the liver damage increases if there is coexistent hepatitis B infection. Diagnosis is by serology. Prevention of vertical transmission of hepatitis B is with immunisation of all neonates born to hepatitis B-infected mothers with the addition of HBIg for all babies <1500 g, those whose mothers had acute hepatitis B infection in pregnancy, those whose mothers are HBsAg positive plus either HBeAg positive or anti-HBe negative.

5.28 Hepatitis A

Answer D: Hepatitis A is an RNA virus

Hepatitis A is an RNA virus. Diagnosis is by detection of the hepatitis A virus IgM. The route of transmission is faeco-oral. There is no carrier state and fulminant hepatic failure is rare (<0.1%). Liver function, however, may be abnormal for up to 1 year. Prevention is by either passive or active immunisation. Passive immunisation is with immunoglobulin and lasts for 3–6 months. Active immunisation is with a live attenuated virus, with booster immunisation being required after 12–18 months. Clinical symptoms are initially non-specific and include anorexia, nausea, fatigue and fever associated with epigastric pain and tender hepatomegaly. The icteric phase then develops with jaundice, pale stools and dark urine. Sometimes there is pruritus, depression and persistent jaundice, with raised transaminases for a prolonged period. The prothrombin time (PTT) should be monitored. A raised PTT raises the possibility of severe hepatic necrosis or decompensation of underlying liver disease.

Hepatitis E is an RNA virus. Epidemics occur in developing countries. In the UK infection is usually seen in travellers from endemic areas. The route of transmission is faeco-oral. The clinical course of hepatitis E infection is similar to hepatitis A. Complete recovery from acute infection occurs. Chronic infection has not been described, although acute fulminant hepatic failure can occur and is more common during pregnancy. Diagnosis is by serology. No vaccine or prophylactic treatment is available.

5.29 Hepatitis C

Answer E: Transmission worldwide is most commonly by the vertical route

Hepatitis C is an RNA virus. The route of transmission is most commonly vertical, otherwise infection occurs via parenteral, sexual or contaminated blood product transfusion. The vertical transmission rate is 9%, higher in HIV-positive mothers. Mode of delivery does not affect the risk of transmission unless coinfection with HIV is present, in which case caesarean section in the developed world may offer some protection.

Diagnosis is usually by serology with the detection of the anti-HCV antibody. Blood and blood products for transfusion have been screened for hepatitis C virus since 1990. Infection is usually asymptomatic or an acute hepatitis can occur. Fulminant hepatitis is uncommon but can occur. HCV RNA detection establishes the presence of viraemia, confirming infection and infectivity. Persistence of HCV RNA indicates continuing infection. Chronic infection is common (prevalence 0.2–0.7% in northern Europe, 1–2% in southern Europe and Japan), with the development of cirrhosis and hepatocellular carcinoma in a number of cases after an interval of 10–15 years. Treatment with pegylated interferon plus ribavirin is the currently recommended treatment for children. Duration of treatment varies depending on the genotype of the infecting virus. Good prognostic factors for antiviral treatment are the absence of cirrhosis, young age at acquisition, and absence or coinfection with HIV and/or hepatitis B. Breastfeeding is not contraindicated for HCV seropositive mothers but, if nipples are cracked and bleeding, caution is advised.

5.30 Colitis

Answer D: Non-typhoid Salmonella sp

Abdominal pain associated with bloody diarrhoea is indicative of colitis. Colitis can be infective or non-infective.

Causes of infective colitis:

- *Salmonella* spp.
- *Shigella* spp.
- *Campylobacter pylori*
- *Escherichia coli* O157 (and other *E. coli*)
- *Clostridium difficile* (pseudomembranous colitis)
- *Yersinia* spp.
- Tuberculosis
- Cytomegalovirus
- *Entamoeba histolytica*
- *Enterobius vermicularis.*

Causes of non-infective colitis:

- Ulcerative colitis
- Crohn disease
- Necrotising enterocolitis

- Vasculitic causes, eg Henoch–Schönlein purpura
- Hirschsprung enterocolitis
- Microscopic colitis
- Allergic enterocolitis.

5.31 *Giardia intestinalis* (formerly *Giardia lamblia*)

Answer B: Infection with Giardia intestinalis can cause chronic diarrhoea, malabsorption, failure to thrive and intestinal histological changes similar to those seen in coeliac disease

It is a protozoal parasite that is infective in the cyst form and can grow in the intestines of humans or animals. Infection in humans is more common in children than in adults; the rates of infection in the UK are highest for the 1- to 4-year age group. It is endemic in areas with poor sanitation and commonly associated with outbreaks secondary to food or water contamination. As relatively low numbers of cysts are required to produce infection, outbreaks in the developed world are often associated with day-care settings and institutions. Children at particular risk are those who have travelled to endemic areas or have contact with those who have travelled to endemic areas, those who are malnourished, those with immunodeficiencies (recurrent infection is seen in those with IgA deficiency) and those with cystic fibrosis. Clinical manifestations include:

- asymptomatic infection
- acute diarrhoeal illness
- chronic diarrhoea and malabsorption (may last weeks to months).

Chronic infection may be associated with partial villous atrophy in small bowel biopsy. Diagnosis is by stool examination for cysts or examination of the duodenal aspirate at small bowel biopsy. Treatment consists of appropriate fluid and nutritional management and/ oral metronidazole for all infected cases who are symptomatic or asymptomatic in non-endemic areas. Good basic hygiene procedures are essential for preventing spread.

5.32 Ulcerative colitis

Answer E: Ulcerative colitis is more common than Crohn disease in younger children and in Asian children

Ulcerative colitis is an inflammatory condition limited to the colon. Most children (90%) have pancolitis; the rest have left-sided colonic disease, or proctitis. Ulcerative colitis is a lifelong illness with 50% of patients relapsing in any 1 year. Children with moderate-to-severe disease at diagnosis have a colectomy rate of 25% at 5 years. The histological changes are mucosal and submucosal inflammation, goblet cell depletion, cryptitis and crypt abscesses, but no granulomas. Twenty-five per cent of cases of inflammatory bowel disease (IBD) present in those aged <16 years; approximately 30% is ulcerative colitis. Ulcerative colitis is the most common form of IBD in the younger child. It is slightly more common in Asian children than in other ethnic groups. The sex distribution in childhood ulcerative colitis is even. A family history of either Crohn disease or ulcerative colitis is common in any index case; breastfeeding appears to be protective and certain GI infections may increase the risk of developing IBD. Most patients with ulcerative colitis present with symptoms of colitis: diarrhoea, abdominal pain and blood per rectum. Rarely the disease can present with extraintestinal manifestations, including arthropathy (10%), ankylosing spondylitis (rare in children) liver disease (sclerosing cholangitis, autoimmune liver disease) and erythema nodosum. Growth failure is much less commonly associated than with Crohn disease and the presenting blood panel may be normal. The peripheral antineutrophil cytoplasmic antibody (pANCA) is positive in 70% of ulcerative colitis and <10% of Crohn disease cases.

Complications include:

- Toxic megacolon
- Osteoporosis
- Colonic cancer
- Increased thrombotic tendency in severe disease.

Treatments include:

- 5-Aminosalicylic acid (ASA) derivatives
- Local or systemic steroids, intravenously in severe colitis
- Antibiotics if infection is suspected
- Azathioprine or 6-mercaptopurine in recurrent–relapse or treatment-resistant disease
- Ciclosporin in resistant disease
- Infliximab in severe non-responding ulcerative colitis to delay surgery
- Surgery.

5.33 Recurrent abdominal pain

Answer C: A family history of migraine is associated with a subset of children with recurrent abdominal pain

Recurrent abdominal pain is common in childhood, affecting 10% of the school-aged population. In the vast majority of cases the aetiology is non-organic. The condition is more common in girls and a family history is common. The pain is usually periumbilical and rarely associated with other GI symptoms. Symptoms suggestive of an organic cause include:

- Age <5 years
- Constitutional symptoms (fever, weight loss, delayed growth, skin rashes, arthralgia)
- Vomiting, especially if bilious
- Nocturnal pain
- Pain away from the umbilicus
- Urinary symptoms
- Family history of organic GI pathology
- Perianal disease
- Blood in the stools.

The ideal management is a thorough initial history and examination, to help to exclude the rare cases of organic disease, followed by limited investigations. Once a diagnosis is made classification into one of four subtypes may aid ongoing management:

1. Functional abdominal pain (syndrome)
2. Functional dyspepsia
3. Irritable bowel syndrome
4. Abdominal migraine.

Many cases respond to the acknowledgement of the symptoms and reassurance about the lack of serious underlying pathology. The acceptance by the child and parents of the bipsychosocial model of illness is an important factor for the resolution of symptoms (butterflies in stomach with exams). Diet and lifestyle changes, including avoidance of trigger factors and improvement of associated constipation, increased exercise and a staged programme of school reintroduction if applicable, can prove helpful. The introduction of the concept of pain management early in the therapeutic relationship is often helpful. There are data to suggest that chronic abdominal pain in childhood is associated with the development of irritable bowel syndrome and anxiety disorders in adult life.

5.34 Portal hypertension

Answer D: Portal vein thrombosis

The portal vein carries about 1500 ml/min of blood from the small and large bowel, spleen, stomach and pancreas to the liver at a pressure of 5–10 mmHg. Any obstruction or increased resistance to flow or, rarely, pathological increases in portal vein blood flow may lead to portal hypertension, defined as portal pressures >12 mmHg.

- Alcoholic and viral cirrhosis are the most common causes in the western world.
- Liver disease due to schistosomiasis is the main cause in other areas of the world.
- Portal vein thrombosis is the most common cause in children.

Aetiology of portal hypertension in children

Prehepatic:

Portal vein thrombosis (accounts for 30% of children with bleeding varices); causes include: sepsis, thrombophilia, umbilical cauterization, pancreatitis.

Intrahepatic:

- Cirrhotic (most common cause of portal hypertension)
  - extrahepatic biliary atresia
  - cystic fibrosis
  - α_1-antitrypsin deficiency
  - Wilson disease
  - schistosomiasis
- Non-cirrhotic: veno-occlusive disease of the liver (sinusoidal obstruction syndrome).

Posthepatic:

- Budd–Chiari syndrome: hepatic vein occlusion, usually secondary to myeloproliferative disease or thrombophilia
- Right ventricular failure
- Constrictive pericarditis.

Clinical features of portal hypertension

- Splenomegaly
- Ascites
- Prominent abdominal vessels (caput medusa)
- Oesophageal varices
- Haemorrhoids
- Rectal varices.

Consequences of portal hypertension

Increased portal pressure causes an increase in portosystemic collaterals, resulting in a disturbed intrahepatic circulation. This may lead to the clinical complications:

- Variceal bleeding
- Hepatic encephalopathy
- Ascites
- Hepatorenal syndrome
- Recurrent infection, spontaneous bacterial peritonitis
- Abnormalities in coagulation.

Hepatorenal syndrome

- Acute oliguric renal failure resulting from intense intrarenal vasoconstriction in otherwise normal kidneys
- Prognosis is poor, treatment often ineffective
- In liver failure avoid nephrotoxic drugs
- Prevented by avoiding excessive diuresis and by early recognition of electrolyte imbalance, bleeding or infection.

5.35 Rectal prolapse

Answer D: It is most common in the pre-school-age group

Rectal prolapse is most common below 4 years of age and most cases occur in the first year of life. It can involve protrusion of the mucosal layer alone or all the layers (procidential).

Causes of rectal prolapse:

- Idiopathic
- Increased abdominal pressure:
  - constipation
  - chronic cough
  - toilet training

- **Diarrhoeal disorders:**
  - **– acute infection**
  - **– malabsorption**
- **Cystic fibrosis (20% of patients with CF have rectal prolapse between 6 months and 3 years and CF accounts for 10% of all cases of rectal prolapse)**
- **Neuromuscular syndromes**
- **Rectal polyps**
- **Malnutrition/anorexia**
- **Child abuse (anal sex).**

In most cases spontaneous reduction has taken place by the time of presentation, so a brief examination in the squatting position is advised to try to visualise a recurrence. It is usually painless, although failure to reduce the prolapsed tissue can result in oedema and ulceration. Parents can be taught to reduce a prolapse at home. Patients with this presentation should be considered for a sweat test if no other explanation is forthcoming. Management should always be conservative in the first instance especially if aged <4 years (90%); will respond by 6 years of age. This involves treating any underlying cause and reducing straining through the use of diet and laxatives to reduce constipation. Surgery is occasionally required for recurrent or resistant prolapse or that associated with ulceration or pain; it can be associated with complications.

5.36 Constipation

Answer C: It can be precipitated by a child's refusal to use school toilets

Constipation is defined (NICE guidelines) as two or more of the following:

- Passage of fewer than complete stools per week
- Hard 'rabbit droppings' or large stools that may block the toilet
- Soiling – the passage of smelly loose stools without sensation
- Poor appetite or abdominal pain that varies with the passage of stools
- Pain associated with defecation
- Evidence of retentive posturing
- Bleeding associated with hard stools.

An extremely common problem in childhood (5–30% of all children), it is rarely associated with any underlying medical problem (5%). A vicious cycle usually develops whereby a child associates pain with defecation and then withholds stool in an attempt to avoid discomfort. This retention of stool causes enlargement of the rectum and distal colon (megacolon) to accommodate the faeces, and the normal urge to defecate is lost. Eventually, faecal incontinence (soiling) may ensue. Parents may be able to identify a trigger to the start of the problem, eg a change in milk, toilet training, after an illness or starting a new school.

All children should undergo examination including growth parameters, perianal, spinal, lumbosacral, lower limbs and abdominal examination to exclude underlying pathology at presentation. An abdominal radiograph should not be used to diagnose idiopathic constipation. Treatment involves disimpaction (ideally via the oral route, although occasionally if oral medications have failed enemas are required), followed by establishing a regular bowel habit (both behavioural modification and maintenance laxatives). Treatment is usually required for many weeks or months and must be continued for some time after the establishment of normal bowel habit. Treatment should be weaned down and never stopped abruptly. Seventy per cent of children will become eventually symptom free off medication, although a significant cohort will continue to have symptoms despite long-term treatment. Education and reassurance of parents are essential.

5.37 Pancreatitis

Answer C: It is a common cause of admission to hospital with abdominal pain in childhood

Pancreatitis is uncommon in childhood. In up to 25% of cases the aetiology is unknown. Unlike adults, the most common identifiable causes are abdominal trauma, viral infection (mumps, rubella, Coxsackie B, cytomegalovirus), medication (azathioprine, steroids, sodium valproate) and congenital abnormalities of the pancreatobiliary system. Pseudocysts, a fibrous, walled cavity filled with pancreatic enzymes, complicates between 10 and 23% of cases and is common in those caused by blunt abdominal trauma. Pancreatitis typically presents with epigastric pain (which can radiate through to the back), nausea and vomiting, and low-grade fever. Elevated serum amylase levels are seen in most cases of acute pancreatitis but can take up to 48 h to reach peak levels. Other abdominal pathologies can cause a rise in serum amylase but rarely to the degree seen in pancreatitis.

Medical management consists of rehydration and analgesia, and may also include a period of being 'nil by mouth', sometimes sufficient to require total parenteral nutrition (TPN) (start at 3 days to prevent catabolism). Antibiotics may also be indicated in some cases to treat systemic infection or sepsis. Ultrasonography and CT are the most commonly used imaging modalities, but MRI and endoscopic retrograde cholangiopancreatography (ERCP) can also be helpful. Findings are variable and include a normal-looking pancreas, initially in up to 20% of cases. The length of the illness is variable but most acute cases resolve after 2–4 days. There is a recurrence rate of approximately 9%. Surgical involvement may be required if necrosis, abscess or pseudocyst formation occurs, although most pseudocysts will spontaneously resolve in 4–6 weeks.

5.38 Gastro-oesophageal reflux

Answer A: Addition of an acid suppressant, eg proton pump inhibitor

Gastro-oesophageal reflux (GOR) is defined as the passage of gastric contents into the oesophagus with or without regurgitation or vomiting. Gastro-oesophageal reflux disease (GORD) is when GOR is accompanied by troublesome symptoms. In addition to irritability and vomiting, affected individuals may present with feeding difficulties, apnoeas, failure to thrive, asthma, aspiration, stridor or haematemesis. Oesophagitis and oesophageal strictures may result from more severe cases of GORD.

If indicated, investigation is ideally done in the form of 24-hour pH probe, increasingly accompanied by multiple intraluminal impedance tests, which give information on acidic, weakly acidic and non-acidic reflux episodes, the severity of which does not necessarily correlate with symptoms.

Treatment involves parental reassurance and advice about lifestyle measures. Medical treatments include:

- Alginates (eg infant Gaviscon), which should not be used as sole agents, long term
- Acid suppression:
  - proton pump inhibitors (PPIs) are superior to H_2-receptor blockers
  - increased risk of community-acquired pneumonia and GI infections, particularly with PPIs
- Prokinetic agents; the routine use of these agents is not currently recommended.

Drug treatment is not indicated in all cases, but should be used when growth is affected or symptoms occur with sufficient frequency to cause distress to the infant and/or caregivers. Medical management, as detailed above, should be the mainstay of treatment. GOR may rarely be associated with cows' milk protein intolerance, in which case a hydrolysed formula can be substituted for a 4- to 6-week trial period. In those cases where medical management fails, surgical intervention by fundoplication should be considered. Potential surgical complications and failure rates mean that this operation should be reserved for only the most severe cases.

In symptomatic individuals, resolution of symptoms is usually seen by the age of 2 years, correlating with developmental maturity including a more upright posture and intake of solids.

5.39 Diarrhoea

Answer D: Advice about dietary intake, especially with regard to the amount and type of fluids being offered with further follow-up to assess weight gain

There are numerous causes of diarrhoea in childhood including the following:

- Infection/inflammation
- Malabsorption: transient or long term, primary or secondary, fat, protein or carbohydrate
- Chronic non-specific diarrhoea of childhood (toddler's diarrhoea)
- Not in fact diarrhoea; overflow constipation, fabricated or induced illness.

Any child presenting with chronic (>14 days) diarrhoea should undergo a thorough assessment including a careful history, head-to-toe physical examination with assessment of growth and visual examination of the stool ± lab microscopy and culture, to help guide appropriate ongoing investigation and avoid unnecessary invasive or excessive procedures where appropriate.

Rotavirus is the most common cause of infective diarrhoea worldwide, followed by adenovirus. *Salmonella, Shigella* and *Campylobacter* spp. are the next most common infecting organisms. Carbohydrate malabsorption is most frequently seen secondary to infective diarrhoea. Pancreatic enzyme deficiency causes fat malabsorption, tested for by stool faecal elastase; false-positive results can occur in conditions with villous atrophy or due to the dilutional effects of excess watery stools. Protein-losing enteropathy should be suspected in any child with low albumin and chronic diarrhoea; it can occur in many different disease processes and can be tested for by measuring stool α_1-antitrypsin. Chronic non-specific diarrhoea of childhood presents with the frequent passage of loose stools, often containing undigested food particles, and is common especially in the run-up to toilet training. The relatively rapid gut transit time in children, in addition to an excessive intake of fruit juices/squash (including fructose-containing apple juice), excess fibre, low dietary fat content and emotional stress, can exacerbate the situation. There are never any additional features of pain, blood in the stools, nocturnal stools or associated faltering growth. Parental reassurance is essential as well as dietary advice, including the type and amount of fluids consumed and follow-up until the condition improves

EMQ Answers

5.40–5.42 Theme: Constipation

The NICE guidelines have highlighted 'red flags' in the history and examination of children presenting with constipation, which should alert the physician to the probability of an underlying organic cause to their problem. Red flags include the following:

- Symptoms from birth/failure to pass meconium in first 48 h
- Locomotor delay or leg weakness
- Abdominal distension and vomiting
- Abnormal position of the anus
- Abnormal examination of the spine, lumbosacral region or gluteal region
- Abnormal examination of the lower limbs including reflexes
- Faltering growth (amber flag).

5.40

Answer B: Hirschsprung disease

Hirschsprung disease is due to congenital aganglionosis of the bowel, always involving the anus and extending proximally to a variable degree. Although 90% of cases of Hirschsprung disease are diagnosed in the neonatal period with failure to pass meconium, it can also be a cause of chronic constipation if a very short aganglionic segment is involved. In these instances, a history of difficulty with passage of stools which has been present since birth should be obtained. It is up to four times more common in boys. Associated abnormalities include cardiac abnormalities (2–5%) and trisomy 21 (5–15%). Diagnosis is confirmed by demonstrating absence of ganglion cells in the rectum. Suction biopsy can be performed at the bedside without a need for an anaesthetic, although the sections can be more difficult to interpret than full-thickness biopsies taken under general anaesthetic.

Medical management in the neonate includes close attention to fluid balance and hydration along with colonic lavage. Surgical care includes identifying the transition zone at laparotomy and formation of a colostomy proximal to this (with presence of ganglion cells being confirmed during the procedure with frozen sections). Definitive repair usually occurs when the child is older. Complications of Hirschsprung disease include enterocolitis (in 10–30%), in which the patient is at risk of bowel perforation. Other complications post-surgery include anastomotic leak and stricture formation.

5.41

Answer G: Meconium ileus

Up to 15% of cases of cystic fibrosis present as meconium ileus. Other surgical presentations of cystic fibrosis include rectal prolapse and nasal polyps. Meconium ileus is caused by production of abnormally viscid and adherent meconium. Characteristically the proximal ileum is greatly dilated and contains thick sticky meconium, whereas distal ileum and colon are collapsed and obstructed by thickly packed, round meconium pellets. Infants are often small for dates but associated malformations are rare. In complicated meconium ileus, the dilated bowel may turn and subsequently perforate, causing meconium peritonitis. Abdominal radiographs in these cases typically show areas of calcification. Up to 20% will have a history of maternal polyhydramnios. Treatment of meconium ileus includes contrast enemas to 'wash out' the inspissated meconium pellets. If this is unsuccessful, and in cases where perforation has occurred, laparotomy will be required. Differential diagnosis includes Hirschsprung disease and neonatal small left colon syndrome (seen with increased frequency in infants of mothers with diabetes).

5.42

Answer C: Tethered cord syndrome (neuro-orthopaedic syndrome)

Spinal dysraphism (aberrations of spinal cord development) may present with a variable constellation of neurological symptoms and signs that reflect dysfunction of the terminal spinal cord. These features may be present at birth or, more rarely, develop over time when differential growth between the bony spine and the spinal cord results in traction of the terminal spinal cord and nerve roots, with consequent neurological dysfunction. Muscle bulk asymmetry (buttocks, thighs or calf), leg-length discrepancy and foot deformity (club foot) are among the more common musculoskeletal manifestations of this syndrome in very young children.

Neurological symptoms include pain, numbness and weakness of the lower limbs. Bowel and bladder symptoms may develop because sacral levels of the spinal cord also control sphincter innervation. Urinary continence is neurologically more complex than bowel continence and so it is almost unheard of for a dysraphism to result in symptoms of soiling or constipation without coincidental absence or abnormal bladder control. It is vital to recognise and treat this pattern of evolving neurological dysfunction in order to minimise further deterioration.

5.43–5.45 Theme: The causes of dysphagia in childhood

The differential diagnosis of childhood dysphagia is varied but can usually be narrowed by taking a detailed history and conducting a thorough examination.

- Congenital defects:
  - choanal atresia
  - cleft palate/velopharyngeal insufficiency
  - laryngeal cleft
  - vascular rings
  - tracheo-oesophageal fistula/oesophageal atresia
- Anatomical obstruction:
  - hypertrophic tonsils
  - tumours: lymphangiomas, haemangiomas and respiratory papillomas
- Trauma:
  - external trauma
  - caustic ingestion
  - foreign body
- Inflammation/Infection:
  - oesophageal candidiasis
  - viral and bacterial pharyngitis
  - anatomical effect of deep neck abscess
  - GORD ± secondary stricture
  - allergic eosinophilic oesophagitis
- Neuromuscular:
  - prematurity
  - cerebral palsy
  - Duchenne muscular dystrophy
  - Guillain–Barré syndrome
- Oesophageal dysmotility:
  - achalasia
  - oesophageal spasm
- Vincristine (chemotherapy) toxicity
- Psychological: globus hystericus.

Symptoms of dysphagia may include:

- eating slowly
- trying to swallow a single mouthful of food several times
- difficulty coordinating sucking and swallowing
- gagging during feeding
- drooling
- a feeling that food or liquids are sticking in the throat or oesophagus
- coughing or choking when eating or drinking

- frequent lower respiratory tract infections
- frequent regurgitation or vomiting
- weight loss.

5.43

Answer G: Eosinophilic oesophagitis

- Symptoms overlap with GOR with predominance in older atopic boys
- Dysphagia is common secondary to oesophageal dysmotility
- Skin-prick testing and IgE RAST (radioallergosorbent test) may be helpful
- Acid reflux may be present on pH study
- Endoscopy in conjunction with clinical picture is diagnostic
- Histology on oesophageal biopsy:
  - reflux oesophagitis – more than seven eosinophils per high power field
  - allergic eosinophilic oesophagitis >20 per high power field
- Treatment options:
  - dietary elimination (milk and soya in the first instance)
  - inhaled corticosteroids – take into the mouth and then swallowed.

5.44

Answer C: Oesophageal obstruction secondary to a swallowed foreign body

Just as with inhaled foreign bodies, a history is not always forthcoming and you have to include this in any differential of sudden onset of dysphagia. There have been case reports of oesophageal foreign bodies presenting in children many months or years after the onset of symptoms. Removal is by endoscopy and resolution of symptoms can be dramatic.

5.45

Answer J: Oesophageal stricture secondary to GORD

Severe GORD that remains unrecognised or untreated for a significant length of time may lead to the development of an oesophageal stricture. This is most common in patients with communication difficulties because symptoms can go unrecognised for prolonged periods of time, allowing the development of late complications such as stricture. Strictures may present with symptoms of dysphagia and regurgitation of food immediately after swallowing. Diagnosis of this condition is through contrast studies, endoscopy and oesophageal biopsy, and treatment with endoscopic balloon dilatation can be remarkably effective in reducing and eliminating symptoms.

5.46–5.48 Theme: Vomiting in childhood

5.46

Answer F: Volvulus secondary to malrotation

Malrotation occurs when the normal embryological development is interrupted, so the whole of the small bowel arises from a narrow pedicle of mesentery rather than the long broad diagonal base that is more normal. This non-rotation of the bowel is prone to volvulus (twisting on itself) at any age, from prenatally to late adulthood. The complications arising from malrotation can be very serious, leading to significant amounts of long-term morbidity, including short gut syndrome and mortality. Mortality rates are increased in infants (2–24%), and further increased by the presence of necrotic gut and associated malformations.

Symptoms of volvulus can occur acutely, leading to complete obstruction and variable amounts of gut ischaemia, perforation and peritonitis. Alternatively the obstruction may be intermittent and partial or complete. Symptoms of chronic intermittent midgut volvulus include vomiting (may be bile stained), abdominal pain, constipation and diarrhoea (malabsorption). Third, the duodenum can be obstructed by extrinsic compression from Ladd bands, abnormal folds of peritoneum that attach the caecum to the abdominal wall in patients with midgut malrotation.

Malrotation is quoted as occurring in about 1 in 500 live births. Approximately 40–60% of midgut volvulus occurs within the first month of life, 75% by age 1 year. Malrotation is associated with duodenal atresia (a third of cases) and stenosis, exomphalos, gastroschiasis, diaphragmatic hernias and congenital cardiovascular disease.

Diagnosis is by barium meal to assess the position of the duodenal–jejunal junction; the 'C' loop of the duodenum fails to cross from right to left across the midline. If not clear a contrast enema can be used to clarify the position of the caecum. Management includes stabilisation of the patient, if acutely unwell, followed by surgical correction with a Ladd procedure.

5.47

Answer D: Pyloric stenosis

Infantile hypertrophic pyloric stenosis is a common cause of infantile vomiting, occurring in 2–3 out of every 1000 live births. It is more common in boys and increased further in firstborn boys; a family history is present in up to 7% of patients and environmental risk factors have been implicated. It appears to be an acquired condition, rather than a true congenital abnormality, but 95% of cases will present within 3–12 weeks of birth, preterm babies becoming symptomatic later than full-term infants, leading to a delay in diagnosis. It results from hypertrophy of the pyloric muscle, producing gastric outlet obstruction.

Presentation is with effortless, non-bilious, projectile vomiting. Onset is most commonly between 3 and 8 weeks. The child appears initially active and alert, is losing weight but appears hungry after vomiting. On examination the pylorus may be palpable (olive sized) in the right upper epigastrium in 60–80% of infants, and visible gastric peristalsis may be seen after a 'test' feed. If diagnosis is delayed the infant may become progressively dehydrated, malnourished and shocked.

Biochemical abnormalities include a hypochloraemic/hypokalaemic metabolic alkalosis and mild hyperbilirubinaemia can be present. Diagnosis is by ultrasound identification of an enlarged pyloric wall. Treatment is by pyloromyomectomy (Ramstedt procedure), after resuscitation, stabilisation and correction of any fluid, electrolyte and acid–base abnormalities. Laparoscopic pyloromyotomy has been shown to be equally effective, when compared with the open procedure, and may be associated with fewer postoperative complications and so is increasingly being employed. Most infants recover rapidly with feeding 6–12 hours postoperatively.

5.48

Answer B: Acute gastroenteritis

Gastroenteritis should be suspected with the sudden change to watery or loose stools or the sudden onset of vomiting. A viral aetiology is common. There are NICE guidelines for the diagnosis, assessment and management of gastroenteritis in children aged <5. A thorough history and examination should be carried out to exclude alternative diagnoses:

- Clinical symptoms, frequency, nature and durations should be noted.
- Diarrhoea normally lasts 5–7 days and resolves within 2 weeks; if blood or mucus is present or prolonged (>2 weeks), further investigation should be considered.
- Vomiting usually lasts 1–2 days and resolves within 3 days; if prolonged or bilious, or haematemesis is present, further investigation should be considered.
- A recent history of antibiotic administration, foreign travel and contact with infective gastroenteritis should be noted.

Assessment of dehydration is essential. The presence of prolonged capillary refill, abnormal skin turgor, tachycardia, tachypnoea, sunken eyes and altered level of consciousness can indicate significant dehydration and shock. Children at increased risk of dehydration include:

- <1 year, especially <6 months
- infants of low birthweight
- more than six diarrhoeal stools in 24 hours
- more than three vomits in 24 hours
- not offered/tolerated supplementary fluids
- stopped breastfeeding during the illness
- malnourished children.

If shock is present it must be corrected with intravenous bolus fluids. If dehydration is present in the absence of shock, oral rehydration solution (ORS) at 50 ml/kg over 4 hours plus maintenance must be attempted in the first instance. Only if oral/nasogastric (NG) rehydration has failed or in the presence of continued deterioration should intravenous rehydration be used. Reassessment is vital.

After rehydration encourage breastfeeding (should not be stopped), other milk feeds and nutrition. Consider 5–10 ml/kg boluses of ORS if ongoing losses. Fruit juices and carbonated drinks should be avoided and isotonic sports drinks are not appropriate.

5.49–5.51 Theme: Milk feed products

5.49 Cows' milk protein (CMP) allergy

Answer E: Nutramigen

This is the most common food allergy in childhood. The underlying immunological mechanisms and the clinical picture can vary greatly. In addition to the much-feared, well-recognised acute IgE-mediated anaphylaxis, a more diverse range of chronic clinical symptoms, which may or may not be IgE mediated, may result from immune reaction to the continued exposure to cows' milk prote'n. Eczema, GOR, colic, enteropathy and constipation are increasingly being recognised as part of this spectrum.

CMP-induced enteropathy presents with protracted diarrhoea and vomiting, which may be accompanied by malabsorption and failure to thrive. Diagnosis is through a combination of endoscopy and small bowel biopsy (which show patchy partial villous atrophy), exclusion and challenge. The natural history is presentation in infancy with resolution in most cases within the first 1–2 years of life. Secondary lactose intolerance is common. It is more common in children with other atopic features but specific IgE to milk is not characteristic. Treatment is with an alternative (often hydrolysed formula with trial of an amino acid [elemental] formula if symptoms persist); soya products should not be used in the first 6 months of life due to concerns about high phytoestrogen content and their potential effects on the reproductive organs. In addition there is a high cross-reactivity with soya protein in these patients.

5.50 Transient lactose intolerance post-gastroenteritis

Answer F: InfaSoy

Intolerance of lactose may occur transiently after a bout of gastroenteritis. Lactase is commonly expressed in mature enterocytes at the tips of the villi. Any condition that increases the enterocyte migration rates, eg gastroenteritis, leads to fewer mature enterocytes at the villous tips. The enterocytes contain less lactase and thus lactose tolerance decreases in the post-enteritis period. Treatment is with a lactose-free formula, eg soy formula, if >6 months or other lactose-free formula, for a short defined period, to allow repletion of mature enterocytes within the villi. Soy formula is a less expensive glucose-based formula that may only be used in children aged >6 months (see above). A 400-g tin of Nutramigen costs £8.61; a 900 g tin of InfaSoy costs £7.47.

5.51 Failure to thrive secondary to insufficient calorie intake

Answer C: Infatrini

Infatrini is a 100 kcal/100 ml feed that is based on a cows' milk protein and is suitable from birth up to a body weight of 8 kg. This child struggles to take in enough calories within a restricted tolerable volume. The most appropriate next step would be to provide a calorie-dense formula to see if feeds of 100 ml/kg per day, providing 100 kcal/kg per day, would lead to the vital weight gain without further compromising cardiac function.

5.52–5.54 Theme: Failure to thrive/faltering growth

There is not a satisfactory definition of this state but in general it refers to children whose current weight or rate of gain of weight is significantly below that of other children of the same age and sex. The presence of underlying organic disease causing the faltering growth in this population of children is around 5% or less, the vast majority of children are constitutionally small but healthy. Low birthweight and preterm birth are associated with failure to thrive but are not its cause. Non-organic faltering growth refers to children who fail to gain weight secondary to an adverse environment including those who suffer from neglect, poor feeding/feeding difficulties and stimulus deprivation. The clear organic/non-organic division of patients is too simplistic, with multiple factors being intertwined often to produce the growth pattern of the child in question.

A thorough history is vital to steer the investigation and management of these patients, which should include the following:

- Birth history, including growth *in utero* and problems associated with the pregnancy
- Feeding history – from birth to date (quality, quantity, drinks and behaviours)
- Developmental history
- Past history of infections, GI symptoms, accidents
- Family history including midparental height calculation
- Social history.

Examination should do the following:

- Ensure accurate growth and nutritional status (thin extremities, narrow face, prominent ribs, wasted buttocks due to loss of subcutaneous fat and muscle wasting)
- Micronutrient deficiencies may be accompanied by pallor and angular stomatitis
- General examination of all systems
- Identify signs of underlying disease
- Dysmorphic features may lead to a genetic diagnosis
- Signs of neglect and abuse
- Observation of feeding while the child is hungry, looking for mechanics of feeding, social interactions with the carer and the developmental stage of the child.

Organic causes of failure to thrive include (note that this is the minority <5%):

- GI causes: coeliac disease, cows' milk protein intolerance, GORD

- Renal causes: UTI (urinary tract infection), renal tubular acidosis
- Cardiopulmonary: cardiac disease, bronchopulmonary dysplasia
- Endocrine: hypothyroidism
- Neurological: cerebral palsy
- Infection/immunodeficiency: HIV, malignancy
- Metabolic: inborn errors of metabolism
- Congenital: chromosomal abnormalities
- ENT: adenotonsillar hypertrophy.

Management of children with faltering growth depends on the cause but almost invariably will require a multidisciplinary assessment and support package for improving all the physical, emotional and behavioural aspects that lead to the suboptimal growth pattern.

5.52

Answer F: Inadequate intake of calories

The most likely cause of this child's faltering growth is a suboptimal supply of nutrients due to suboptimal breastfeeding. This is a common situation because support for breastfeeding first-time mothers can be lacking. To treat this child will probably involve support to maximise breastfeeding, including the input of a specialised breastfeeding adviser to help with positioning, appropriate length of feeds and optimising milk supply. In the meantime additional nutrition is required to ensure the health of this baby, often in the form of top-up milk as either formula or expressed breast milk. Further monitoring and intensive support should be able to turn the situation around.

5.53

Answer H: Coeliac disease

This is a classic presentation of coeliac disease, although a minority of the children who are diagnosed with coeliac disease present in this way. This child appears to have been thriving until the introduction of gluten-containing foods at the time of weaning. He appears to have very well-educated parents who have gone to a lot of trouble to ensure that his diet is nutritionally adequate and have followed the WHO guidelines for weaning very closely. A more detailed discussion of coeliac disease can be found elsewhere in this chapter.

5.54

Answer C: Neglect leading to malnutrition

This is most likely to be a case of the child taking too few calories because she is offered too few calories. This is probably due to a combination of factors rather than malicious calorie restriction. The treatment for this child may include a period in hospital to ensure that weight gain occurs when adequate calories are provided, and then support and very close monitoring to ensure that the situation at home for this child and her four other siblings is improved.

5.55–5.57 Theme: Neonatal jaundice

The investigation and management of neonates presenting with jaundice is the subject of NICE guidelines published in May 2010.

5.55

Answer H: Glucose 6-phosphate dehydrogenase deficiency

This is an X-linked disorder, most common in those of African, Asian and Mediterranean origin. Haemolysis can be precipitated by oxidative drugs or chemicals, infection or fava bean ingestion. Heterozygote females can develop haemolytic attacks. Deficiency can vary from mild (>60% normal enzyme activity detected) to severe (<10%). In neonates, phototherapy and exchange transfusion may be required. Advice about avoidance of known precipitants is important for future management.

5.56

Answer A: Biliary atresia

Biliary atresia is characterised by obliteration of the extrahepatic biliary system and should be considered in all neonates with conjugated (direct) hyperbilirubinaemia. Incidence is higher in Asian and black races than in white races, and more females are affected than males. Stools may be pigmented normally at birth and become gradually paler over the first few weeks of life. Appetite, growth and weight gain may be normal. Hepatomegaly may be present early and an enlarging spleen can suggest cirrhosis and portal hypertension. Surgical treatment in the form of portoenterostomy (the Kasai procedure) before the age of 2 months has been shown to reduce the likelihood of developing irreversible biliary cirrhosis and need for transplantation. Complications after the Kasai procedure include cholangitis, portal hypertension and cirrhosis.

5.57

Answer G: Congenital cytomegalovirus infection

If primary infection with cytomegalovirus (CMV) occurs during pregnancy, there is a 40% risk of transmission to the fetus. As only approximately 50% of women of childbearing age in the developed world are seropositive for CMV (compared with nearly 100% in developing countries), there is a substantial risk of congenital infection in this population. Congenital CMV infection may be symptomatic or asymptomatic, although the latter are still at risk of neurological sequelae (especially sensorineural deafness).

Symptomatic congenital CMV infection is characterised by intrauterine growth retardation, hepatosplenomegaly, thrombocytopenia, microcephaly, ventriculomegaly, chorioretinitis and sensorineural deafness. Over 90% of survivors have neurological or neurodevelopmental sequelae. Infection occurs via contact with infected body secretions and hence infection can also occur parentally (during birth or via breast milk). Prenatal acquisition may lead to lymphadenopathy, hepatitis and pneumonitis. Viral culture for CMV can be performed on most body fluids, including blood, urine, saliva and cerebrospinal fluid. CT brain imaging is imperative for all infants with suspected congenital CMV because the presence of calcification has a positive predictive value of identifying those at risk of neurological sequelae.

5.58–5.60 Theme: Rectal bleeding

5.58

Answer H: Henoch–Schönlein purpura

As well as renal complications, this IgA-mediated, small vessel vasculitis of unknown aetiology can also cause purpura, arthralgia/arthritis (most commonly affecting the knees and ankles), abdominal pain, and GI bleeding, testicular swelling and central nervous system involvement including seizures and mononeuropathies. The median age of onset is 4–5 years, with approximately 75% of cases occurring between 2 and 14 years of age. Gastrointestinal complications include intussusception, bowel wall perforation and infarction. Pain is secondary to vasculitic involvement of small mesenteric or bowel mucosa vessels. Systemic symptoms may precede the onset of the rash, which typically appears on the buttocks, thighs, feet and ankles. The appearances of this rash vary from erythematous, macular or urticarial, to blanching papules, palpable purpura or bullae, or necrotic and ulcerating lesions.

5.59

Answer F: Meckel diverticulum

This is the most common congenital abnormality of the small intestine and is formed due to the incomplete obliteration of the vitelline duct. It is located in the distal ileum on the anti-mesenteric border within 100 cm of the ileocaecal valve. It is present in about 2% of the population, but only 5% of cases ever have complications. In 50% it contains ectopic gastric, pancreatic or colonic tissue. The two most common paediatric complications are bleeding from ectopic gastric tissue (secondary to peptic ulceration) and bowel obstruction (secondary to intussusception). Classically the child aged <2 years will present with the unheralded sudden onset of painless, massive rectal bleeding which often spontaneously subsides. Pain may accompany the presentation and many cases may present later in childhood; most children present with rectal bleeding between age 2 and 8 years; bleeding as a presentation in adults is rare, where abdominal obstruction or inflammation of the diverticulum is more common. The diagnosis is often a clinical one but may be confirmed in some cases with a technetium scan which will highlight the ectopic gastric mucosa (sensitivity of 80–90% and specificity of 95%). Management of an acute bleed depends on the stability of the patient. Bleeding may be severe enough to cause shock and patients may require stabilisation and resuscitation before investigation and/or definitive surgical management.

5.60

Answer D: Intussusception

This is a process in which a segment of bowel invaginates into the adjoining segment's lumen, causing bowel obstruction. Intussusception is usually ileocaecal, the origin being either the ileocaecal valve or the terminal ileum. There are two age groups that present with intussusception: most (two-thirds) present under a year (5–10 months) with idiopathic intussusception. Children aged >3 years presenting often have an underlying lead point (Meckel diverticulum, small bowel polyp, cystic fibrosis, duplication cyst, lymphosarcoma, Henoch–Schönlein purpura). The typical history is of an infant presenting with a preceding URTI, leading to spasmodic abdominal pain, vomiting, lethargy, passage of blood and mucus (red currant jelly) per rectum, and a palpable abdominal mass. The presentation is more often atypical, however, leading to a delay in diagnosis and so a high index of suspicion should be maintained for any child aged <5 years presenting with acute abdominal pain because it is more common in this population than acute appendicitis.

Diagnosis is usually clinical with confirmation using plain abdominal radiograph ± abdominal ultrasonography ± air enema, which can be therapeutic by inducing reduction. Treatment includes resuscitation and bowel decompression with nasogastric tube insertion and definitive management by either air enema reduction or definitive surgery (for cases with evidence of perforation or peritonitis). Prognosis in idiopathic intussusception is excellent. Recurrence rates of up to 10% have been observed post-reduction with air enema, most of which occur within 72 h of the initial presentation. Of recurrences 95% will respond to a non-surgical reduction again; two or more recurrences are indicative of a lead point that may require surgical intervention.

CHAPTER 6

Haematology, Oncology and Poisoning Answers

MTF Answers

6.1 Sickle cell disease

Answers: A B C D E

Sickle cell disease is due to synthesis of an abnormal haemoglobin. There are various forms; HbSS is the most common and the most severe. Sickling occurs during hypoxia which causes the abnormal haemoglobin to crystallise, making the red cell stiff. This then blocks the microcirculation, causing infarction. Clinical expression is varied, some patients leading an almost normal life. *In utero* diagnosis can be made by chorionic villous sampling at 10 weeks. Diagnosis at birth can be made on heel-prick or cord blood. This allows early follow-up and treatment.

Crises due to sickling are precipitated by anoxia, cold, infection and dehydration. Painful vascular occlusive crises occur in bone, the common sites being hips, shoulders, vertebrae, and the bones of the hands and feet. Sickling can also result in pulmonary infarction, splenic infarction (causing hyposplenism), gut infarction and cerebrovascular accidents. Treatment of a crisis involves intravenous antibiotics, intravenous fluid, oxygen, analgesia and sometimes blood transfusion. Acute sequestration of blood may occur in the spleen or lung (acute chest syndrome), causing an acute anaemia. An aplastic crisis can occur secondary to infection with parvovirus B19.

There is functional hyposplenism. Prophylactic penicillin needs to be given. Although often large in the first few years, the spleen reduces in size throughout childhood as a consequence of autoinfarction. Nocturnal enuresis is common (45% of 8 year olds). Growth rate is reduced but puberty delayed, resulting in a reasonable final height in most cases. Mortality is low in the first 6 months, peaks between 6 and 12 months, and falls after the first year. In Jamaica, mortality rate is 5% by first year and 25% by 20 years. The most common cause of death is infection.

6.2 Neonatal thrombocytopenia

Answers: A C D E

Causes of neonatal thrombocytopenia are:

- congenital
- TAR (thrombocytopenia, absent radii) syndrome
- Fanconi anaemia
- Bernard–Soulier syndrome
- Wiskott–Aldrich syndrome
- immune-mediated platelet destruction
- maternal ITP (idiopathic thrombocytopenic purpura)
- neonatal isoimmune thrombocytopenia
- maternal systemic lupus erythematosus
- due to congenital infection
- TORCH
- congenital syphilis
- sepsis
- polycythaemia
- drugs, eg tolazoline.

Neonatal isoimmune thrombocytopenia

This occurs in neonates who are platelet antigen (PL A1) positive born to PL A1-negative mothers. Sensitisation occurs *in utero* and first pregnancies can be affected. Maternal antibodies can be monitored during pregnancy, and platelet transfusion of PL A1-negative platelets given to infants at risk. Two per cent of the population are PL A1 negative, 98% are PL A1 positive but only 6% of PL A1-negative mothers with positive fetuses will develop antibodies, and 10% of affected fetuses will have intraventricular haemorrhage with a high associated morbidity and mortality. As a result of this risk cranial ultrasonography can be indicated particularly in these infants, although may not be undertaken in all causes of neonatal thrombocytopenia.

6.3 Neutropenia

Answers: A B D E

Neutropenia is classified as either $<1.0 \times 10^9$/l or $< 0.5 \times 10^9$/l neutrophils. Causes of neutropenia are as follows.

Congenital

- Reticular dysgenesis – failure of development of stem cells
- X-linked hypogammaglobulinaemia – neutropenia in a third of cases
- Kostmann syndrome – severe neutropenia ($< 0.2 \times 10^9$/l)
- Schwachman syndrome

- Cartilage–hair hypoplasia
- Fanconi anaemia.

Neutropenia associated with metabolic disorders

- Propionic acidaemia
- Isovaleric acidaemia
- Methylmalonic acidaemia
- Hyperglycinaemia.

Immune mediated

- Neonatal isoimmune
- Autoimmune neutropenia, eg systemic lupus erythematosus
- Drugs
- Others:
  - infection
  - drugs – chemotherapy
  - Felty syndrome (neutropenia, leukopenia, rheumatoid arthritis and splenomegaly)
  - cyclical neutropenia.

Fanconi anaemia

Autosomal recessive disorder presenting between 3 and 10 years of age with thrombocytopenia and variable pancytopenia. There are many associated features which include abnormal pigmentation, short stature, renal anomalies and learning disability. There is an increased risk of leukaemia.

Chronic granulomatous disease

Chronic granulomatous disease (CGD) is a primary immunodeficiency affecting phagocytes of the innate immune system and is characterised by an increased susceptibility to severe bacterial and fungal infections; it can be life threatening. CGD is caused by mutations in any one of four genes that encode the subunits of phagocyte NADPH oxidase, the enzyme that generates microbicidal (and proinflammatory) oxygen radicals. The condition can be confirmed by the nitroblue tetreazolium test (NBT). The disorder leads to chronic recurrent infections, frequent skin infections, and bone and joint infections. Acute infections need prompt aggressive treatment with antibiotics and prophylactic antibiotics may be used. Bone marrow transplantations can be preformed to treat the underlying cause.

6.4 Causes of bone pain and anaemia

Answers: A B C D E

Vitamin C deficiency (scurvy)

Most cases occur between 6 and 24 months of age. Deficiency results in impairment of the formation of collagen. Symptoms are of irritability, loss of appetite, tachypnoea and generalised bone tenderness due to subperiosteal haemorrhages. Haemorrhage may also occur in the skin, bone, subdural space and gut. Other features include poor wound healing, bluish purple spongy swelling of the gums and haematuria. Radiological changes may be seen in the long bones around the knee, with white lines seen on the ends of the shafts of the femur and tibia. Areas of bone destruction may also be seen.

Langerhans cell histiocytosis

Langerhans cell histiocytosis is the condition previously described histiocytosis X, which encompasses Letterer–Siwe disease, Hand–Schüller–Christian disease and eosinophilic granulomas. Syndromes are identified according to the degree or number of organ systems involved, eg Langerhans cell histiocytosis, solitary skull lesion instead of eosinophilic granuloma. In children presenting with generalised Langerhans cell histiocytosis many organ systems can be involved.

6.5 Acute lymphoblastic leukaemia

Answers: A B C E

Acute lymphoblastic leukaemia (ALL) accounts for one-third of childhood malignancies in the UK. The overall risk of ALL is 1 in 3500 in the first 10 years of life. There is a peak incidence between 2 and 6 years of age with boys affected more than girls (ratio 1.2:1.0). In affected individuals the risk of an identical twin developing ALL is 14–20%; the risk of a sibling developing ALL is 1 in 900. Clinical symptoms at presentation include fever (60%), lethargy, bone pain, bruising, abdominal pain, anorexia and central nervous system (CNS) involvement (2.5%).

Signs include pallor and bruising, lymphadenopathy and hepatosplenomegaly. An anterior mediastinal mass is present in 5–10%. Investigations show anaemia (70%), thrombocytopenia (70%), neutropenia in nearly all patients and a high white count (>50 × 10^9/l in 20%). Chest radiograph may show mediastinal mass, pleural effusions or cardiomegaly. Cerebrospinal fluid (CSF) examination shows leukaemic cells in 5% and implies CNS involvement. The white count at diagnosis is the most important prognostic indicator, with white count >50 × 10^9/l indicating a worse prognosis. Other poor prognostic features include age <2 years at diagnosis, CNS involvement, presence of a mediastinal mass and being a boy. Long-term survival has improved hugely over the last two decades and is now on average 80%.

6.6 Aplastic anaemia

Answers: A B C D E

Aplastic anaemia is pancytopenia resulting from aplasia of the bone marrow with no evidence of extramedullary disease. The following are causes of aplastic anaemia.

Congenital

- Schwachman diamond syndrome
- Dyskeratosis congenita.

Acquired

- Idiopathic (majority)
- Drugs (chloramphenicol, sulphonamides, gold, cytotoxics)
- Ionising radiation, chemicals and toxins (eg benzene, organic solvents, insecticides)
- Viral infections (eg hepatitis A and C, parvovirus, human immunodeficiency virus [HIV], Epstein–Barr virus)
- Pre-leukaemic states
- Pregnancy.

Acquired aplastic anaemia has an incidence of 1 per 100 000 with a male:female ratio of 2:1. Onset is often acute and prognosis can be poor.

6.7 Diseases with an increased risk of malignancy

Answers: A B C D E

- Ataxia telangiectasia: leukaemia or lymphoma in 10%
- Bloom syndrome: risk of leukaemia or other malignancy in 25%
- Down syndrome: risk of leukaemia in 1 in 74
- Fanconi anaemia: leukaemia in 1 in 12
- Hemihypertrophy and Beckwith–Wiedemann syndrome: adrenal carcinoma, Wilms tumour, hepatoblastoma
- Chédiak–Higashi syndrome: risk of lymphoma
- Gardner syndrome/familial adenomatous polyposis coli: carcinoma of colon
- Xeroderma pigmentosum: increased risk of skin cancer
- Neurofibromatosis: CNS tumours in 5–10%
- Tuberous sclerosis: rhabdomyoma of heart, astrocytomas
- Von Hippel–Lindau syndrome: phaeochromocytoma, cerebellar haemangioblastoma and retinal angiomas
- Klinefelter syndrome: breast cancer.

6.8 Bleeding time

Answers: A D E

The bleeding time assesses platelet function, platelet number and vascular integrity. It is extremely sensitive to platelet number. Normal bleeding time is between 4 and 8 minutes. The technique is very precise and the most common cause of a prolonged bleeding time is that this has been done incorrectly, eg too deep a cut has been made or the cuff pressure is too high. Causes of a prolonged bleeding time include:

- Poor technique
- Aspirin
- Platelet function disorders
- Glanzmann thrombasthenia

- Bernard–Soulier disease
- Thrombocytopenia from any cause
- Von Willebrand disease.

If the prolonged bleeding time is not due to a low platelet count then a defect of platelet function should be suspected. Platelet counts of >50 × 10^9/l are usually associated with normal bleeding times.

BOF Answers

6.9 TAR (thrombocytopenia, absent radii) syndrome

Answer E: Digit deformities

Inheritance is autosomal recessive, although autosomal dominance with incomplete penetrance has been postulated.

Clinically:

- Absent radii and other limb abnormalities
- Thrombocytopenia
- Variable other manifestations including cardiac, renal, gastrointestinal and skeletal.

The bone marrow shows myeloid hyperplasia with an absence of megakaryocytes. Haemorrhagic manifestations can range from petechiae to fatal intracranial haemorrhages, but for patients who survive the first year the platelet count tends to stabilise and the prognosis is better.

6.10 Tumour lysis syndrome

Answer C: Treatment includes hyper hydration

Tumour lysis syndrome is an oncological emergency. It most commonly occurs in patients with a high tumour burden such as ALL or lymphoma. It may be precipitated by starting chemotherapy or a single dose of steroids but can occur spontaneously. Rapid cell proliferation accompanied by lysis and cell death leads to release of intracellular metabolites in quantities that saturate the body's usual renal and physiological buffering mechanisms.

Laboratory finding include:

- Hyperuricaemia
- Hyperkalaemia
- Hyperphosphataemia
- Hypocalcaemia
- Renal failure.

Management includes:

- Hyperhydration: potassium should not be administrated until the tumour lysis is under control
- Diuretics if necessary to maintain good urine output
- Allopurinol to treat hyperuricaemia and reduce urate precipitation
- Infusion of insulin/dextrose, salbutamol to treat hyperkalaemia
- Dialysis may be required.

6.11 Hodgkin disease

Answer D: Mediastinal masses can lead to airway obstruction

Hodgkin disease is characterised by progressive painless lymph node enlargement. Lymphadenopathy occurs in more than 80% of cases and mediastinal adenopathy in 60%. Patients may also present with a non-productive cough or complications of a mediastinal mass such as superior vena caval and airway obstruction.

Histopathology of the lymph nodes shows Reed–Sternberg cells which are multinucleated giant cells. Bone marrow involvement is rare, with dissemination to other organs being a late complication.

Associations:

- Epstein–Barr virus (EBV) infection
- Systemic lupus erythematosus (SLE)
- Rheumatoid arthritis
- Ataxia telangiectasia.

Prognosis is good with a >90% 5-year survival rate.

6.12 Chemotherapy

Answer C: Cyclophosphamide leads to late effects on fertility

Although knowing the side effects of all chemotherapy agents is neither possible nor necessary, having knowledge of some of the more commonly used agents and side effects can be useful.

- Cyclophosphamide: alkylating agent; causes myelosuppression, nausea and vomiting. Also can cause cystitis and late effects on fertility.
- Cisplatin: platinum compound; causes myelosuppression (mild), nausea and vomiting. Also can cause renal impairment, neurotoxicity and ototoxicity.
- Asparaginase: causes hypersensitivity reactions, coagulopathy, pancreatitis, neurotoxicity.
- Vincristine: plant alkaloid; causes neurotoxicity, alopecia.
- Bleomycin: anti-tumour antibiotic; causes pulmonary toxicity and hypersensitivity reactions.

6.13 Glanzmann thrombasthenia

Answer B: Its gene locus is known

This is autosomally recessively inherited, with the gene locus on chromosome 7. Pathogenesis is a failure of platelet aggregation in response to ADP, collagen and thrombin. This is due to a defect in glycoprotein IIb and IIIa, both being part of the platelet membrane and deficiency resulting in a failure of the platelet to bind fibrinogen. It is a rare condition and presents in early childhood with recurrent bleeding. Platelet count and morphology are normal. The only possible long-term treatment is bone marrow transplantation. In the short term tranexamic acid can be used to control acute bleeding.

Bernard–Soulier syndrome

This is an autosomal recessive condition. The characteristic features are giant platelets with a reduced life span and hence thrombocytopenia, and a prolonged bleeding time. Platelet aggregation is normal.

6.14 Hereditary spherocytosis

Answer A: Splenomegaly

The incidence of hereditary spherocytosis is 1 in 5000 people of northern European extraction. It is inherited as an autosomal dominant with variable penetrance. It usually presents in childhood with the classic triad of anaemia, jaundice and splenomegaly. The jaundice is unconjugated and worsens with viral infections. Pigmented gallstones are present in 85% by the second decade. Neonatal jaundice is common. Aplastic crises can occur. The diagnosis is made on clinical grounds, by observing the spheroidal cells on a blood film and by the increased osmotic fragility of red cells when tested. Treatment is symptomatic or by splenectomy usually done laparoscopically. The spleen is the site of red cell destruction. Removal of the spleen will reduce haemolysis and the incidence of gallstones. There is, however, an increased risk of pneumococcal and other infections with splenectomy, and therefore it should be ensured that the patient has had pneumococcal immunisation as part of the routine schedule and receive lifelong prophylactic penicillin.

6.15 Vitamin B_{12} deficiency

Answer A: Deficiency can cause ataxia

To be absorbed vitamin B_{12} must combine with intrinsic factor which is secreted by the parietal cells of the stomach. The complex is then absorbed in the terminal ileum. Symptoms and signs of vitamin B_{12} deficiency are:

- megaloblastic anaemia
- smooth tongue
- ataxia
- hyporeflexia
- upgoing plantars.

Pernicious anaemia is the most common cause of vitamin B_{12} deficiency in adults. It is due to deficiency of intrinsic factor and is associated with either parietal cell or intrinsic factor antibodies. These are usually not detected in children with juvenile pernicious anaemia. The Schilling test can be used to assess the absorption of vitamin B_{12} from the gut.

Causes of vitamin B_{12} deficiency include the following:

- Nutritional, e.g. vegans
- Infants of vegan mothers particularly if breastfed
- Inflammatory bowel disease
- Tuberculosis affecting the terminal ileum
- Surgical resection of the terminal ileum, eg necrotising enterocolitis
- Bacterial overgrowth (blind loop syndrome)
- The mean corpuscular volume is raised in vitamin B_{12} deficiency.

Vitamin B_{12} deficiency is rare in coeliac disease at presentation.

6.16 Rhesus haemolytic disease

Answer D: It can present as hydrops fetalis

Haemolytic disease of the newborn occurs as a consequence of the transplacental passage of anti-D antibodies (IgG) from the rhesus-negative mother to the rhesus-positive fetus. This can occur only if the mother has been sensitised. Other rhesus antibodies (eg anti-C and -E) can occur and produce less severe disease. The use of anti-D passive immunisation in mothers within 72 hours of delivery has reduced the incidence of the disease. Sensitisation in the mother (rhesus negative) can occur after miscarriages, abortions and previous deliveries of rhesus-positive fetuses.

Haemolytic disease can occur *in utero* and may produce hepatosplenomegaly, ascites and hydrops (which can be detected on ultrasonography). Screening is done on rhesus-positive mothers at booking, 28 weeks, 34 weeks and at time of delivery. If anti-D antibodies are found the tests are repeated every 2 weeks. If titres are high (>10 IU/ml) referral to a specialist centre is indicated. Titres >100 IU/ml indicate severe disease. If the anti-D antibody titres are high then *in utero* monitoring of the fetus is carried out by amniocentesis to measure bilirubin levels in the amniotic fluid. If amniotic bilirubin levels indicate that a high degree of haemolysis is present, cord blood sampling is performed. Fetal anaemia will be the consequence of severe haemolysis and can be treated with *in utero* blood transfusions. Severe disease is an indication for premature delivery (at 34–36 weeks), the infant being likely to require exchange transfusion after birth. The severity of disease will increase with successive pregnancies.

ABO haemolytic disease

This usually occurs in mothers with blood group O who have IgG anti-A or anti-B antibodies, which will cross the placenta and react if the baby is blood group A or B and cause haemolysis. The degree of haemolysis is generally only mild. It occurs in 3% of births. Phototherapy usually controls the jaundice. Diagnosis is by measuring anti-A or anti-B antibodies in a blood group O mother with a blood group A, B or AB neonate with a positive direct Coombs test.

6.17 Anaemia secondary to chronic disease

Answer C: The anaemia is usually normocytic

Anaemia can occur in any disease with chronic inflammation. Characteristic features include:

- normal MCV (mean corpuscular volume)
- normochromia
- normal or low reticulocyte count
- low serum iron
- low iron-binding capacity and transferrin saturation
- normal or raised ferritin
- increased reticuloendothelial stores of iron.

Several factors are thought to contribute to the anaemia, including decreased red cell survival, inflammatory mediators suppressing erythrocyte production, a blunting of the erythropoietin response to anaemia and trapping of iron by macrophages, reducing utilisation for new red cells. Anaemia is usually not <9 g/dl. Although most cases will not respond to iron, supplements are given if serum ferritin is <50 μg/ml and may improve anaemia if there is coexistent iron deficiency. Anaemia secondary to chronic renal failure is due to absence of erythropoietin production and responds to treatment with recombinant erythropoietin. Ferritin can also be raised and serum iron low as part of the acute phase response

6.18 Blood transfusion

Answer B: Back pain may be a symptom of severe transfusion reaction

Transfusion reactions can be immediate or delayed. Immediate reactions occur in:

- haemolysis
- reaction to infected blood
- allergic reactions to platelets or white cells (causing urticaria)
- pyrogenic reactions to plasma proteins or transfused antibodies
- clotting abnormalities after large transfusions
- circulatory overload
- citrate toxicity
- hyperkalaemia.

Late reactions:

- Transmission of infection, eg hepatitis A, B and C, HIV
- Cytomegalovirus, *Brucella*, *Salmonella*, *Toxoplasma* spp., malaria
- Iron overload
- Immune sensitisation.

Reactions can be mild with pyrexia normally due to reactions to white cells, platelets or transfused plasma proteins, and usually occurring in patients receiving multiple transfusions. Treatment is with intravenous hydrocortisone and antihistamines. If the reaction is more severe the transfusion should be stopped. Adrenaline may occasionally be required. Using white cell-depleted blood or white cell filters can reduce transfusion reactions; this is done in patients receiving multiple transfusions. Clinical features of severe reactions include abdominal pain, back pain, flushing, headache, shortness of breath, pyrexia, rigors, chest pain, vomiting and shock.

6.19 Thrombocytosis

Answer E: Juvenile idiopathic arthritis

Thrombocytosis may be physiological (preterm infants) or rebound thrombocytosis after thrombocytopenia (eg due to disseminated intravascular coagulation, chemotherapy).

Physiological

- Primary:
  - Down syndrome (transient)
  - myeloproliferative disorders
- Secondary:
  - infection
  - malignancy
  - post-splenectomy (absent splenic pooling)
  - chronic inflammatory disease (juvenile idiopathic arthritis, ulcerative colitis, Crohn disease)
  - Kawasaki disease, platelet count raised in second to third week of illness
  - iron deficiency
  - vitamin E deficiency.

6.20 X-linked agammaglobulinaemia

Answer D: IgA, IgG and IgM are all reduced

This is also known as Bruton disease. It is more common in boys. The gene is localised to the long arm of chromosome X. Prenatal diagnosis is possible. The disorder is characterised by absent or low IgA, IgG and IgM. T-cell function is normal. It presents after 3–6 months as the fall in transplacentally acquired IgG occurs. Presentation is with recurrent bacterial infection. There is an increased risk of malignancy as with most other immunodeficiencies. Screening is by doing the serum immunoglobulins in children with recurrent infection Blood group antibodies and the antibody response to immunisations given will also be absent. Regular intravenous immunoglobulin (IVIG) is indicated in addition to prompt treatment of infections with appropriate antibiotics. In some patients prophylactic antibiotics are indicated. Bone marrow transplantation is the treatment of choice.

6.21 Di George syndrome (22q deletion syndrome)

Answer C: It is associated with cardiac defects

This is usually sporadic although familial clustering has been reported. The gene has been localised to chromosome 22.

Clinical features of Di George syndrome are as follows:

- Thymic aplasia/hypoplasia (hypoplasia is more common than aplasia)
- Hypoparathyroidism
- Presents with hypocalcaemic seizures (neonatal tetany)
- Absent parathyroid hormone
- Congenital heart disease
- Right-sided aortic arch
- Truncus arteriosus
- Interrupted aortic arch
- Atrioventricular septal defect
- Ventricular septal defect
- Hypoplastic pulmonary artery
- Pulmonary atresia
- Facial abnormalities
- Hypertelorism
- Cleft lip or palate
- Low-set ears
- Anti-mongoloid slant
- Others:
  - imperforate anus, oesophageal atresia
  - failure to thrive
  - chronic infection (otitis media, pneumonia, diarrhoea)
  - deafness.

The total lymphocyte count can be low, normal or raised. Assessment needs to be made of the percentage of circulating mature lymphocytes by assessing their response to phytohaemagglutinin (PHA). Treatment first aims to deal with manifestations of the syndrome (hypocalcaemia, cardiac defects). In the long term, bone marrow transplantation is the treatment of choice. Graft-versus-host disease can occur after cardiac bypass and irradiated blood products need to be given to try to avoid this.

6.22 Osteosarcoma

Answer C: Usually occurs in the metaphyseal region of growing bones

The male:female ratio of osteosarcoma is 1.5:1.0, with a peak incidence in the second decade. There is an increased risk associated with retinoblastoma, previous chemotherapy and radiotherapy. Tumours occur in the metaphyseal region of long bones, with the distal femur being the most common site followed by the proximal tibia and proximal humerus. It usually presents with pain, and metastases (lung and bone) are present at presentation in 20%. Diagnosis is by radiology and biopsy, with bone appearing sclerotic on a plain radiograph. Treatment is with chemotherapy and surgery. Prognosis is 60% cure if metastases are not present at diagnosis and 20% if they are. The differential diagnosis includes Ewing sarcoma and osteomyelitis.

Ewing sarcoma

This has a male:female ratio of 1.5:1.0. It usually presents in the second decade and there are no known risk factors. Tumours may arise in any bone but are found most often in flat bones (pelvis, chest wall, vertebrae) and the diaphyseal region of long bones. The presentation is with local pain and swelling. Fever and a raised erythrocyte sedimentation rate (ESR) are common. The appearance on a radiograph is of a lytic lesion affecting the medullary cavity and cortical bone. The tumour elevates the periosteum giving an 'onion skin' appearance. Metastases are present in 25% at presentation. Treatment is with radiotherapy and chemotherapy; surgery is not always needed. Survival depends on whether metastases are present at diagnosis and is 20% cure if they are and 70% if not.

Differential diagnosis of a lytic bone lesion

- Ewing sarcoma
- Langerhans cell histiocytosis
- Osteomyelitis
- Lymphoma
- Neuroblastoma
- Metastatic sarcoma.

6.23 Iron poisoning

Answer C: Haematemesis within 2 hours of ingestion

Ingestion of 60 mg/kg of iron may result in systemic iron toxicity. An abdominal radiograph may be useful to confirm iron ingestion because the tablets are radio-opaque. The effects of iron toxicity are dependent on the time after ingestion:

- Stage 1 (30 min–2 h): local effects of gastrointestinal irritation including diarrhoea and vomiting. Haematemesis and hypotension may occur.
- Stage 2 (2–6 h): apparent recovery during which iron absorption and accumulation of iron in tissues and mitochondria occur.
- Stage 3 (12 h): cellular and mitochondrial damage occurs with hypoglycaemia and lactic acidosis.
- Stage 4 (2–4 days): severe hepatic necrosis with raised aspartate aminotransferase, alanine aminotransferase, bilirubin and abnormal prothrombin time.
- Stage 5 (2–4 weeks): late effects with scarring and stenosis of the pylorus.

Investigation of iron poisoning includes free iron levels in serum and an abdominal radiograph. Although investigations are useful, it is important to consider the child's symptoms as a guide to toxicity. The treatment is general and specific. Emesis and gastric lavage are not useful. Desferrioxamine (iron chelator) is the main therapeutic agent available. Supportive treatment needs to be given for hypotension or shock. If free iron is >50 mg/dl or total iron is >350 mg/dl then parenteral desferrioxamine is indicated. Desferrioxamine can cause anaphylaxis; it causes the urine to turn red while chelated iron is being excreted. Oral desferrioxamine may actually promote iron absorption and should not be used.

6.24 Carbon monoxide poisoning

Answer A: CO combines with haemoglobin to form carboxyhaemoglobin

Carbon monoxide is a tasteless, odourless, colourless and non-irritant gas. It binds to haemoglobin to form carboxyhaemoglobin, which reduces the oxygen-carrying capacity of the blood and shifts the oxygen dissociation curve to the left. The affinity of haemoglobin for carbon monoxide is 250 times greater than that for oxygen. Endogenous production occurs and maintains a resting carboxyhaemoglobin level of 1–3%. Smoking increases carboxyhaemoglobin levels. Other sources of raised levels include car exhaust fumes, poorly maintained heating systems and smoke from fires.

Clinical features of carbon monoxide poisoning occur as a result of tissue hypoxia. PaO_2 is normal but the oxygen content of the blood is reduced. Toxicity relates loosely to the maximum carboxyhaemoglobin concentration. Other factors include duration of exposure and age of the patient. Maximum carboxyhaemoglobin concentration:

- 10%: not normally associated with symptoms
- 10–30%: headache and dyspnoea
- 60%: coma, convulsions and death.

Neuropsychiatric problems can occur with chronic exposure. Treatment of carbon monoxide poisoning is with 100% oxygen, which will reduce the carboxyhaemoglobin concentration. Hyperbaric oxygen is said to reduce the carboxyhaemoglobin level quicker.

6.25 Tricyclic poisoning

Answer E: Multiple doses of charcoal therapy can be used

Mortality of deliberate tricyclic antidepressant overdose is 7–12%. Effects of tricyclic antidepressants include the following:

- Anticholinergic: causing tachycardia, pupil dilatation, dry mucous membranes, urinary retention, hallucinations and flushing
- Adrenergic (early): causing hypertension and tachycardia
- α-Adrenergic receptor blocking: causing prolonged hypotension
- Central inhibition of neuronal re-uptake of noradrenaline, 5-hydroxytryptamine, serotonin and dopamine: leading to convulsions and coma
- Cardiac: mainly ventricular tachycardia and fibrillation.

Arrhythmias are the main cause of death.

Treatment of overdose

Initial treatment is aimed at preventing absorption of the drug. Emetics should be used only if there is no CNS depression. Activated charcoal should be given every 2–4 hours. Arrhythmias may respond to correction of hypoxia and correction of acidosis with sodium bicarbonate, aiming for a pH of 7.45–7.55. Anti-arrhythmics are best avoided. Convulsions should be treated with intravenous diazepam. Diazepam can also be used to treat delirium and agitation during recovery. Hypotension may respond to treatment with intravenous fluids and colloid. In overdosage, tissue concentrations quickly rise, giving tissue:plasma ratios of between 10:1 and 30:1. The drug in plasma is extensively bound to plasma proteins and removal by dialysis is ineffective.

6.26 Aspirin poisoning

Answer E: Deafness is a recognised complication

Clinical features

In young children there is dehydration and tachypnoea. Older children and adults have tachypnoea and vomiting with progressive lethargy. There is tinnitus and deafness, and hypoglycaemia or hyperglycaemia can occur. There are three phases.

Phase 1

- May last up to 12 hours
- Salicylates directly stimulate the respiratory centre, resulting in a respiratory alkalosis with a compensatory alkaline urine with bicarbonate sodium and potassium loss.

Phase 2

- May begin straight away, particularly in a young child, and last 12–24 hours
- Hypokalaemia with, as a consequence, a paradoxical aciduria despite the alkalosis.

Phase 3

- After 6–24 hours
- Dehydration, hypokalaemia and progressive lactic acidosis, the acidosis now predominating
- Can progress to pulmonary oedema with respiratory failure, disorientation and coma.

Management

- Gastric lavage up to 4 hours. Activated charcoal for sustained-release preparations.
- Level at 6 hours plotted on a nomogram.
- Alkalisation of the urine to aid drug excretion, adequate fluids including bicarbonate sodium and potassium, with close monitoring of acid–base and electrolytes.
- Discuss with poisons centre.

6.27 Lead poisoning

Answer B: Encephalopathy

Lead poisoning is uncommon but potentially very serious. It often results from pica (persistent eating of non-nutritive substances, eg soil) and is therefore more common in pre-school-age children. Other causes include sucking/ingesting lead paint, lead pipes, discharge from lead batteries and substance abuse of leaded petrol. Lead intoxication can be divided into acute and chronic effects, and results from its combination with and disruption of vital physiological enzymes. In acute intoxication there is a reversible, renal, Fanconi-like syndrome.

In chronic intoxication:

- Failure to thrive
- Abdominal upset: pain/anorexia/vomiting/constipation
- Lead encephalopathy: behavioural and cognitive disturbance drowsiness, seizures, neuropathies, coma
- Glomerulonephritis and renal failure
- Anaemia: microcytic/hypochromic, basophilic stippling of red cells.

Haematemesis occurs in iron poisoning; skin and hair changes are very common in arsenic intoxication.

6.28 Sickle cell anaemia

Answer B: Short stature

Sickle cell disease causes chronic anaemia with multisystem manifestations aside from the typical 'crises' (sequestration, aplastic, haemolytic). First presentation is usually a sequestration crisis in the pharyngeal bones at about 6 months, a dactylitis. The continual ischaemic insults to the spleen result in 'autoinfarction' (and hyposplenism) in the first few years, and a palpable spleen beyond this age suggests another diagnosis. The hyposplenism increases susceptibility to polysaccharide-capsulated organisms particularly pneumococci. It is thought that the relative deformability of the cell membrane protects against malaria.

6.29 Acute lymphoblastic leukaemia

Answer D: Common cell type ALL

Good prognostic signs are:

- female sex
- age >2 years at presentation
- normal white cell count
- common cell type
- normal chest radiograph.

6.30 Iron deficiency

Answer E: Dietary review

Although this could be the picture of small bowel gastrointestinal loss (eg through a Meckel diverticulum), the likeliest (and still surprisingly common) cause is over-consumption of cows' milk which has a poor bioavailability of iron and fills children up, reducing their appetite for high iron-containing foods. Transfusion is not usually required unless the child is significantly compromised or it is contraindicated because by definition the iron deficiency is long-standing and well compensated. Treatment is a change in diet with oral iron supplements at least until the haemoglobin starts to rise to reasonable levels. Untreated iron deficiency has adverse developmental consequences.

6.31 Lymphadenopathy

Answer B: Single supraclavicular node

Isolated lymphadenopathy is generally benign in children. It may be related to infection in the area of local drainage. If multiple areas are involved the illness is likely to be systemic, eg a mononucleosis-like illness, but it is rare even in these cases for diagnosis to require histology. The main exception to this rule is enlargement of a supraclavicular node (due to its regional drainage), which cannot be ignored and is much more likely to herald serious (especially malignant) pathology. In such cases a chest radiograph should be undertaken to look for a possible mediastinal mass.

6.32 Lead poisoning

Answer E: Delayed developmental milestones

Lead poisoning is rarely seen nowadays due to house paints being lead free. Above a certain concentration it is neurotoxic and the developmental effect is only partially reversible by chelation.

Classic features of lead poisoning are:

- microcytic anaemia
- developmental delay
- constipation
- vomiting.

A coexisting iron deficiency is common which first further exacerbates the anaemia and second contributes to increased lead absorption. Basophilic stippling is due to inhibition of pyrimidine 5-nucleotidase and results in accumulation of denatured RNA.

Treatment involves:

- removing source
- chelation
- mild oral D-penicillamine
- severe intravenous sodium calcium edetate (EDTA)
- very severe-intramuscular injections of dimercaprol to increase effect of EDTA.

EMQ Answers

6.33–6.35 Theme: Thrombocytopenia

6.33

Answer D: Wiskott–Aldrich syndrome

Wiskott–Aldrich syndrome is an X-linked inherited cause of thrombocytopenia. The gene is located to the short arm of X chromosome.

Clinical features of Wiskott–Aldrich syndrome:

- Recurrent infections secondary to immunodeficiency
- Eczema
- Thrombocytopenia with reduced platelet size
- Malignant potential.

Laboratory investigations:

- Reduced platelet number and reduced platelet size
- Low serum IgM, normal IgG, and raised IgA and IgE
- T-cell defect.

Acute haemorrhage is a significant cause of death (20%), other causes being infection and malignancy. Survival beyond the teenage years is rare. Bone marrow transplantation offers a potential cure. Prenatal diagnosis and carrier detection are possible in 98%.

6.34

Answer A: Acute idiopathic thrombocytopenic purpura

The incidence is 4/100 000 children per year. Peak age is 2–4 years, and incidence in boys and girls is equal. It is most common in the winter and spring, and often preceded by an upper respiratory tract infection. It is thought to be immune mediated although the precise mechanism is not known. In general ITP is a benign self-limiting illness; in its acute form platelet count returns to normal within 6 months. Management is controversial with US/UK differences in approach. Investigations are determined by the clinical history and physical examination. An FBC and blood film are essential in all cases. Other investigations are as appropriate. A bone marrow biopsy is required if there is doubt about the diagnosis and leukaemic infiltration is a possibility. If performed, this will show increased megakaryocytes. Bed rest is not helpful. Treatment options include steroids, IVIG or nothing. Steroids and IVIG will increase the platelet count in about 12 hours if treatment is required. Chronic idiopathic thrombocytopenia occurs more commonly in girls and is defined as the persistence of the thrombocytopenia beyond 6 months. Treatment options include steroids, regular IVIG and splenectomy. Intracranial haemorrhage is a rare complication of ITP.

6.35

Answer H: Disseminated intravascular coagulopathy

Disseminated intravascular coagulopathy (DIC) is characterised by the consumption of platelets and plasma clotting factors. It is a thrombohaemorrhagic disorder that can be triggered by a variety of clinical situations. With the deregulation of both coagulation and fibrinolysis, widespread coagulation occurs within the vasculature, leading to the exhaustion of clotting factors and subsequent haemorrhage.

Diseases associated with DIC:

- Trauma, eg head injury
- Burns
- Respiratory distress syndrome
- Infection
- Malignancy.

6.36–6.38 Theme: Anaemia

6.36

Answer B: β Thalassaemia

β Thalassaemia is an autosomal recessive condition that is more prevalent in the eastern Mediterranean population. Point mutations in one or both of the major β-globin genes on chromosome 11 lead to ineffective haematopoiesis and increased haemolysis. Loss of one of the β-globin chains leads to β-thalassaemia trait, whereas the loss of both will lead to β thalassaemia major. The severity of the disease depends on the nature of the mutation. Due to the presence of fetal haemoglobin during the first 6 months, presentation is not usually until after the first 6 months of life.

Presenting signs and symptoms:

- Anaemia: microcytic/normochromic
- Failure to thrive
- Developmental delay
- Recurrent infection
- Extramedullary haematopoiesis
- Hepatosplenomegaly.

Teatment involves regular blood transfusions to maintain haemoglobin at a level to ensure adequate growth and development. Iron overload due to recurrent transfusions may need to be managed with the use of chelating agents.

6.37

Answer A: Iron deficiency anaemia

Laboratory features:

- Microcytosis
- Hypochromia
- Low serum iron
- Increased total iron-binding capacity
- Low serum ferritin
- Thrombocytosis (occasional thrombocytopenia).

The most common cause of iron deficiency anaemia in childhood is dietary. Iron is absorbed in the proximal small intestine. It is usually the case that about 10% of the ingested load is absorbed. This can be increased by the simultaneous administration of vitamin C. Iron deficiency anaemia is particularly common in the first year of life. Both breast and cows' milk are low in iron and iron-rich foods such as fortified cereals and infant formula milks need to be taken. The symptoms and signs of iron deficiency include pallor, fatigue, pica and poor appetite, the last exacerbating the problem. Splenomegaly is present in 10–15%. There is much recent evidence to suggest that iron deficiency even in the absence of anaemia is a cause of reduced intellectual performance and that this responds well to therapy.

Treatment is with oral iron. A reticulocyte response should be seen within a few days, and 6 mg/kg per day of elemental iron is required. Chronic blood loss needs to be considered as an alternative cause of iron deficiency anaemia particularly if stools are positive to blood or there are suggestive features in the history.

6.38

Answer D: Glucose 6-phosphate dehydrogenase deficiency

Glucose 6-phosphate dehydrogenase deficiency (G6PD) is an X-linked recessive disorder. It is more common and more severe in boys but girls can be affected. The enzyme protects the red cell membrane from oxidant stress, keeping glutathione in its reduced state. It can present either with an acute haemolytic crisis or as a chronic haemolytic anaemia. Infection, eg hepatitis A and diabetic ketoacidosis, may also provoke a crisis. Neonatal jaundice is common.

Diagnosis is by estimation of the G6PD level (can be normal during a crisis). Its management includes avoidance of precipitating factors and substances/drugs to avoid include:

- Broad beans (fava)
- Aspirin
- Antimalarials
- Sulphonamides
- Dapsone
- Nitrofurantoin
- Nalidixic acid
- Methylene blue
- Naphthalene.

6.39–6.41 Theme: Common childhood cancers

6.39

Answer D: Neuroblastoma

This tumour arises from primitive neural crest cells and can arise anywhere in the sympathetic nervous system. The most common site is the adrenal medulla. Other sites include the cervical and thoracic sympathetic chains.

It accounts for 8% of childhood cancer, and the incidence is 1 per 100 000. Median age at onset is 20 months.

Metastasis can occur anywhere with bone pain, cord compression, mediastinal mass, metastasis to skin, liver and bone marrow, with bone marrow suppression and pancytopenia. Production of catecholamines may cause hypertension and products detected on urine testing include vanillylmandelic acid (VMA) and homovanillic acid (HVA). Prognosis depends upon staging and the age at presentation.

6.40

Answer F: Wilms tumour (nephroblastoma)

Wilms tumour is an embryonic kidney tumour. It most commonly affects young children with >90% being under the age of 7. It most commonly occurs sporadically, although can be genetic, particularly if bilateral, and presents with a painless abdominal mass. Prognosis and treatment depend on staging, with stage 1 having >90% 5-year survival rate. Genetic typing of tumours can also now provide further prognostic information.

- **Stage 1**: affecting one kidney and has not begun to spread. It can be completely removed with surgery.
- **Stage 2**: spread beyond the kidney to nearby structures, but it is still possible to remove it completely with surgery.
- **Stage 3:** spread beyond the kidney, during surgery, lymph nodes or incomplete removal by surgery.
- **Stage 4**: metastases.
- **Stage 5**: bilateral Wilms tumour.

Associated conditions include:

- Beckwith–Wiedemann
- Denys–Drash syndrome
- Aniridia.

6.41

Answer E: Medulloblastoma

Medulloblastoma is the most common malignant brain tumour in children, accounting for 10–20% of primary CNS neoplasms and approximately 40% of all posterior fossa tumours.

Medulloblastomas have a peak incidence between the ages of 3 and 8. It is an invasive embryonal neuroepithelial tumour that arises in the cerebellum and has a tendency to disseminate throughout the CNS early in its course.

Signs and symptoms are usually those of raised intracranial pressure:

- Headache – early morning
- Lethargy
- Irritable
- Clumsiness and ataxia
- Change in behaviour.

If spread occurs to the spinal cord, symptoms of spinal cord compression can occur, eg pain, bladder and bowel dysfunction.

6.42–6.44 Theme: Coagulopathy

6.42

Answer B: Von Willebrand disease

This has autosomal dominant inheritance; chromosome 12 carries the defect. The pathogenesis is under-production of von Willebrand protein, the role of which is platelet aggregation and carriage of factor VIII.

Laboratory features include:

- Prolonged bleeding time
- Normal platelet count
- Normal prothrombin time
- Prolonged partial thromboplastin time.

Diagnostic features include a reduced level of von Willebrand protein, von Willebrand activity and factor VIII activity.

Clinical features reflect the bleeding tendency and include bruising, nose bleeds, bleeding from the gums, menorrhagia and prolonged bleeding after injury. Haemarthrosis is rare but can occur in severe disease. Treatment of bleeding episodes is with fresh frozen plasma or cryoprecipitate, the latter being more effective. DDAVP (desmopressin) can be used for mild episodes.

6.43

Answer D: Factor V Leiden

Factor V Leiden is the most commonly found disorder predisposing to thrombosis in the white population. It occurs due to a single point mutation within the factor V gene; this makes the factor V relatively resistant to inactivation by protein C and thus excessive clotting occurs. In children it has been associated with both cerebral infarction and venous thrombosis.

6.44

Answer C: Haemophilia A

Haemophilia A is an X- linked bleeding disorder caused by decreased levels of factor VIII. It is one of the most common coagulation disorders, with an incidence of 1 in 5000 live male births.

Laboratory investigations show:

- Normal prothrombin time
- Normal bleeding time
- Prolonged activated partial thromboplastin time.

Clinical manifestations relate directly to the plasma level of factor VIII that any patient has; this itself is usually related to the gene involved.

Severe haemophilia A: <1% of factor VIII

- Spontaneous haemorrhages
- Haemathroses
- Deep soft-tissue haemorrhages.

Moderate: 1–5% of plasma levels

- Bleeding after mild-to-moderate trauma
- Some haemathroses.

Mild: 5–25%

- Haemorrhage after moderate-to-severe trauma
- Haemorrhage with surgery.

Haemophilias

- Haemophilia A: factor VIII deficiency (X linked)
- Haemophilia B: factor IX deficiency (X linked), Christmas disease
- Haemophilia C: factor XI deficiency (autosomal recessive).

6.45–6.47 Theme: Presenting symptoms of paediatric malignancies

6.45

Answer C: ALL

An acute limp is a classic presentation of ALL and is due to small vessel obstruction in bones or bony metastases. A good rule of thumb is to always take an FBC and film in a child presenting with an acute painful limp.

6.46

Answer E: Rhabdomyosarcoma

The orbital muscles are a common primary site for this tumour.

6.47

Answer H: Histiocytosis X

Protean symptoms but a hard-to-define rash with bone pain, lytic lesions (skull particularly) and lymphadenopathy are very suspicious. Skin biopsy can help make the diagnosis.

As for the other malignancies:

- hepatoblastoma and Wilms tumour tend to present with an abdominal mass/pain
- medulloblastoma with signs of raised intracranial pressure and cerebellar signs (infratentorial)
- osteosarcoma with bone pain (long bones).

6.48–6.50 Theme: Signs of poisoning

6.48

Answer C: Haematemesis

Iron poisoning goes through several phases if sufficient (>60 mg/kg elemental iron) has been ingested. In the first few (<2) hours there is abdominal pain, hypotension and haematemesis followed by a 'purple patch'. If untreated liver function progressively deteriorates thereafter. Treatment is by resuscitation and parenteral desferrioxamine.

6.49

Answer F: Hyperventilation

Often forgotten but the first phase of salicylate poisoning is a respiratory alkalosis. Caused by a direct effect of the salicylate on the respiratory centre, resulting in tachypnoea. Tinnitus and metabolic acidosis (later) are additional features.

6.50

Answer A: Mydriasis

This is a classic anticholinergic effect. Other signs include:

- dry mouth
- retention of urine
- tachycardia
- abdominal cramps
- flushing
- hallucinations.

CHAPTER 7

Infectious Diseases and Immunology Answers

MTF Answers

7.1 IgE-mediated food allergy

Answers: A B C D E

The National Institute for Health and Clinical Excellence (NICE – www.nice.org.uk – Feb 2011give web reference) have issued guidance on food allergy in children and young people. There are three main categories of food allergy:

1. IgE mediated
2. Non-IgE mediated
3. Mixed.

IgE mediated (main symptoms)

- Skin: pruritus:

– erythema
– acute urticaria (localised and generalised)
– acute angio-oedema (lips, face and eyes typically)

- Gastrointestinal system:

– angio-oedema of lips, tongue, palate
– oral pruritus
– nausea
– vomiting
– diarrhoea
– colicky abdominal pain

- Respiratory system:
  - – upper respiratory tract:
    - – nasal itching
    - – sneezing
    - – rhinorrhoea or congestion (with or without conjunctivitis)

  - lower respiratory tract:
    - cough
    - chest tightness
    - wheezing
    - shortness of breath
- Signs or symptoms of anaphylaxis or other severe allergic reaction.

7.2 Low-level immunoglobulins

Answers A B C D E

Newborns rely on maternal IgG for 4–6 months; adult levels are achieved at different ages for the various immunoglobulins (hence transient hypogammaglobulinaemia of infancy). IgG is the only antibody that crosses the placenta. The transplacental transfer occurs after 30 weeks' gestation. (IgM antibody found in cord blood or at birth can be assumed to be due to intrauterine infection.)

Causes of low immunoglobulins

- Prematurity (<36/40 – transfer is low)
- Excessive loss:
  - nephrotic syndrome
  - burns
  - enteropathy (GI loss)
- Transient hypogammaglobulinaemia of infancy
- Infections:
  - congenital toxoplasmosis
  - congenital cytomegalovirus (CMV)
  - Epstein–Barr virus
  - HIV
- Neoplasia
- Autoimmune, eg systemic lupus erythematosus (SLE)
- Drugs:
  - carbamazepine
  - antimalarials
  - phenytoin
  - captopril
  - gold salts.

The broad functions of immunoglobulins are to bind antigens and set about series of reactions to destroy antigens. They consist of two heavy and two light polypeptide chains, divided into the antigen-binding fragment (Fab) and the complement-binding fragment (Fc). It is the structure of the latter that varies between different immunoglobulin classes. The Fc portion binds to cell-based Fc receptors on complement, basophils, phagocytes, etc. Immunoglobulins in descending order of serum concentration.

IgG

- Most abundant Ig (70–80%)
- Involved in secondary immune response
- Crosses placenta by active transport
- Fc receptors bind to and activate complement via classic pathway and also bind to phagocytic cells
- Four subgroups:
  - – IgG1 and -3 – responses to protein antigens
  - – IgG2 – responses to bacterial polysaccharides
  - – IgG4.

IgA

- Present in secretions – protects mucosal surfaces
- Produced in lymphoid tissue
- Exists as monomer in plasma; dimer in secretions (joined by J chain)
- Activates complement via alternative pathway
- IgA deficiency is associated with:
- Autoimmune disorders, eg coeliac disease
- Infections of mucosal surfaces, eg gastroenteritis, lower respiratory tract infection
- Food allergy.

IgM

- Involved in primary immune response
- Exists as pentamer (joined via J chain)
- Does not cross the placenta
- Activates complement via classic pathway
- Extremely effective against bacteria
- Antibodies to ABO blood group antigens are usually IgM.

IgD

- Expressed on B cells
- Involved in regulating B-cell activation together with IgM.

IgE

- Present in very low concentration in normal individuals
- Binds to and activates basophils/mast cells via Fc receptor, and once bound causes the release of histamine and other mediators
- Levels rise in:
  - – atopic patients, eg asthma, eczema
  - – type I hypersensitivity responses, eg anaphylaxis, acute asthma
  - – parasitic infections.

Hypersensitivity reactions

- Type I – immediate
- Type II – cell-bound antigen and extracellular matrix (eg basement membrane)
- Type III – immune complexes (eg systemic lupus erythematosus)
- Type IV – delayed (eg contact dermatitis).

7.3 Notifiable diseases

Answer: E

As of April 2010, it is no longer a requirement to notify the following diseases:

- Dysentery
- Ophthalmia neonatorum
- Leptospirosis (Weil disease)
- Relapsing fever (*Borrelia* spp.).

Clinicians and diagnostic laboratories have a requirement to notify the Health Protection Agency (HPA) of notifiable diseases. Notification requires completion of a form but also notification of urgent cases by phone. There is no longer a fee payable for notification. There are separate departments for notification in Scotland and Wales.

Notifiable diseases (April 2010):

- Acute encephalitis
- Acute poliomyelitis
- Acute viral hepatitis
- Anthrax
- Cholera
- Diphtheria
- Enteric fever (typhoid or paratyphoid)
- Food poisoning (all sources)
- Haemolytic uraemic syndrome
- Infectious bloody diarrhoea
- Invasive group A streptococcal disease and scarlet fever
- Legionnaires disease
- Leprosy
- Malaria
- Measles
- Meningitis (viral, bacterial, other or unspecified)
- Meningococcal septicaemia without meningitis
- Mumps
- Plague
- Rabies

- Rubella
- SARS (severe acute respiratory syndrome)
- Smallpox
- Tetanus
- Tuberculosis
- Typhus
- Viral haemorrhagic fever
- Whooping cough
- Yellow fever.

7.4 Anaphylaxis in children

Answers: A B D

Anaphylaxis is an extreme and severe allergic reaction, potentially fatal. A very useful website is www.anaphylaxis.org.uk.

Anaphylaxis occurs because the body reacts inappropriately to the presence of a substance that is perceived as a threat. A reaction between the allergen (food, drugs, venom, etc.) and IgE causes a sudden release of histamine and other cell mediators, resulting in an anaphylactic reaction.

Anaphylaxis is characterised by:

- acute and rapid onset of symptoms
- life-threatening airway, and/or breathing, and/or circulation problems
- usually skin changes.

Life threatening problem:

- Airway: swelling, hoarseness, stridor
- Breathing: tachypnoea, wheeze, cyanosis, confusion
- Circulation: pale, clammy, drowsy/coma.

The treatment for anaphylactic shock is:

- removal of allergen
- giving oxygen if available
- giving intramuscular adrenaline (either 10 μg/kg or 0.15 mg for age <6 years). Preloaded injection kits are available eg Junior EpiPen 0.3 mg adrenaline (6–12 years) and adult EpiPen 0.5 mg adrenaline (>12 years).
- Assess airway, breathing and circulation.

In addition to intramuscular adrenaline:

- Nebulised adrenaline may be given to treat stridor
- Nebulised salbutamol will alleviate wheeze
- Hydrocortisone is usually given
- Antihistamine (eg chlorpheniramine) is usually given.

Children with anaphylaxis should wear a MedicAlert bracelet/card and carry their adrenaline with them at all times. After giving intramuscular adrenaline, 999 should be called and the patient should be observed in hospital because there may be a rebound with clinical deterioration after some hours. Those with asthma and multiple allergies are most at risk of anaphylaxis.

Tryptase may be raised after anaphylaxis. Levels of tryptase, a mast cell specific protease, peak at 1 hour after an anaphylactic reaction and remain elevated for 6 hours (in contrast, histamine levels decrease within 30 minutes). Elevated serum tryptase implies either massive mast cell degranulation (eg anaphylaxis) or too many mast cells (mastocytosis). It should be noted that NOT all cases of anaphylaxis result in elevated tryptase (eg may work through basophil-mediated histamine release).

7.5 Schistosomiasis

Answers: A C D E

Schistosomes are trematodes that have a mammal as the definitive host and a snail as an intermediate host.

Schistosomiasis is a very common infection worldwide, which particularly affects children and young adults in endemic areas.

Humans are infected through contact with fresh water contaminated with cercariae, the free-living infective stage of the parasite. Infection is usually asymptomatic.

The manifestations of acute infection:

- Fever
- Arthralgia
- Lymphadenopathy
- Hepatosplenomegaly
- Rash.

This is immune complex mediated.

More serious is chronic infection with retention of eggs in the host and chronic granulomatous injury. The organs affected are the urinary tract and intestine (directly), and liver, lungs and central nervous system (CNS) by haematogenous spread. Granulomas surround the eggs. Cell-mediated responses play a role.

Renal

S. haematobium usually affects the renal tract and can cause haematuria, frequency and dysuria, and obstructive uropathy. Chronic renal failure and bladder carcinoma can result.

Intestinal

S. japonicum, *S. mansoni*, *S. intercalatum* and *S. mekongi* usually cause intestinal symptoms, the most common being abdominal pain and bloody diarrhoea. Other manifestations include chronic liver disease and cirrhosis, chronic lung disease and cor pulmonale, and spinal cord lesions such as transverse myelitis. Seizures can occur secondary to CNS disease.

Diagnosis is by the identification of the eggs in excreta. Eosinophilia is common.

Treatment is by eradication of the parasite using praziquantel.

7.6 Unpasteurised milk, milk products

Answers: A C D E

The HPA website is very useful resource: www.hpa.org.uk.

Brucellosis

Also known as undulant Mediterranean fever (as high fevers spike every afternoon, classically). Caused by the bacterium *Brucella* spp. and treated with antibiotics. It is a zoonosis (acquired from animals). Humans become infected by drinking or eating unpasteurised milk products or by contact with infected animals. Sheep and goats most commonly affected. Cattle and pigs also affected.

Endemic in Africa, the Middle East, south-east Asia, south America and some Mediterranean countries. May cause a chronic septic arthritis.

Listeriosis

Rare but potentially fatal. Pregnant women, and elderly and immunocompromised people are more susceptible to listeriosis. The illness is unlikely to be serious to the mother (flu-like illness) but may result in miscarriage, premature delivery or severe illness in the neonate.

The Gram-positive *Listeria monocytogenes* bacterium is killed by cooking food and pasteurisation. Likely foods contaminated with *Listeria* sp. include: cheese, cold cuts of meat, pâtés and smoked fish, or ready meals that have been pre-cooked and then chilled for some time before consumption.

Meconium-stained amniotic fluid is common, particularly post-term. (However, beware 'thick meconium staining' at <40 weeks' delivery because this may be listeria infection). Consider listeriosis in cases of neonates (or immunocompromised children) with sepsis or meningitis.

Treatment: ampicillin as *Listeria* sp. is not susceptible to cephalosporins of any generation.

Atypical mycobacteria

These are acid-fast mycobacteria that do not cause tuberculosis (non-tuberculous, NTB) or leprosy:

- *Mycobacterium avium-intracellulare* (*Mycobacterium avium* complex or MAC)
- *M. marinum* (fish tank granuloma)
- *M. kansasii.*

They are ubiquitous organisms in soil, food, water and animals, and the infection typically presents as lymphadenitis (often cervical), pulmonary infections and cutaneous infections. Diagnosis is usually by culture (PCR in some labs).

May have weakly positive Mantoux (with no signs of TB) but usually negative Mantoux.

Treatment

This is by surgical excision alone for lymphadenitis. If excision is incomplete or there are multiple sites two drugs need to be taken for 3–6 months.

***Campylobacter* sp.**

This is the most commonly reported bacterial cause of infectious intestinal disease in England and Wales. Infection with *C. jejuni* and *C. coli* is characterised by severe diarrhoea (may be bloody) and abdominal pain and fever. It can develop in undercooked meat (especially poultry), unpasteurised milk and untreated water. Symptoms usually appear 1–7 days after ingestion.

Supportive treatment ensuring adequate hydration is usually sufficient. Antibiotic treatment is rarely necessary. Indications include very young children, and severe or persistent symptoms.

Legionnaires disease

This is an uncommon infection caused by the bacterium, *Legionella* sp. It may cause a lung infection, sometimes fatal, or the milder Pontiac fever (flu-like illness). Outbreaks are usually from artificial water distribution systems (air conditioning, jacuzzis, etc.). Immunocompromised people and those with chronic lung disease are most susceptible.

7.7 Enteroviruses

Answers: A B C D

Group of RNA viruses

- Polioviruses
- Coxsackie A and B viruses
- Echoviruses.

Enteroviruses isolated more recently are named with a system of consecutive numbers. They are the most common cause of aseptic meningitis in children (group B Coxsackie virus and echovirus account for 90% of cases in children aged <1 year). Most common route of transmission of enterovirus is faeco-oral.

- Coxsackie A virus and enterovirus 71: hand, foot and mouth disease
- Coxsackie B virus: the common 'cold'
- Coxsackie virus may also cause myocarditis, pericarditis and pancreatitis.

7.8 Recurrent bacterial meningitis

Answers: A B C D

Cranial defects, spinal dural defects, asplenia and complement deficiencies are all risk factors for recurrent bacterial meningitis.

Increased risk of recurrent bacterial meningitis:

- Cranial dural defect: pneumococcal and *Haemophilus influenzae* b (Hib) meningitis
- Spinal dural defects: coliform meningitis
- C5–9 complement deficiency: meningococcal meningitis
- Asplenia: risk of infection from encapsulated organisms such as a *Streptococcus pneumoniae* (pneumococcus). Other common organisms include Hib, meningococci and group A streptococci.

Consider the following in the management of recurrent bacterial meningitis:

1. CT of the bones and anterior skull base including paranasal sinuses (may also require more sophisticated imaging techniques).
2. Consider immunodeficiency investigations (rare without history of recurrent infection).
3. Note that salmonella meningitis and brain abscesses may require more prolonged courses of treatment.

7.9 Humoral immunodeficiency

Answer: D

Defects in humoral immunity/B-cell immunity result in susceptibility to bacterial infection and are the result of an absolute or qualitative deficit in B lymphocytes. Cell-mediated/T-cell immunodeficiency renders the 'host' susceptible to viral and fungal pathogens. Classic defects of acquired cell-mediated immunity problems are HIV and TB. Inherited defects reduce T-cell mobility, phagocyte function and cytokine production. Candidiasis, chronic diarrhoea and failure to thrive all suggest a serious cell-mediated immune problem. Urinary tract infections and hepatitis simplex virus type 1 (HSV1) cold sores usually have no immune implications. Recurrent abscesses are an indication to check immunoglobulins as well as, of course, fasting glucose.

7.10 Cerebrospinal fluid

Answers: C D

The normal values for CSF cell count, protein, glucose and pressure at different ages should be known and can be found in any standard reference text.

Normal values (from Royal children's Hospital, Melbourne – www.rch.org.au)

	White cell count		Biochemistry	
	Neutrophils (x 106/l)	Lymphocytes (x 106/l)	Protein (g/l)	Glucose (CSF:blood ratio)
Normal (>1 month)	0	≤5	<0.4	≥0.6 (or ≥2.5 mmol/l)
Normal neonate (<1 month)	0	<20	<1.0	≥0.6 (or ≥2.5 mmol/l)

The presence of any neutrophils in the CSF is unusual in normal children and should raise concern about bacterial meningitis. Meningitis can occur in children with normal CSF microscopy and CSF glucose.

If clinically indicated, children who have a 'normal' CSF should still be treated with intravenous antibiotics pending cultures.

The CSF white cell count (WCC) and protein levels are higher at birth than in later infancy and fall fairly rapidly in the first 2 weeks of life. In the first week, 90% of normal neonates have a WCC <18, and a protein level <1.0 g/l.

Red cells are not a normal finding in the CSF of older children, although they may be present as a consequence of the tap being traumatic. CSF pressure rises with age. There are many causes of a raised CSF WCC including tumours.

BOF Answers

7.11 Parvovirus infection

Answer B: Avoid pregnant women, immunocompromised patients and those with haematological conditions

Avoid immunocompromised patients, pregnant women and those with haematological conditions. Parvovirus can cause a transient aplastic crisis (and thrombocytopenia and neutropenia).

Slapped cheek is a mild illness with a rash and mild fever, and occurs in mainly in the spring. It is also known as Fifth disease or human parvovirus infection.

The face rash (reddening of the cheeks) is followed by a lace-like rash on the trunk and limbs; 25% of patients are asymptomatic.

The incubation period is 4–20 days. Children are NOT contagious after the appearance of the rash. Unless the child is obviously unwell, there is no need for school/nursery exclusion after the onset of the rash.

Parvovirus in pregnancy

Most women who are infected with parvovirus B19 in pregnancy have a satisfactory outcome. However, infection before 20 weeks' gestation may result in hydrops or death. Mortality rate from untreated hydrops is 50% (reduced to 18% by transfusion); >20/40 no risk of hydrops.

Other groups are at risk of serious sequelae (haemolytic anaemia and immunocompromised individuals).

Replication of parvovirus in the bone marrow can lead to red cell aplasia. Parvovirus can cause transient aplastic crisis in patients with chronic anaemias, eg sickle cell, β thalassaemia and hereditary spherocytosis. Red cell aplasia and chronic anaemia may occur in immunodeficient patients.

7.12 Kawasaki disease

Answer C: Kawasaki disease

Kawasaki disease is an acute, self-limiting, systemic vasculitis of unknown aetiology that affects infants and young children. The vasculitis involves medium and small vessels. Clinical and epidemiological characteristics suggest toxin-induced superantigen stimulation. Person-to-person transmission has not been documented.

Diagnostic criteria for Kawasaki disease:

- Fever persisting for 5 days or more
- Four of the following:
  - bilateral non-suppurative conjunctivitis
  - polymorphous exanthema
  - cervical lymphadenopathy
  - inflammation of the tongue, lips and oral mucosa
  - oedema and erythema of the hands and feet
  - illness not explained by a known disease process.

Atypical Kawasaki disease implies that not all the diagnostic criteria are met but clinically the child is felt to have Kawasaki disease, and later coronary artery dilatation or other pathognomonic criteria develop. Atypical Kawasaki disease is more common in infants than in older children.

There are no diagnostic tests for Kawasaki disease and, although not part of the clinical criteria, the following findings may aid diagnosis:

- Perianal erythema
- Children are very miserable
- Induration at site of BCG
- Gallbladder hydrops.

There are three stages:

1. Acute stage (1–11 days): fever, conjunctivitis, oral changes, irritability, rash and lymphadenopathy. There is usually a leukocytosis, raised C-reactive protein (CRP), raised erythrocyte sedimentation rate (ESR) and a transient disturbance of liver function in the acute stage.
2. Subacute stage (11–30 days) lasts for 21 days and is when skin peeling, thrombocytosis and coronary artery aneurysms occur. Thrombocytosis is a late feature after week 1.
3. Convalescent phase (>30 days): expansion of aneurysm and possible myocardial infarction. Smaller aneurysms may resolve (60% cases).

   Complications: coronary artery aneurysms occur in 10–40% of untreated patients. Most patients do well, but 1–2% die of cardiac complications, eg myocardial ischaemia. Infants have a higher incidence of coronary artery aneurysms.

Treatment: intravenous immunoglobulin and aspirin

Intravenous immunoglobulin (IVIG) is given within the first 10 days of the illness at a dose of 2 g/kg. This is associated with a reduction in symptoms and the incidence of coronary artery aneurysms.

Aspirin: anti-inflammatory and anti-platelet effects. A high dose of 100 mg/kg per day is used in the acute phase, with a maintenance dose of 5 mg/kg per day in the convalescent phase.

Follow-up: all children in whom the diagnosis of Kawasaki disease is suspected should be referred for an echocardiogram.

7.13 Pneumococcal infection

Answer C: Immunise with 23-valent PPV (Pneumovax)

There should be continued vigilance and early use of intravenous antibiotics for suspected bacterial sepsis.

Pneumococci (*Streptococcus pneumoniae*) are Gram-positive diplococci and there are more than 80 distinct serotypes. More than 60% of the population carry pneumococci in their nasopharynx, most of these being strains of low virulence.

Diseases caused by *S. pneumoniae*:

- Otitis media
- Sinusitis
- Scarlet fever
- Impetigo
- Pneumonia
- Septicaemia
- Peritonitis
- Septic arthritis
- Osteomyelitis
- Meningitis
- Brain abscess.

Pneumovax or 23-valent PPV accounts for 96% of the pneumococccal isolates that cause serious infection in the UK (information from the HPA 2003). Children aged >2 years who are at risk and adults >65 years should receive the 23-valent PPV. Re-immunisation is recommended every 5 years.

The Department of Health has a wealth of information available online (previously referred to as the Green immunisations book) – www.dh.gov.uk and www.immunisation.nhs.uk.

Clinical at-risk group:

- Asplenia or splenic dysfunction
- Chronic respiratory disease: cystic fibrosis, cerebral palsy or neuromuscular disorder with risk of aspiration, bronchopulmonary dysplasia

- Chronic heart disease
- Chronic renal disease (nephrotic, chronic renal failure and renal transplantation)
- Chronic liver disease
- Diabetes requiring medication
- Immunosuppression (antibody deficiency, immunodeficiency, HIV, leukaemia)
- Individuals with cochlear implants
- Individuals with CSF leak (after trauma or major skull surgery).

The childhood immunisation schedule:

- The original Prevenar (was 7-valent): PCV introduced in 2006
- The latest Prevenar 13x is now 13-valent (six extra strains) and to be used by all surgeries from April 2010.

7.14 Immunisation

Answer B: Immunise now = at 8/52 chronological age

Preterm babies may be at increased risk of infection. They should be immunised in line with the recommended schedule from 2 months of age after birth, no matter how preterm they are (www.dh.gov.uk and www.immunisation.nhs.uk).

7.15 MMR

Answer A: Vaccinate with the MMR immunisation

MMR should be offered to unimmunised individuals if there is contact with suspected measles, mumps or rubella. If the individual is already incubating measles, mumps or rubella, MMR immunisation will not exacerbate the symptoms. If there is doubt about an individual's MMR status, MMR should be given. The diagnosis of measles, mumps and rubella can be confirmed by non-invasive means from saliva samples. Notification to the Health Protection Unit (HPU) should be based on clinical suspicion and should not await lab confirmation.

Common events after MMR

Mumps component:

- Malaise, fever and/or rash a week after immunisation (lasting 2–3/7)
- Parotid swelling (1% of those aged <4 years) usually in third week.

Rubella component is likely to cause the following:

- Idiopathic thrombocytopenia (ITP) within 6/52 – resolves spontaneously
- Arthropathy D14-21 (arthralgia or arthritis) – rare.

There is overwhelming evidence that MMR does not cause autism, and there is no evidence that it causes inflammatory bowel disease.

7.16 Menigococcal infection

Answer D: Meningococcal PCR

The sensitivity of meningococcal PCR is not affected by prior antibiotic treatment. Meningococci are Gram-negative diplococci. *Neisseria meningitidis* group B is the most common cause of infection (85%) since introduction of the immunisation against group C in 1999.

Group C used to account for 40% of infection in the UK before vaccine introduction, but is now responsible for <10% of cases.

Group A: 1–2% of cases in UK but is common in other parts of the world.

Peak ages are 0–5 and 15–19 years. Meningococcal carriage rate is 5–15%. Transmission is by droplet spread, and the incubation period is 2–7 days. Symptoms vary from fulminant disease to insidious with mild prodromal symptoms. Mortality rate is around 10% (higher in septicaemia). Early on the rash may be non-specific, but later it may be petechial or purpuric and does not blanch with pressure. One in eight people who recover from meningococcal disease will experience long-term effects – headaches, joint problems, epileptic fits, deafness and learning difficulties. Antibiotics are recommended for close contacts of the index case.

There is a new NICE guideline on the a management of bacterial meningitis and meningococcal septicaemia (September 2010) – an evolving and rapidly progressing rash is a contraindication to lumbar puncture (www.nice.org.uk).

Immunisation

- No vaccine available against group B organisms.
- Meningococcal plain polysaccharide A and C vaccine is effective against A and C. Young infants respond less well than older children. Immunity lasts 3–5 years. Immunity to C group is only transitory.
- Meningococcal conjugate group C vaccine is effective against group C. It is protective in younger children. It was introduced as part of the routine child immunisation programme in autumn 1999.

Schedule

See websites www.immunisation.nhs.uk and www.dh.gov.uk for up-to-date immunisation schedule in the UK.

7.17 10-year-old with rash after New Forest trip: Lyme disease (*Borrelia burgdorferi*)

Answer B: Prescribe amoxicillin (if there is no allergy to penicillin)

The standard treatment course is 2 weeks.

This history is typical of Lyme disease (www.hpa.org.uk). Lyme borreliosis is an infection caused by spirochaete bacteria carried by ticks. The ixodid tick is often found on deer. Late spring, early summer and autumn are peak times for tick feeding (and camping!). At least 50% of infections acquired in the UK are known to have occurred in the southern counties. High-risk areas in the UK include the New Forest, Exmoor, the Lake District and the Scottish highlands.

Avoidance of tick-infested areas, the use of insect repellents and early removal of ticks are important because there is no vaccine against *Borrelia* spp.

Symptoms

The most common symptom is a rash (may appear after 3–30 days, spreading from the site of the bite). The 'bull's eye' rash or erythema migrans (formerly erythema chronicum migrans) may be seen with Lyme disease; it may be painless or can feel itchy and hot. Flu-like symptoms, facial (Bell) palsy, nerve damage, meningitis, chronic fatigue, headaches, myalgia and arthritis may also occur.

Empirical treatment with antibiotics is advised. Blood should also be taken to confirm the diagnosis (with acute and convalescent samples taken for borrelia serology). IgM antibodies usually occur 3 weeks after infection, IgG after 4–6 weeks. Usually the acute phase is indicated by high titres of IgM antibodies.

Treatment with antibiotics is useful for all stages of Lyme disease but is most successful early in the course of the illness.

In general:

- Oral amoxicillin (children >12 years: doxycycline)
- 2/52: erythema migrans and isolated facial palsy (Bell palsy)
- 4/52: Lyme arthritis.

The standard treatment is two weeks

Antihistamines may be tried. Doxycycline is prescribed in those aged >12 years or on an individual basis after microbiology advice.

7.18 Necrotising fasciitis

Answer B: Group A streptococcus

Necrotising fasciitis should be suspected in any child with a history of varicella infection and an increasing complaint of pain and swelling in an extremity or other body area, associated with increasing fever, erythema and lethargy.

Management of necrotising fasciitis to prevent muscle necrosis, major limb dysfunction and death:

- Resuscitate appropriately
- Early and aggressive surgical debridement
- Intensive antibiotic therapy (usually including clindamycin).

Clinicians should be alert to the possibility of increased risk of necrotising fasciitis when ibuprofen (non-steroidal anti-inflammatory drug or NSAID) is administered for varicella virus infection. The mechanism may be by either impairment of the immune response or masking the symptoms of secondary infection, leading to delayed diagnosis and treatment. NSAIDs are cyclo-oxygenase inhibitors and may have adverse effects on neutrophils, cell-mediated immunity and cytokines.

7.19 Orbital cellulitis

Answer C: Commence intravenous antibiotics and organise urgent CT scan of head

Although I do agree with your question I do think in reality you would give the antibiotics before you do the CT scan and so you may want to re wordOrbital cellulitis (may cause blindness and is potentially fatal). The following may be associated with fever, headache and systemic malaise:

- Proptosis
- Pain associated with blurred vision – painful ophthalmoplegia
- Evidence of optic neuropathy (optic disc oedema).
  - Orbital cellulitis may occur as a result of either extension of periorbital (preseptal cellulitis – secondary to sinusitis) or orbital trauma.

Management of orbital cellulitis:

- CT of the sinuses and orbit if intracranial abscess is suspected
- Refer to ophthalmologists and ENT surgeons
- Broad-spectrum intravenous antibiotics ± surgery if there is evidence of an orbital infection.

7.20 Sickle cell disease

Answer E: Salmonella osteomyelitis

Children with sickle cell disease are at risk of vascular occlusive crises (and the long-term complication of avascular necrosis), septic arthritis and osteomyelitis of the joints. This child had a fever, making infection most likely. A normal ultrasound scan excludes a septic arthritis. Post-streptococcal arthritis typically occurs at least 10 days (usually 2–3/52) after the infection has cleared and is felt to be an autoimmune response.

There is some debate as to whether *Salmonella* sp. or *Staphylococcus aureus* causes the most common presentation of osteomyelitis in patients with sickle cell. Salmonella osteomyelitis is rare in children; however, in patients with sickle cell disease it is the responsible pathogen in more than 50% of cases. The differentiation between the much more common bone crisis due to vascular occlusive crises and osteomyelitis is difficult to make. Antibiotic therapy should cover for *Salmonella* sp. and *Staph. aureus*. Adequate analgesia and fluid hydration are important aspects in the management of sickle cell disease.

7.21 Epstein–Barr virus infection

Answer: C: EBV serology

Epstein–Barr virus

Infectious mononucleosis (glandular fever) is caused by infection with the EBV. An infectious mononucleosis-like illness can be caused by other agents including CMV, adenovirus and toxoplasmosis. EBV infection is often subclinical. Clinical infection is rare in the preschool group. Spread is by transmission of oral secretions ('kissing disease'). The clinical features are of fever, pharyngitis and lymphadenopathy. The syndrome often persists for some weeks and a postviral fatigue syndrome can occur. The appearance of a maculopapular rash after the administration of ampicillin is quite characteristic. Splenomegaly is seen in 50%. A smaller number of patients develop mild jaundice and hepatomegaly. Laboratory features include an atypical lymphocytosis, mild thrombocytopenia and a transient elevation of the transaminases. Confirmation is by the Paul Bunnell test or EBV serology/PCR. It is important to realise that, particularly in children <5 years, the Paul Bunnell test can be negative in glandular fever due to EBV infection. In such cases the presence of IgM antibody to viral capsid antigen or PCR is diagnostic. Complications are rarely seen but include splenic rupture, airway obstruction, Guillain–Barré syndrome, nerve VII palsy, agranulocytosis and pancarditis. Treatment is supportive.

Infections commonly associated with an atypical lymphocytosis:

- CMV
- Malaria
- Toxoplasmosis
- TB
- Mumps.

EBV is associated with:

- Nasopharyngeal carcinoma
- Burkitt lymphoma
- B-cell-driven lymphomas.

Differential diagnosis of cervical lymphadenopathy:

- Cervical abscess
- TB
- Cat-scratch fever
- Mumps
- Salivary stone.

7.22 Erythema nodosum

Answer D: Cat-scratch disease (Bartonella henselae)

The oral contraceptive pill does cause erythema nodosum but, with cervical lymphadenopathy and history of a kitten, cat-scratch disease is the most likely diagnosis in this case (www.hpa.org.uk).

Cat-scratch disease often begins with a small papule developing at the site of a cat (often kitten) scratch. Nearby lymph nodes become swollen and can persist for months. Other symptoms include fever, malaise, headache and poor appetite. A blood test for *Bartonella henselae* antibodies confirms the diagnosis. In healthy individuals antibiotics are not recommended.

Causes of erythema nodosum:

- Idiopathic
- Streptococcal infection
- TB
- Leptospirosis
- Histoplasmosis
- EBV infection
- Herpes simplex virus
- *Yersinia* sp.
- Sulphonamides
- Oral contraceptive pill
- Systemic lupus erythematosus (SLE)
- Crohn disease
- Ulcerative colitis
- Behçet syndrome
- Sarcoidosis
- Hodgkin disease.

7.23 Atypical mycobacterial infection (ATB)

Answer D: Atypical mycobacterial infection (ATB)

The key point is that of fistula formation in a previously well-child with no response to antibiotics. Needle aspiration and incomplete excision of atypical mycobacteria result in chronic sinus or fistula formation.

Important differentials of persistent cervical lymphadenopathy

- Tuberculous adenitis
- EBV
- Adenovirus
- CMV
- Cat-scratch disease
- Brucellosis
- Actinomycosis
- Toxoplasmosis

- Malignancies (especially lymphoma)
- Cystic hygroma.

Generalised lymphadenopathy is associated with most viral causes. Kawasaki disease is an important cause of cervical lymphadenopathy. Ultrasonography may be helpful in the work-up.

- TB: often a history of TB contact, weight loss or fevers. Mantoux/other TB testing indicated.
- Cat-scratch disease: history of scratch from kitten (check for *Bartonella henselae* antibodies).
- Lymphoma/leukaemia: usually associated with larger nodes (>3 cm diameter), may be firm, fixed and painless. Look for associated hepatosplenomegaly, pallor and bruising.
- Adenovirus: often associated with flu-like illness and generalised lymphadenopathy (check serology/PCR for adenovirus).

Atypical mycobacteria

These are acid-fast mycobacteria that do not cause TB (non-tuberculous). In children, the most common site of clinically significant atypical mycobacterial infection is the superficial lymph nodes of the head and neck, often the submandibular area or anterior superior cervical chain.

Infected children are usually healthy with no underlying immunological impairment, although there is increased incidence of atypical bacilli in immunosuppressed hosts, in particular those with HIV in the adult population.

Typically presents with a non-tender unilateral swelling in a systemically well child. There is often a delayed diagnosis – initial medical management fails.

- *Mycobacterium avium-intracellulare* (*Mycobacterium avium* complex or MAC)
- *M. marinum* (fish tank granuloma)
- *M. kansasii*
- Ubiquitous organisms – in soil, food, water and animals.

Typically presents as lymphadenitis (often cervical), pulmonary infections and cutaneous infections.

Diagnosis: depends on isolation of organism. Usually by culture (PCR in some labs) – may take weeks (eg 8/52 with 12/52 for sensitivities), and culture may be negative even when atypical mycobacterial infection is present.

May have weakly positive Mantoux test (with no signs of TB) but usually negative.

Treatment: complete surgical excision for lymphadenitis with or without chemotherapy.

If incomplete excision occurs or there are multiple sites, need two drugs for 3–6 months. Clarithromycin and ciprofloxacin have been used.

7.24 Congenital infection

Answer C: Congenital toxoplasmosis

The TORCH screen (toxoplasmosis, rubella, cytomegalovirus and herpes) is often used for the investigation of unexpected small-for-date babies. It is better to test for specific conditions depending on clinical presentation.

Hydrocephalus is a characteristic of congenital toxoplasmosis and not seen in congenital rubella or CMV infections. Microcephaly and growth retardation may be seen in all three infections.

Congenital rubella

- Sensorineural hearing loss
- Microcephaly
- Cataracts
- Growth retardation
- Hepatosplenomegaly
- Petechiae ('blue berry muffin' rash
- Cardiac anomalies
- Bony involvement.

Congenital CMV

- Sensorineural hearing loss
- Microcephaly
- Periventricular calcification (compare with congenital toxoplasmosis: widespread calcifications)
- Chorioretinitis
- Pronounced growth retardation.

Congenital syphilis

High transmission rate; 40% mortality rate if untreated. Consider in a very 'snuffly' child with hepatosplenomegaly and rash. Osteochondritis and periostitis.

Congenital herpes simplex virus

Cutaneous scars or vesicles. Microcephaly and intracranial calcifications.

Congenital toxoplasmosis

When previously uninfected women become infected with *Toxoplasma* sp. for the first time in pregnancy, the infection can be passed on to the fetus and cause congenital toxoplasmosis. There is a 40% risk of transmission if the mother is infected during pregnancy. The risk of infection is higher the more advanced the pregnancy. However, manifestations are more serious the earlier infection occurs. The classic triad of retinochoroiditis, hydrocephalus and intracerebral calcification is uncommon, and the clinical manifestations are usually non-specific. If infection is diagnosed during pregnancy then termination is an option; alternatively spiramycin has been given (see www.hpa.org.uk for flow chart of management in pregnancy). Neither pyrimethamine nor sulfadiazine can be given during the first trimester of pregnancy because both are teratogenic. They are used later in pregnancy. Of congenitally infected infants 90% are asymptomatic in the neonatal period. The infant may develop clinical symptoms months or years after birth, usually with eye lesions.

7.25 Febrile convulsion

Answer C: Human herpesvirus 6 (HHV-6)

HHV-6 (roseola infantum or exanthem subitum)

This is a common cause of febrile seizures in children aged 6 months to 2 years. Sudden onset of high fever (up to 40°C), which abruptly stops at day 3–4, at which point a rash may appear. The rash starts on the trunk and spreads to the face and limbs. This rash is found in a minority of patients. Children can contract primary HHV-6 without a rash. Encephalitis may develop in children with HHV-6 infection.

HHV-6 may increase the severity of CMV infection in immunocompromised individuals and transplant recipients. It induces bone marrow suppression, respiratory failure and other problems in transplant or stem cell recipients.

7.26 HIV

Answer D: HIV

This child has signs of immunodeficiency and the key point in the history that points to HIV is the bilateral parotitis.

Children with HIV can present as failure to thrive or pyrexia of unknown origin, and have generalised lymphadenopathy and/or hepatosplenomegaly with candidiasis and parotitis. They may present with infections secondary to immunodeficiency.

Diagnosis (WHO recommendations)

In infants exposed to HIV, the mother's antibodies to HIV may be found in the child's blood up to age 18 months. Accurate HIV testing <18/12 requires specialised testing. The appropriate resource depends on availability of resources and expertise.

- Age <9 months PCR
- Age >9 months, consider antibody testing.

Note that antibody testing may not be diagnostic in children <18/12. Virology testing is recommended for children <18/12.

Management principles

- Avoid live vaccines including live polio and BCG
- Co-trimoxazole prophylaxis when CD4 counts low (to protect against *Pneumocystis* sp.)
  - highly active antiretroviral therapy (HAART) – nucleoside analogues (eg zidovudine) and non-nucleoside inhibitors (eg nevarapine) and protease inhibitors
  - regular follow-up for growth and development, side effects of treatment.

Of children with AIDS in the UK, 85% acquire the disease vertically. This can occur during pregnancy, during childbirth or through breastfeeding. Current data show that HIV is passed on to 25% of babies born to untreated HIV-infected mothers, but only 4% of treated HIV-infected individuals in the USA. Internationally, the risk of transmission is up to 48% in breastfed infants, but 24% if no breastfeeding occurs.

Risk factors for vertical transmission of HIV:

- Advanced maternal disease
- Symptomatic AIDS
- Low CD4 count
- Presence of other sexually transmitted infections
- Higher viral load.

In the perinatal period:

- Amnionitis
- Vaginal delivery
- Preterm and post-term delivery
- Low birthweight
- Prolonged rupture of membranes
- Invasive procedures
- Breastfeeding
- Maternal immunity
- Cigarette smoking.

Factors that reduce the transmission rate:

- Delivery by caesarean section
- Avoidance of breastfeeding
- Antiretroviral therapy
- Zidovudine (nucleoside reverse transcriptase inhibitor)
- Orally from second trimester onwards
- Intravenously during delivery
- Orally to newborn for 6 weeks.

- Combination antiretroviral therapy to women with more advanced disease or higher viral load (zidovudine plus second nucleoside reverse transcriptase inhibitor plus non-nucleoside reverse transcriptase inhibitor or protease inhibitor). Other antiretroviral therapy is undergoing evaluation.
- Avoidance of rupturing of membranes if possible
- Avoidance of invasive procedures, eg fetal scalp blood sampling
- Passive immunisation of mother and child with HIV hyperimmune immunoglobulin
- Vitamin A supplementation to mother.

Chronic granulomatous disease

This is a rare genetic disorder resulting in abnormality of neutrophil membrane and inability to produce superoxide radicals. It is most susceptible to catalase-positive bacteria (eg *Staph. aureus, Salmonella* sp., *E. coli, Candida* and *Aspergillus* spp. Most common presentation is with severe infections of the skin and lymph nodes with abscess formation. Chronic diarrhoea, hepatosplenomegaly, pneumonia and faltering growth are common.

Di George syndrome

Syndrome caused by 22q11 deletion affecting third and fourth pharyngeal pouches. Features vary widely. Characteristic features: congenital heart defect (especially conotruncal malformations such as truncus arteriosus), palate defects, learning disability and recurrent infections. Thymic hypoplasia (absent thymus on neonatal chest radiograph) results in reduced T cells and increased infections. Hypocalcaemia results from absent parathyroid glands and may cause hypocalcaemic tetany.

Wiscott–Aldrich syndrome

X-linked disorder of B cells (resulting in *Haemophilus* sp. and *Strep. pneumoniae*) and T cells (resulting in herpes, CMV and *Pneumocystis* sp.) causing:

- immunodeficiency
- chronic eczema
- thrombocytopenia (very small platelets).

7.27 Hepatitis B

Answer D: The baby should receive only hepatitis B immunisation (at birth, 1 and 6 months)

Vertical transmission is thought to account for 40% of hepatitis B worldwide. The hallmark of ongoing infection is the presence of HBsAg. The presence of antibody to HBsAg alone suggests successful immunisation; its presence along with anti-HBcAg suggests resolved infection. This is mainly thought to occur around the time of birth.

The risk of transmission is increased to >90% if the mother is hepatitis B 'e' antigen positive: advise immunisation and hepatitis B immunoglobulin.

Hepatitis B immunoglobulin given at birth alone reduces the risk of vertical transmission. The effect of giving active immunisation (hepatitis B vaccine at birth, 1, 2 and 12 months) and passive immunisation with hepatitis B immunoglobulin is additive.

Protection is achieved in 93% of neonates.

Active immunisation does not seem to be affected by transmitted maternal IgG.

Hepatitis B is spread by an infected mother passing it to her baby or by sexual contact or from blood/blood products or sharing of needles, etc. It is important to prevent transmission and be immunised.

Hepatitis B immunisation is indicated for anyone at increased risk of infection, eg workers who will be exposed to blood through their occupation (healthcare workers), people who live in close contact with someone infected with hepatitis B. Also:

- Those with haemophilia requiring treatment
- Prison inmates
- Travellers to countries where hepatitis B is common.

7.28 Visceral leishmaniasis

Answer B: Visceral leishmaniasis

This clinical picture is similar to that of malaria but the key point in the history is the dry, DARK skin – blackening of the skin gave visceral leishmaniasis its common name in India: kala-azar, 'black fever'.

Causes of massive splenomegaly:

- Visceral leishmaniaisis
- Tropical splenomegaly
- Malaria (hyper-reactive malarial splenomegaly)
- Schistosomiasis: symptoms vary with species of the parasite; invasion of the skin may cause a rash – 'swimmer's itch'
- Gaucher syndrome (genetic disorder resulting from glucocererosidase enzyme deficiency – storage diseases. Fatty substance accumulates in spleen, liver and bone marrow)
- (Myelofibrosis)
- (Chronic myeloid leukaemia).

Leishmaniasis

Leishmaniasis is a zoonotic infection caused by a protozoon that belongs to *Leishmania* sp. Leishmaniasis is transmitted by sandflies (not found on beaches but in forests/stone or mud walls). Reported by US troops stationed in Saudia Arabia and Iraq, and also soldiers in Afghanistan.

- Cutaneous (*Leishmania tropica* and *L. brasiliensis*):
  - 90% in Afghanistan, Iran, Peru, Saudia Arabia
  - presents as skin lesion that develop weeks or months after infection; round ulcers to granulation-based ulcers
  - diagnosis: skin smear with Giemsa stain and microscopy
- Diffuse cutaneous:

– mucocutaneous: 90% in S. America
– visceral (*L. donovani, L. infantum* and *L. chagasi*): the most serious and potentially fatal; presents with fevers, weight loss, splenomegaly (may be massive), thrombocytopenia, anaemia, leukopenia and hypergammglobulinaemia
– disease of reticuloendothelial system – mainly India, Bangladesh, S . America, Middle East and Africa.

Visceral and cutaneous are the types most commonly diagnosed in the UK.

The incidence of leishmaniasis is increasing because of environmental changes (urbanisation) that increase exposure to the sandfly. Co-infection with HIV has led to the spread of leishmaniasis, typically a rural disease, to cities. Leishmaniasis accelerates the onset of AIDS in those with HIV.

Diagnosis

By direct visualisation of Leishman–Donovan bodies, stains with Giemsa or culture. PCR and serology may be helpful.

Prevention

No vaccine for prevention currently. Insect avoidance measures. Impregnate mosquito net with permethrin.

Treatment

Refer to specialist tropical centre. Several treatment options including sodium stibogluconate (pentivalent antimonial) and amphotericin have been used.

7.29 Farm visits and hand washing/gels

Answer D: Handwashing with hot running water and soap, drying followed by sanitising hand gels may provide extra benefit

Washing hands in hot running water with soap followed by careful drying and the application of hand gels is recommended.

The HPA (April 2010) reviewed infections between 1992 and 2009. Diarrhoea, and even haemolytic uraemic syndrome, have been linked with petting farms. Hand gels and wipes are not effective in killing *E. coli* or *Cryptosporidium* sp., which can be found in animal droppings and on contaminated surfaces around farms.

7.30 Malaria

Answer E: Thick and thin films

Flu-like symptoms of lethargy, headache and myalgia, with diarrhoea and fever are malaria until proven otherwise in a child who has been to an infected area. Malaria should be suspected if symptoms occur within a year of return from infected area.

Malaria is a potentially fatal disease caused by the bite of an infected female (*Anopheles*) mosquito with the protozoon, *Plasmodium* sp. Malaria is one of the leading causes of death in the world.

- Thick film = quick diagnosis
- Thin film = species identification.

The gold standard is a thick film because it screens a greater quantity of blood than a thin film but the appearance of the organism is distorted. Thin films allow species identification. The film should be repeated if there is any doubt. Blood cultures are important because the malaria screen may prove negative.

Malaria

Fever along with flu-like symptoms are common. Be aware of the predominance of gastrointestinal symptoms. Incorrect or delayed diagnosis is often made assuming viral illnesses, influenza, gastroenteritis and hepatitis. Pallor, splenomegaly and thrombocytopenia are late presentations.

Poor prognostic features for malaria:

- Altered conscious level
- Seizures
- Prostration (inability to sit/stand normally)
- Respiratory distress
- Metabolic acidosis
- Haemoglobin <5 g/l.

Hypoglycaemia is common and is exacerbated by quinine treatment (which stimulates insulin secretion).

Treatment of falciparum:

- Broad-spectrum intravenous antibiotic cover
- Intravenous quinine
- Then oral quinine for 1/52
- + Fansidar (sulfadoxine pyrimethamine).

7.31 Vivax malaria

Answer A: Contact specialist for advice

Tropical medicine or Infectious disease units should guide management because this is a rare condition in the UK. The recommended treatment for vivax is to start chloroquine and test for G6PD (before starting primaquine which prevents hepatic relapse).

The WHO estimates that half the world's population (3.3 billion people) are at risk from malaria with almost a million deaths a year.

Of malaria cases in the UK 90% are acquired in Africa, the majority in West Africa; 55% are from Nigeria. The rest of the cases are mainly from the Indian subcontinent. There is a seasonal peak coinciding with school holidays. Most cases in England are in children of African descent, born in the UK, who travel to Africa to visit family.

Falciparum is the most severe and potentially fatal and requires quinine therapy (intravenous, if severe). In London, 80–90% of cases are due to falciparum, whereas in Birmingham more cases are due to vivax.

Incubation

Falciparum: symptoms can occur within a week of being bitten. Usually present within 1 month. Note that vivax and ovale may have an incubation period of years. Think of malaria even if antimalarial treatment was taken. Nothing guarantees 100% protection against malaria.

Advice to patients:

- Bite avoidance
- Malaria prevention treatment and finish course
- See doctor immediately with any symptoms (fever) while abroad or for a year after return.

Mistaking malaria for influenza and delay in seeing a doctor increase risk of dying from malaria.

7.32 Chédiak–Higashi syndrome

Answer B: Partial oculocutaneous albinism

Chédiak–Higashi syndrome

This is a rare autosomal recessive disease of the immune and nervous systems characterised by pale hair, eyes and skin. Children have albinism due to lack of melanocytes in skin and hair (silvery hair), often complain of photophobia, may bruise easily and have recurrent infections.

Giant granules disable chemotaxis and bactericidal properties in skin and white cells.

Diagnosis: confirmed by bone marrow smears that show 'giant inclusion bodies'. Prenatal diagnosis is also possible (examination of hair from fetal scalp biopsy and of fetal blood).

Genetic testing may show mutations on the *CHS1* gene. There is no specific treatment. Bone marrow transplantations have been successful in several patients. Death often occurs in the first 10 years of life, from chronic infections or accelerated disease that results in lymphoma-like illness (thought to be triggered by a viral, eg EBV, infection).

Cherry-red spots (macula)

The cherry-red spot sign was first used to describe the findings in Tay–Sachs disease (lipid storage disorder). The relative transparency of the macula allows the red choroid below to be seen.

Cherry red spots are seen in a number of conditions:

- Metabolic storage diseases (Tay–Sachs disease, Niemann–Pick disease, etc.)
- Central retinal artery occlusion
- Drug toxicity (quinine, dapsone)
- Poisoning (carbon monoxide, methanol).

7.33 Liver abscess

Answer C: Nitroblue tetrazolium test (NBT).

When liver abscesses are seen in children and adolescents, an underlying immunodeficiency, severe malnutrition or trauma often co-exists.

Immunodeficiency should be suspected with osteomyelitis and a hepatic abscess. Chronic granulomatous disease is likely in this case and is confirmed by the NBT test.

Neutrophil defects

Neutrophil defects may be congenital (see below) or acquired (due to bone marrow dysfunction). Defects may occur in any of the various steps: recognition, chemotaxis, adherence, ingestion, degranulation and killing.

Qualitative congenital disorders, ie neutrophil function disorders include the following.

Chronic granulomatous disease

Neutrophils ingest but not are able of killing bacteria (catalase positive, including *Staph. aureus*, *Salmonella* sp., *E. coli*, *Candida* and *Aspergillus* spp.). Due to abnormalities in NADPH (nicotinamide adenosine dinucleotide phosphate) oxidase (reduced form), cells are unable to generate the respiratory burst (which normally produces oxygen radicals for bacterial killing). The incidence of 1 in 1000 000, and it is X linked in 50–70% and autosomal recessive (chromosome 7) in 30–40%.

Presentation: first 3 years of life with skin infections, pneumonias, osteomyelitis (especially of small bones), abscesses, persistent lymphadenopathy and hepatosplenomegaly, and uncommon organisms.

Investigation: NBT test (yellow dye fails to turn blue when added to neutrophils due to failure of respiratory burst). The actual neutrophil numbers may be normal or increased.

Management: prophylactic antibiotics and antifungals with aggressive treatment of infections. Bone marrow transplantation is an option.

Liver abscesses in children should raise the possibility of immunodeficiency. Surgical, radiology and infectious disease/microbiology input is vital.

Leukocyte adhesion deficiency (lazy leukocyte syndrome)

This is autosomal recessive with defects in adherence, chemotaxis and phagocytosis.

T-cell cytotoxicity

- Delayed separation and infection of umbilical cord.
- Recurrent infections with absent pus (neutrophils do not accumulate at infection site)
- gingivitis
- neutrophilia that may resemble a leukaemoid reaction (chemotaxis failure).

Myeloperoxidase deficiency

This is an autosomal recessive condition with defects in activity against bacteria and fungi. There is persistent candidiasis.

7.34 Infliximab and Crohn disease

Answer E: If you develop a fever, bruise or bleed easily or look very pale, call a doctor urgently

It is important that patients and their families are aware of the potential complications of infliximab: infliximab is a drug that blocks a protein called TNF. TNF is produced by cells of the immune system to allow inflammation. Infliximab is given as a drip (infusion) into the vein which usually takes 2 hours. The complete course of treatment is spread out over several weeks. The more common side effects are a blocked or runny nose, headache, dizziness and abdominal pain. In some people taking infliximab, the body may be unable to produce enough cells to fight infection or stop bleeding – urgent medical attention should then be sought.

Most centres provide an extensive patient information leaflet.

Tumour necrosis factor

TNF is one of a number of cytokines involved in the inflammatory process, having a wide range of functions, many in combination with other cytokines especially interleukin (IL)-1. Its name originates from early studies of its cytotoxic effect on tumours, although it can, in fact, encourage tumour growth.

It exists in two forms.

TNF-α is synthesised by many cells including macrophages, T and B lymphocytes, eosinophils, natural killer cells, astrocytes and Kupffer cells. Key role in immune responses to bacteria, viruses, immunocomplexes, C5a, other cytokines, oxygen intermediates, and in Crohn disease, rheumatoid arthritis and multiple sclerosis. Together with interferon-γ it is cytotoxic to many tumours (used as chemotherapy in melanomas). Plays a part in the processes of septic shock, multiorgan failure and cerebral malaria.

TNF-β is synthesised by activated T and B lymphocytes. It has a wide range of functions including actions on lymphocytes, and endothelial, neuronal and bone cells.

Infliximab is the monoclonal antibody against TNF. It binds to TNF-α and is used in Crohn disease, juvenile idiopathic arthritis (JIA) and rheumatoid arthritis (RA). Infliximab may make a person more susceptible to food-borne infections such as those caused by *Salmonella* and *Listeria* spp. Live vaccines should be avoided when a patient is on infliximab therapy. There is an increased risk of lymphoma and other cancers associated with Infliximab.

Etanercept inhibits the action of TNF-α by targeting the TNF-α receptor; used in JIA and RA.

7.35 SLE

Answer D: Anti-double-stranded DNA: SLE

The history of fever, weight loss and lack of appetite could fit with Crohn disease, for which upper and lower endoscopy with biopsy are indicated. The lethargy may be secondary to hypothyroidism. The history could fit with JIA (positive antinuclear antibodies or ANAs); however, the key point in the history is the photosensitive rash. SLE is the diagnosis that encompasses all the symptoms in this case.

SLE

Anti-double-stranded DNA is highly specific for SLE; it has 60% sensitivity for lupus nephritis and CNS lupus, and correlates with disease activity. Anti-cardiolipin antibody is often present and reflects a thrombotic tendency. The combination of a high ESR and low CRP is highly suggestive of SLE (and Sjögren syndrome). (Note that in the presence of a coexisting infection CRP will also be raised.)
Twenty per cent of SLE cases begin in childhood. There is a higher incidence in dark-skinned racial groups. The female:male ratio is 8:1. HLA (human leukocyte antigen) associations are HLA-B8, HLA-DW2/DR3 and HLA-DW2/DR2. The onset can be insidious or acute.

Early features usually include fever, malaise, arthralgia and a rash. There are many other manifestations and many organ systems can be involved.

Neonatal lupus erythematosus (NLE) is a rare disorder caused by transplacental passage of maternal autoantibodies. Only 1% of infants with maternal autoantibodies develop NLE. If a mother with anti-Ro autoantibodies has one child with NLE, the incidence in subsequent pregnancies is approximately 25%. The incidence of congenital heart block is 15–30% in infants with NLE. The presence of maternal anti-Ro and anti-La antibodies increases the risk of having neonatal lupus.

Drug-induced SLE

Certain drugs can induce SLE and ANA positivity and these include anticonvulsants, hydralazine, sulphonamides and procainamide. The disease tends to run a milder course. CNS and renal involvement are unusual.

Causes of ANA positivity in children:

- Juvenile chronic arthritis (particularly the pauciarticular type, ANA positivity associated with eye disease)
- Chronic active hepatitis
- Scleroderma
- Mixed connective tissue disease
- Drugs
- EBV infection
- Chronic active hepatitis.

Causes of antineutrophil cytoplasmic antibodies (ANCAs):

- Ulcerative colitis
- Crescentic glomerulonephritis
- Cholangitis
- Wegner granulomatosis
- Churg–Strauss syndrome
- Drug-induced vasculitis

7.36 Anaphylaxis

Answer E: Give intramuscular adrenaline

This child has severe respiratory complications in her upper airway and has generalised urticaria indicating anaphylaxis. She needs urgent intramuscular adrenaline. The likely allergen is a food – possibly nuts in a cake or chocolate eaten at the party.

Anaphylaxis is an extreme and severe allergic reaction that is potentially fatal. It is caused by degranulation of mast cells mediated by IgE. Anaphylaxis can be triggered by any of a very broad range of allergens, the most common being food (children), drugs (adults) and venom.

Features of anaphylaxis

- Acute and rapid onset of symptoms:
  - life-threatening airway, and/or breathing, and/or circulation problems
  - usually skin changes
- Life-threatening problems requiring intramuscular adrenaline
- Life-threatening airway: swelling, hoarseness, stridor
- Life-threatening breathing: tachypnoea, wheeze, cyanosis, confusion
- Life-threatening circulation: pale, clammy, drowsy/coma.

For a more detailed algorithm of anaphylaxis management refer to www.aplsonline.com.

Antihistamines and hydrocortisone are recommended in the treatment of anaphylaxis.

Dial 999 after administration of adrenaline because there may be a return of symptoms requiring further treatment.

A very useful is website anaphylaxis.org.uk.

Children with anaphylaxis should wear a MedicAlert bracelet/card and carry their adrenaline with them at all times.

The most commonly prescribed autoinjector is the EpiPen (there is also an Anapen autoinjector):

- EpiPen junior: 0.15 mg adrenaline (<6 years)
- EpiPen: 0.3 mg adrenaline (6–12 years)
- Intramuscular adrenaline 0.5 mg (>12 years).

Blood test for tryptase may be helpful in diagnosing anaphylaxis.

7.37 Hyper-IgE syndrome (HIES)

Answer C: Hyper-IgE syndrome (HIES)

Failure to shed primary teeth is a consistent finding in HIES.

Eosinophilia is a common finding with more than 90% patients having an eosinophil count >2 SD (standard deviations) above the normal mean. An IgE of >2000 IU/ml (normal adult value is <100 IU/ml) has been used as a cut-off level for HIES when other features including boils and pneumonia are present. In infants, in whom normal IgE levels are very low, an IgE of 10 times the age-appropriate level is a reasonable guide for HIES. Pneumatoceles and bronchiectasis are recognised complications in HIES.

A common mnemonic is FATED:

- Facies: coarse
- Abscess: cold staphylococcal
- Teeth: retained primary
- Increased IgE
- Dermatological problems.

In patients with autosomal dominant HIES, pathological fractures occur. Scoliosis may be seen. There is also an autosomal recessive form.

7.38 Varicella Zoster Immunoglobin (VZIG)

Answer A :Varicella Zoster Immunoglobin (VZIG)

The immunosuppressed children need protection because this child is infectious. Infectivity is from 5 days before the rash appears until the last crop. Aciclovir is indicated only once there are signs of infection. VZIG given intramuscularly is the appropriate measure as well, of course, as keeping the child from visiting until non-infectious.

EMQ Answers

7.39–7.41 Theme: Primary immunodeficiencies

7.39

Answer H: Severe combined immunodeficiency (SCID)

Faltering growth, chronic diarrhoea and the absence of thymus (absence of lymphoid tissue – hence no lymphadenopathy in response to infections) are characteristic of severe combined immunodeficiency (SCID). This is also known as 'bubble boy' disease after the boy with X-linked SCID, who lived for 12 years in a plastic, germ-free bubble.

Compare with: Di George (22 q11) – absent thymus also.

Compare with: Bruton disease (X-linked hypogammaglobulinaemia) – little lymphoid tissue but thymus present.

SCID

There is a failure of differentiation into B (humoral immunity) and T cells (cell-mediated immunity). There are multiple genetic defects, the most common being:

- X linked
- Autosomal recessive (50% have an adenosine deaminase [ADA] deficiency).

It presents at age <3/12 with faltering growth. *Pneumocystis* sp. infection and CMV are common.

Lymphopenia, reduced T cells, reduced CD4-helper cells. Reduced IgG, IgA and IgM antibodies.

Treat infections aggressively. Prophylaxis with amphotericin (against *Candida* sp.) and co-trimoxazole (against *Pneumocystis* sp.) often used ± intravenous immunoglobulins.

No live vaccines and only CMV-negative and irradiated blood products used to prevent graft-versus-host disease.

Curative option is bone marrow transplantation.

X-SCID gene therapy and enzyme replacement (for ADA SCID) are available.

7.40

Answer J: X-linked agammaglobulinaemia (Bruton disease)

Absent B cells and very low levels of all immunoglobulins. IgM and IgA are usually undetectable in patients of any age. Low Ig G (note maternal IgG present up to 6 months of age). Absent or low (<1%) CD19+ B cells confirm the diagnosis of X-linked agammaglobulinaemia in boys.

Onset is after a few months, with recurrent lung and paranasal infections. *Staph. aureus, Streptococcus pneumoniae* and *Haemophilus influenzae* are common pathogens. Poor or no response to vaccines. There is little lymphoid tissue.

Early diagnosis to prevent lung disease. Treatment with intravenous immunoglobulin most commonly (subcutaneous immunoglobulin may also be used). Antibiotics to treat infections.

7.41

Answer D: Common variable immunodeficiency (CVID)

The key clue here is the normal IgM with recurrent infections. The chronic diarrhoea with malabsorption is suggestive of *Giardia* sp. which is common in CVID.

Reduced IgG and IgA with normal IgM may be seen in CVID; 50% of cases will have low IgM. There is abnormal T-cell function.

It presents in later childhood with chronic sinopulmonary infections, diarrhoea, lymphadenopathy and splenomegaly. The diagnosis should be considered in any patient with recurrent infections and alopecia.

Diagnosis: reduced immunoglobulins, absent isohaemagglutinins and poor vaccine responses.

Increased autoimmune disease (20% of patients will develop autoimmune problems) – RA, ITP, pernicious anaemia, etc.

Increased risk of malignancies – non-Hodgkin lymphoma, gastric carcinoma (50 × more common in patients with CVID).

7.42–7.44 Theme: Respiratory infections

7.42

Answer H: RSV bronchiolitis

RSV

Respiratory syncytial virus (RSV) is an enveloped RNA virus that belongs to the Paramyxiviridae family within the *Pneumovirus* genus. RSV is a common cause of respiratory tract infections. It can be severe in infants who are at increased risk of acute lower respiratort tract infections. Predisposing factors for infection include prematurity, cardiopulmonary disease and immunodeficiency. Bronchiolitis is a common cause of hospitalisation in children aged under a year. RSV is the most common cause of bronchiolitis. Occurs in October–February. Diagnosis is by nasopharyngeal aspirate (NPA). The Scottish Intercollegiate Guidelines Network (SIGN) guidelines are a useful tool to aid with RSV management (see www.sign.ac.uk).

Green book: Synagis (palivizumab) is a humanised monoclonal antibody (see www.dh.gov.uk). This passive immunisation has been shown to be safe and effective in reducing hospital admission rates and serious complications among high-risk children:

- Children born at 35 weeks or less gestation and under 6/12 of age at onset of the RSV season
- Children <2 years requiring treatment for bronchopulmonary dysplasia within the previous 6/12
- Children <2 years and with haemodynamically significant congenital heart disease
- All children <24 months who have SCID
- All children who are on long-term ventilation aged <12 months at the start of the RSV season
- All children on long-term ventilation aged <24 months at the start of the RSV season with additional co-pathology (heart disease/pulmonary hypertension, intrinsic lung disease (as reflected by oxygen dependency).

Synagis should be given as a maximum of five doses given 1 month apart from the start of the RSV season (beginning calendar week 40, ie beginning of October). Where the course of treatment begins later in the season, treatment should be given until the end of the calendar week 8 (ie the end of February).

7.43

Answer A: Chlamydia trachomatis

Chlamydia trachomatis

Conjunctivitis is the most common presentation. The cough is pertussis like with fine crepitations and eosinophilia in an afebrile child. Diagnosis is by chlamydia swab from the eye (Giemsa stain with chlamydia inclusion bodies in epithelial cells), culture and serology. It is important to screen and treat parents because infertility is a common complication.

Chlamydia spp. are Gram-negative obligate intracellular bacteria. There are four species: *C. trachomatis, C. pneumoniae, C. psittaci* and *C. pecorum*. Infections caused by *C. trachomatis* include trachoma, the most important preventable cause of blindness worldwide. It is endemic in the Middle East and south-east Asia. It starts as a conjunctivitis and spreads from eye to eye. Flies are a frequent vector.

Other manifestations of infection with *Chlamydia trachomatis* include:

- Pneumonia
- Non-specific urethritis
- Epididymo-orchitis
- Proctocolitis
- Reactive arthritis (Reiter syndrome)
- Pelvic inflammatory disease (endometritis, salpingitis)
- Lymphogranuloma venereum.

Vertical transmission from a mother with an infected genital tract occurs in up to 50% of cases. Most infants will present with conjunctivitis at 1–2 weeks. A smaller proportion (10–20%) may present with pneumonia (age 1–3 months). Treatment is with erythromycin or tetracyclines (older children and adults). *C. pneumoniae* is a cause of bronchitis and pneumonia in children and young adults. *C. psittaci* causes psittacosis, a flu-like illness in humans. It mainly infects parrots and birds. *C. pecorum* primarily infects cattle and sheep. There is no evidence of human infection.

7.44

Answer G: Pneumocystis jiroveci/carinii

The key points here are the marked cyanosis with raised lactate dehydrogenase (LDH). LDH levels are elevated in 90% of patients with PCP who are infected with HIV.

PCP

Pneumocystis jiroveci (*carinii*) (new name but 'PCP' is still acceptable as abbreviation).

PCP is often the first clinical indication of HIV. Beware the child whose clinical presentation is typical of RSV bronchitis outside the bronchiolitis season (October–February) with RSV-negative NPA. In older children there is often marked exertional dyspnoea.

LDH may be raised in patients with PCP. The chest radiograph usually looks worse than clinical findings. Co-trimoxazole/pentamadine with steroids is a recognised treatment – for up to 3 weeks.

7.45–7.47 Theme: Rashes

7.45

Answer F: Measles

Koplik spots in the mouth are pathognomonic.

Worldwide, measles infection is very common and is associated with significant morbidity and mortality. Measles is caused by an RNA virus, with transmission person to person and by droplet infection. Humans are the only host. It is a notifiable disease. Infection is rare under the age of 6 months due to the presence of maternal antibodies. Second attacks can occur. Incubation is 14 days from exposure to the appearance of the rash. Infectivity is greatest during the prodromal period and persists for 5 days after the appearance of the rash. The initial symptoms are fever, cough and coryza. The rash is an erythematous maculopapular one. It is widespread and classically starts behind the ears. Diagnosis is clinical and by serology.

Complications of measles can be divided into:

- early:
  - – otitis media
  - – laryngotracheobronchitis
  - – myocarditis/pericarditis
  - – encephalitis
  - – primary or secondary (bacterial) pneumonia
- late – subacute sclerosing panencephalitis.

Prevention of measles is by immunisation. Measles immunisation is given as part of the MMR at around 14 months of age. Since October 1996 a pre-school booster has also been given because a single dose of vaccine does not confer life-long immunity.

7.46

Answer E: Herpes simplex virus

Neonatal herpes simplex virus disease is associated with high morbidity and mortality.

Herpes simplex virus type 1 (HSV-1) typically causes infection above the waist and the infections are localised to the mouth and oropharynx, whereas herpes simplex virus type 2 (HSV-2) usually causes genital infections and can also cause CNS or disseminated disease in neonates.

Most cases (85%) occur during birth when the baby comes in contact with infected genital secretions in the birth canal. This is most common with mothers who have been newly exposed to the virus (mothers who had the virus before pregnancy have a lower risk of transmission). Five per cent are infected *in utero*, and approximately 10% of cases are acquired postnatally.

There are three forms of herpes infection:

1. SEM: skin, eyes, mouth: likely to occur on trauma sites such as fetal electrode sampling, forceps, around eyes or even circumcision area; 75% cases progress to disseminated disease if not treated with prompt antiviral therapy.
2. DIS: disseminated herpes affects internal organs especially the liver. Usually presents in first few days of life with hepatic, pulmonary and neurological problems. High morbidity if not treated early.
3. CNS causes encephalitis and has a high mortality. May present with lethargy, irritability and focal seizures. Most children with CNS die or survive with severe neurological impairment.

Treatment is with aciclovir. Early diagnosis is difficult because only 20–40% neonates have skin lesions. Elective caesarean section is recommended for mothers with primary or active genital herpes to reduce risk of infection to neonate.

Herpes simplex virus

Herpes simplex virus is a common precipitating factor for erythema multiforme. Steven-Johnson syndrome is the extreme form of erythema multiforme with oral, eye and genital involvement.

7.47

Answer J: Varicella virus

Varicella zoster immunoglobulin (VZIG) is recommended for infants whose mothers develop chickenpox in the 7 days before to 7 days after delivery.

If maternal varicella status is negative, VZIG should be given to the baby within 10 days of exposure (ideally within 7 days). About half the neonates exposed to maternal varicella will become infected despite VZIG prophylaxis. In up to a third of these infants, infections are mild. Fatalities occur with the onset of maternal chickenpox in the period 4 days before and 2 days after delivery. Early treatment with intravenous aciclovir is recommended for infants in this exposure category who develop varicella despite VZIG prophylaxis

7.48–7.50 Theme: Fever

7.48

Answer E: Influenza B

All these symptoms are compatible with a flu-like illness. Most people recognise the myalgia and lethargy symptoms. It is important to note that vomiting and diarrhoea may be seen with influenza.

Common symptoms include a high fever, headache, myalgia, fatigue, sweating and chills. Subsequently, respiratory symptoms follow (sore throat, cough). Care is supportive and a particular contraindication is aspirin in those aged <16 years because of the association with Reye syndrome. Influenza B is less serious than type A. Type C has symptoms similar to a cold.

7.49

Answer I: Rubella

Transmission of rubella is by droplet spread. The incubation period is 14–21 days. The infection can be asymptomatic; however, rubella infection is now rare as a consequence of the immunisation programme. Prodromal symptoms may or may not be present and precede the rash by 1–5 days. These include fever, coryza, conjunctivitis and lymphadenopathy (suboccipital, postauricular and cervical). The rash is macular and lasts for 3–5 days. Complications include persistent lymphadenopathy, arthritis, neuritis, thrombocytopenic purpura and encephalitis (associated with a CSF lymphocytosis). Differential diagnosis of rubella includes the following:

- Infectious mononucleosis
- Toxoplasmosis
- Enteroviral infection
- Roseola, scarlet fever
- Mycoplasma infection
- Parvovirus infection.

Viral isolation is difficult and diagnosis is by serology. Treatment is supportive. Prevention is by immunisation with the MMR vaccine.

Congenital rubella occurs secondary to maternal infection in the first trimester. Clinical manifestations are variable and include:

- jaundice
- thrombocytopenia
- growth retardation
- cardiac abnormalities
- eye problems (cataracts, blindness, microphthalmia)
- deafness
- microcephaly
- fetal death
- stillbirth.

7.50

Answer D: Scarlet fever (sometimes called scarletina)

Scarlet fever is caused by the exotoxin released by group A streptococci.

The rash is fine, red and rough textured. It is worse in the axilla and groin. It starts on the chest, then moves to the axilla and behind the ears. Desquamation may occur (compare Kawasaki disease). There is usually a positive throat culture, with blood culture often being negative.

Immune complications include acute glomerulonephritis, rheumatic fever and erythema nodosum:

- Malignancy
- Infectious mononucleosis
- Toxoplasmosis
- Brucellosis.

7.51–7.53 Theme: Treatments

7.51

Answer F: Ganciclovir (congenital CMV)

CMV is a significant cause of morbidity in neonates and of mortality in immunocompromised patients.

If primary maternal infection occurs during pregnancy, the average rate of transmission to the fetus is 40%; approximately 65% of these have CMV at birth. (90% will have neurological sequelae).

Maternal recurrent infection (pre-existing immunity) protects against severe disease; approximately 15% of these infants will have sequelae, especially sensorineural hearing loss.

Cytomegalic inclusion disease (CID)

The most severe form of congenital CMV infection is referred to as CID:

- Intrauterine growth retardation
- Hepatosplenomegaly
- Haematological abnormalities (thrombocytopenia)
- Microcephaly
- Cerebral atrophy
- Chorioretinitis
- Sensorineural hearing loss.

Periventricular calcification: predictive of cognitive and audiological deficits in later life and of a poor neurodevelopmental outcome.

To make a diagnosis of congenital CMV, culture of the virus is necessary before 3 weeks of age. Viral culture after 3 weeks of age may represent perinatal acquisition.

Ganciclovir may result in improvement in hearing in symptomatic infants with congenital CMV.

7.52

Answer G: Isoniazid, rifampicin, ethambutol and pyrazinamide (TB)

TB is the leading cause of death among curable infectious diseases. It is the most common cause of infection-related death worldwide. In 1993, the WHO declared TB to be a global public health emergency. It is more common in those who are malnourished, homeless and living in overcrowded areas.

Infants, elderly people, those infected with HIV and those on immunosuppressive treatments are at higher risk for disseminated TB. Incomplete treatment of TB infections contributes to the development of drug-resistant strains of mycobacteria.

Disseminated (including miliary TB) should be tested for CNS involvement (NICE guidelines – see www.nice.org.uk)

Diagnosis

TB is diagnosed definitively by identifying the causative organism (*Mycobacterium tuberculosis*) in a clinical sample (eg sputum).This may take 4–12 weeks to culture.

Other means to diagnose TB include:

- Imaging (X-rays or scans)
- Tuberculin skin test (Mantoux test)
- ± an interferon-γ release assay (IGRA).

Tuberculin skin tests (Heaf, Mantoux)

Until 2005 The Heaf test (tuberculin skin test) was used in the UK. Now, we use the Mantoux test. The Mantoux intradermal injection of tuberculin (purified protein derivative, PPD) is given in the forearm and read 48–72 hours later. The reaction is read by measuring the diameter of induration across the forearm. A positive result indicates TB exposure.

A positive (>10 mm) reaction in a Mantoux test (even with a previous BCG) is diagnostic for children generally. However, Mantoux testing in BCG-immunised people may be less reliable.

There may be false negative tuberculin skin test in the following:

- Immunosuppressed children
- Severe malnutrition
- Advanced HIV
- Sarcoidosis
- Lymphoma
- Active TB disease.

IGRAs, eg QuantiFERON-TB Gold and T-SPOT.TB

These are whole blood tests that can help diagnose *Mycobacterium tuberculosis* infections and have fewer false-positive results than skin tests. Used to diagnose:

- TB disease
- Latent TB infection (LTBI).

White blood cells from most people who have been infected with *M. tuberculosis* will release interferon-γ when mixed with *M. tuberculosis* antigens. IGRAs measure a person's immune reactivity to *M. tuberculosis*. Blood samples are mixed with antigens and controls. After incubation of the blood with the antigens, the interferon-γ is measured.

Benefits of IGRAs

- Single visit for blood test (but blood must be processed soon after collection)
- Results available in 24 hours.
- Prior BCG immunisation does not cause a false-positive IGRA test result.

Positive IGRA result: *M. tuberculosis* is likely.

Negative IGRA result: *M. tuberculosis* infection unlikely.

NICE

The NICE guidance suggests that a study is needed to assess whether interferon-γ tests are acceptable to patients and are more effective than tuberculin skin tests when undertaking TB screening in the following:

- New entrants from high TB prevalence countries
- Healthcare workers
- Children in high-risk areas who missed neonatal BCG
- Contacts of people with sputum smear-positive TB
- HIV positive patients.

Indications for IGRA testing may include:

- BCG-immunised people
- Those with positive Mantoux results.

7.53

Answer H: Praziquantel (schistosomiasis)

Travellers are at risk if they wade or swim in fresh water in endemic areas. In travellers, schistosomiasis is almost exclusively acquired in Africa – swimming in Lake Malawi is an important risk factor.

7.54–7.56 Theme: Investigations

7.54

Answer B: Bronchoscopy (foreign body)

The recurrent pneumonias most likely to be secondary to aspiration of a foreign body after a choking episode. Bronchoscopy (usually after further imaging, eg CT of the chest) will confirm the diagnosis. The foreign body acts as a persistent focus for infection, if not removed.

Immunoglobulins

Without the history of choking, one may consider a diagnosis of hypogammaglobulinaemia. Ig levels are confirmatory. The most common type (Bruton disease) is X linked. Treatment is regular (approximately 6 weekly) immunoglobulin transfusion and antibiotic prophylaxis.

Sweat test

Recurrent chest infections may be the result of cystic fibrosis. These days, children with cystic fibrosis may be picked up after neonatal screening. The newborn screen initially measures for raised blood concentration of immunoreactive trypsinogen, along with the Guthrie test. Infants with an abnormal newborn screen need a sweat test in order to confirm the cystic fibrosis diagnosis. The gold standard investigation to confirm the diagnosis is a sweat test.

7.55

Answer G: Oral fluid (saliva) swab for serology/PCR mumps

Mumps is an acute contagious RNA paramyxovirus spread by droplet infection. Typically, it involves the parotid glands but may cause meningitis and orchitis.

Presentation:

- Parotitis: swelling and local pain, especially when chewing; may be unilateral but is bilateral in 90% cases
- Fever
- Headache
- Orchitis: postpubertal males have 30% risk of orchitis; subfertility and infertility may result.

Diagnosis

Usually made clinically. Mumps is a notifiable disease in the UK. Oral fluid (saliva) testing on all cases of measles, mumps and rubella was introduced in 1995 by the HPA (see www.hpa.org.uk). Samples are tested for IgM, IgG and viral RNA.

Note that it is also possible to send viral culture of saliva, CSF and urine to confirm mumps.

7.56

Answer F: Meningococcal PCR

Meningococcal infection is the most common cause of bacterial meningitis in the UK. Over the last 50 years, most cases have been due to Men B and Men C. However, now that there is a very effective Men C vaccine, 85% of cases are caused by Men B. Septicaemia (blood infection causing purpura) in the absence of meningitis (inflammation of meninges) is more likely to be fatal than meningitis.

Meningococcal PCR is a rapid, sensitive test that may be used to confirm a diagnosis of meningococcal disease. Preadmission antibiotic treatment, which reduces mortality and is recommended by the Chief Medical Officer, reduces the chances of a positive culture to 5% or less. Only 50% of untreated patients with meningococcal disease will have positive blood cultures. Prompt treatment with high-dose antibiotics is imperative and should not be delayed if blood culture/CSF for lumbar puncture is not possible.

Note that lumbar puncture is contraindicated in the presence of a rapidly evolving purpuric rash.

Close contacts of the index with meningococcal disease are given antibiotic prophylaxis. Public health doctors arrange contact tracing (refer to the BNF for current choice of antibiotic prophylaxis).

Theme: Diagnosis

7.57

Answer I: Typhoid (enteric fever) – Salmonella typhi

Typhoid is characterised by a progressive fever, profuse sweating and gastroenteritis:

- First week: there may be malaise, cough and headache.
- Second week: delirium and 'rose spots' on the lower chest and abdomen. 'Pea soup' diarrhoea may occur.
- Third week: intestinal haemorrhage, encephalitis and neuropsychiatric problems.

Diagnosis of typhoid:

- Blood, bone marrow or stool culture
- Widal test (salmonella antibodies against antigen)
- Prevented by typhoid vaccine – recommended to those travelling to high-risk areas. Oral rehydration to treat diarrhoea and antibiotics. Death occurs in 10–30% of untreated cases.

7.58

Answer C: Hepatitis A

Campylobacter sp. causes diarrhoea, EBV can cause jaundice, but hepatitis A can result in diarrhoea and jaundice.

Hepatitis A

Caused by an RNA virus, usually spread by faeco-oral route. Incubation of 2–6 weeks. High incidence in developing countries.

Can be mistaken for influenza. There may be fatigue, fever, nausea, loss of appetite and jaundice. Diagnosed by IgM antibodies in blood. IgM is present in acute infections and persists for up to 14 weeks. IgG antibody is found after immunisation or after the acute phase (when the patient is immune). Alanine aminotransferase (ALT) may be elevated.

Hepatitis A is prevented by immunisation, good hygiene and sanitation. Hepatitis A does not cause chronic hepatitis (unlike hepatitis B and C).

There is no specific treatment for hepatitis A, other than rest and good diet and hydration.

***Campylobacter* sp.**

Gram-negative bacterium usually transmitted by the faeco-oral route. It produces diarrhoea with cramps/abdominal pain and fever. Symptoms usually last for 5–7 days.

Good hygiene to prevent spread and adequate rehydration are generally all that is needed. Antibiotics are rarely indicated

7.59

Answer H: Strep. pyogenes (group A streptococcal or GAS infection)

The other main differential to consider is Kawasaki disease. Kawasaki disease is a diagnosis of exclusion. In this case the anti-streptolysin O titre (ASOT) is elevated. Anti-DNase B is also elevated in GAS infection. Throat swabs are another useful investigation.

Many people carry GAS in the throat or on the skin and are asymptomatic. Most GAS infections such as 'strep throat' and impetigo are mild illnesses. Rare complications of GAS infections include acute rheumatic fever and post-streptococcal glomerulonephritis. Occasionally, these bacteria can cause life-threatening illnesses.

Severe life-threatening disease occurs with invasive GAS. The HPA estimates that 15–25% of people diagnosed with invasive GAS infections will die.

Invasive GAS infections:

- Necrotising fasciitis ('flesh-eating bacteria')
- Streptococcal toxic shock syndrome (STSS – not to be confused with staphylococcal toxic shock syndrome)

CHAPTER 8

Neonatology Answers

MTF Answers

8.1 Amniotic fluid

Answers: B C D

Amniotic fluid is predominantly produced by fetal urination, and fetal swallowing recycles this fluid. The volume of amniotic fluid varies with gestation and can be defined as an amniotic fluid volume greater than the 95th centile for gestational age. Polyhydramnios occurs in approximately 0.5% of pregnancies and is associated with an increased risk of preterm labour, preterm rupture of the membranes, cord prolapse and placental abruption.

Polyhydramnios occurs most commonly with maternal diabetes and this should be excluded.

Fetal causes of polyhydramnios become increasingly likely with increasing severity of polyhydramnios.

Causes can be grouped into categories as follows.

Obstructive

- Intestinal atresia (oesophageal, duodenal)
- Intestinal obstruction due to extrinsic compression (diaphragmatic hernia, mediastinal masses).

Neurological (impaired swallowing)

- Neuromuscular disorders
- Cleft lip and palate
- Anencephaly
- Chromosomal abnormalities (trisomies).

Fetal polyuria

- Congenital nephrotic syndrome
- Twin-to-twin transfusion
- High-output cardiac failure (severe anaemia, arteriovenous [AV] malformation).

Congenital infection

- Cytomegalovirus, rubella, toxoplasmosis.

Oligohydramnios is defined as an amniotic fluid index of less than the 5th centile for gestational age. This is most commonly associated with amniotic fluid leak secondary to preterm rupture of the membranes and it is associated with pulmonary hypoplasia, contractures and postural deformities.

Other causes include:

- Intrauterine growth restriction (placental insufficiency)
- Renal causes (agenesis – Potter syndrome, dysgenesis)
- Posterior urethral valves, urethral obstruction
- Prune belly syndrome.

8.2 Nitric oxide

Answers: A C

Nitric oxide is a potent vasodilator and is used in the neonatal population as therapy for conditions associated with increased pulmonary vascular resistance, such as persistent pulmonary hypertension of the newborn (PPHN), secondary to poor perinatal adaptation, meconium aspiration, congenital pneumonia and respiratory distress syndrome. Nitric oxide is synthesised in vascular endothelium from L-arginine and oxygen, catalysed by nitric oxide synthase.

At birth nitric oxide is involved in the conversion to normal postnatal respiration and lowering of pulmonary vascular resistance. Inhibition or failure of synthesis of endogenous nitric oxide leads to development of PPHN. Inhaled nitric oxide acts to:

- relax smooth muscle and vasodilate pulmonary vasculature
- reverse hypoxaemia
- improve ventilation–perfusion mismatching.

Nitric oxide diffuses rapidly through alveoli with rapid onset of action. As nitric oxide is an inhaled gas vasodilatation is largely selective and systemic hypotension is rarely a problem. An added advantage over other vasodilators is its very short half-life (3–6 seconds). Nitric oxide, is however, rapidly metabolised to toxic metabolites (NO^{2-}) and these combine with haemoglobin to form methaemoglobin, which should be monitored in patients.

Caution is advised currently in the routine use of inhaled nitric oxide in preterm (<34 weeks) babies because the body of evidence for improved long-term neurological outcome or decreased bronchopulmonary dysplasia or death in this population is lacking. There are, however, promising animal model trials and clinical trials under way to help to define the risk–benefit balance of the use of low-dose nitric oxide in this population of neonates.

8.3 Assessment of gestational age

Answers: B D E

Gestational age assessment can be done in various ways listed in decreasing order of accuracy:

- Known date of conception or embryo transfer (usually in vitro fertilisation related)
- First trimester ultrasonography between weeks 6 and 13(+6) (using crown–rump length [CRL])
- Second trimester ultrasonography between 18 and 22 weeks (using head circumference)
- Other ultrasonography up to 24 weeks (using head circumference)
- Certain last menstrual period (LMP) with regular menstrual cycle.

Gestational age can be estimated after birth by careful physical and neurological examination. This should be done on the first day because some signs change rapidly after birth. Physical signs used include the following:

- Skin colour, texture and opacity
- Lanugo hair and hair development
- Plantar creases
- Ear form and firmness
- Breast and genital development.

There is a variety of scoring systems, which have been used to assess an infant's gestational age, eg the Dubowitz or Ballard scores.

Neurological criteria depend on posture (increasingly flexed), muscle tone (increases with gestation) and passive joint mobility. The scarf sign refers to when the arm is pulled across the supine infant to wrap it around the opposite shoulder. The elbow reaches the opposite axilla in very preterm infants but does not reach the midline in term infants.

8.4 Infants of mothers with diabetes

Answers: C D E

Mothers can have pre-existing diabetes or develop impaired glucose tolerance in pregnancy, which may resolve after the pregnancy (gestational diabetes) or may be permanent.

Clinical features of babies of diabetic mothers include the following:

- General:
  - macrosomia secondary to fetal hyperinsulinaemia in response to hyperglycaemia
  - but also can be small for gestational age secondary to placental insufficiency
  - increased adiposity
  - increased risk of shoulder dystocia, obstructed labour, hypoxic ischaemic injury and birth trauma if macrosomic
- Central nervous system:

– jitteriness
– hyperexcitability
– hypotonia
– increased seizures (secondary to hypoglycaemia and hyperviscosity)

- Respiratory: increased risk of respiratory distress syndrome
- Cardiovascular:
  – cardiomegaly (up to 30%)
  – transient hypertrophic cardiomyopathy with disproportionate septal hypertrophy which, when severe, may cause outflow tract obstruction
  – persistent fetal circulation
- Metabolic:
  – hypoglycaemia (usually within the first few hours)
  – hypocalcaemia
  – hypomagnesaemia
- Haematological:
  – polycythaemia and hyperviscosity
  – jaundice
  – renal vein thrombosis
- Congenital malformations (infants of mothers with diabetes have a three- to fivefold increased risk):
  – cardiac (ventricular septal defect, atrioventricular septal defect, transposition of the great arteries, coarctation of the aorta)
  – neural tube defects including anencephaly and meningomyelocele
  – holoprosencephaly
  – sacral agenesis, vertebral dysplasia
  – hydronephrosis
  – renal agenesis
  – duodenal atresia
  – anorectal malformations
  – small left colon syndrome.

8.5 Problems associated with preterm gestation

Answers: A B C D E

There are multiple problems associated with prematurity, the most common of which are listed here:

- Respiratory:
  – respiratory distress syndrome
  – pneumothorax
  – chronic lung disease
  – pulmonary haemorrhage

- Cardiovascular:
  - hypotension
  - patent ductus arteriosus
- Gastrointestinal:
  - necrotising enterocolitis
  - feed intolerance
  - poor nutrition and growth
- Metabolic:
  - hypo-/hypernatraemia
  - hypo-/hyperglycaemia
  - acidosis
  - jaundice
- Neurological:
  - intraventricular haemorrhage
  - periventricular leukomalacia
- Other:
  - infection
  - retinopathy of prematurity
  - anaemia
  - apnoea of prematurity.

Details of these problems should be revised and can be found in any of the pocket books of neonatal intensive care.

8.6 Chickenpox

Answer: B

The incubation period for varicella is 10–21 days; an infected person is infective 48 hours before the appearance of a rash, until the vesicles crust over completely. As chickenpox is a common childhood disease, most pregnant women are immune. In non-immune pregnant women, however, primary infection with varicella-zoster virus (VZV) may cause severe morbidity or even death. It may also cause fetal varicella syndrome or varicella infection of the newborn.

Infants born to mothers who develop chickenpox 4 days before to 2 days after delivery should be given varicella-zoster immunoglobulin (VZIG). This reduces the severity of neonatal disease but does not prevent infection; it may also increase the period of incubation from 11 to 30 days. In some centres prophylactic aciclovir is given in addition to VZIG prophylaxis. Regardless of the prophylaxis regimen, it is important to maintain vigilance and treat with aciclovir early should symptoms develop because delay may lead to increased morbidity and mortality.

Any baby felt to be at high risk from varicella (eg preterm infants and those with co-morbidities) and those developing vesicles should be treated with intravenous aciclovir. Babies born more than 7 days after onset of maternal rash receive some transplacental transfer of immunity, do not require treatment and generally have a good prognosis.

Breastfeeding should be encouraged. Without prophylaxis or treatment infection rates are up to 50% with a 30% mortality rate.

If a baby of a seronegative mother is exposed to chickenpox in the first 7 days of life he or she should be offered VZIG.

If a mother develops chickenpox during early pregnancy the infant is at risk of developing congenital varicella syndrome, the risk being 1–2%. The congenital varicella syndrome includes limb hypoplasia, microcephaly, cataract, growth retardation and skin scarring.

8.7 Cataracts

Answers: A B C

Cataract describes a total or partial opacity of the lens. Congenital cataracts are often diagnosed soon after birth with the finding of leukocoria (white reflex) or abnormal, irregular, red reflex during the first newborn examination. If cataracts go undetected, permanent visual loss may occur as a consequence, as early as 6 weeks after birth. Metabolic or systemic disease is found in up to 60% of patients presenting with bilateral cataracts in the neonatal period. Unilateral cataracts are more likely to be sporadic events. Cataracts may be static or progressive and so can develop after birth in a variety of conditions. Surgery is the treatment of choice to ensure minimal visual disruption in the long term. Surgery can be associated with the development of glaucoma (up to 10%). The following may be causes of neonatal cataract:

- Idiopathic/sporadic
- Hereditary: mostly dominantly inherited (up to 23%)
- Congenital infection:
  - rubella
  - cytomegalovirus
  - syphilis
  - herpes zoster virus
  - herpes simplex virus
  - toxoplasmosis
  - infectious mononucleosis
  - measles
- Metabolic: galactosaemia
- Syndromes:
  - trisomies 21, 13 and 18
  - Lowe syndrome
  - Turner syndrome (occasional)
  - Conradi syndrome
  - Cockayne syndrome
  - Zellweger syndrome
- Myotonic dystrophy.

Corneal clouding

Clouding of the cornea results in reduced visual acuity and an inability to visualise structures within the eye clearly on examination.

Causes include:

- Congenital glaucoma
- Metabolic:
  - mucopolysaccharidosis (Hurler syndrome NOT Hunter syndrome)
  - tyrosinaemia
  - mucolipidoses
- Infections: congenital rubella
- Birth trauma
- Corneal dystrophies
- Corneal dysgenesis, eg sclerocornea
- Exposure: any condition leading to excessive dry eyes, facial nerve palsy, Möbius syndrome
- Familial dysautonomia
- Prematurity: clouding of the cornea is present in fetuses until approximately 27 weeks' gestation.

8.8 Sudden infant death syndrome (SIDS)

Answers: A B C D E

Cot death/SIDS/sudden unexpected death in infancy (SUDI) are terms used to describe the death of a baby where no medical or forensic cause can be identified after full investigation. Rates have fallen substantially in the UK over the last 20 years from almost 2 per 1000 live births to 0.5 per 1000 live births. This fall has been greater in the less deprived groups of society and has been attributed to national awareness campaigns such as the 'Back to sleep' and 'Reduce the risk' campaigns. Risk factors associated with increased rates of SIDS include:

- Maternal and paternal smoking (during pregnancy and after)
- Prematurity/Low birthweight
- Lower parental age
- Lower maternal education
- 'Not in a cot' sleeping (sleeping with a sleeping adult on a sofa, armchair, bed or bean bag), increased further with adult alcohol/drug intoxication or extreme tiredness
- Prone sleeping
- Maternal drug abuse in pregnancy even when babies are removed at birth
- Over-heating
- Family history of SIDS
- Antecedent respiratory infection

- Antecedent weight loss.

Breastfeeding appears to be protective although evidence of specific effect is hard to separate from other confounders.

The use of dummies during sleep appears to be protective.

BOF Answers

8.9 Pathophysiology of perinatal asphyxia

Answer D: Hypothermia has been shown to improve neurological outcome in neonates after moderate hypoxic ischaemic injury

- The brain has high energy consumption and little capacity for storage/production of glucose/glycogen.
- Primary neuronal injury secondary to hypoxia → deprivation of glucose metabolite ATP →:
  - failure of Na^+/K^+ pump
  - ↑ Na^+ and water into cell (cell swelling → cell death)
  - ↑ intracellular calcium
  - ↑ extracellular glutamate (excitatory amino acid neurotransmitter released secondary to depolarisation).
- Reperfusion/Reoxygenation injury → cascade of toxic free radicals within hours of the insult.
- Secondary neuronal injury (secondary energy failure after a latent phase of around 6 hours despite resuscitation):
  - ↑ intracellular calcium
  - ↑ extracellular glutamate (correlating with onset of seizures)
  - ↑ free radicals
  - inflammation.
- Cell death after brain injury/insult occurs via two mechanisms:
  - necrosis – occurs early secondary to failure of Na^+/K^+ pump and calcium accumulation
  - apoptosis – triggered by excitotoxicity, ↑ intracellular calcium, oxidative stress, loss of trophic factors and inflammation.

Neuroprotection

Moderate systemic hypothermia to 33.5°C is now the standard of care for neuroprotection post-neonatal hypoxic ischaemic brain injury. It works to prevent/reduce the secondary neuronal injury by lowering cellular metabolism, inhibiting glutamate and free radical accumulation, attenuating inflammation and inhibiting apoptosis. Trials have shown (actually no reduction in death) improved neurodevelopmental outcome in survivors and reduced incidence of cerebral palsy at 18 months. A patient should be registered on the

TOBY online register to allow ongoing data collection and monitoring.

Inclusion criteria for cooling:

- Gestational age ≥36/40
- Within 6 hours of insult
- Apgar ≤5 at 10 minutes
- Continued need for resuscitation at 10 minutes after birth
- Acidosis pH <7 and/or base deficit ≥16 mmol/l within 60 minutes of birth (cord gas, arterial or capillary sample)
- **PLUS** evidence of moderate-to-severe encephalopathy by clinical assessment:
  - altered consciousness, lethargy, stupor, coma
  - abnormal tone
  - abnormal primitive reflexes (grasp, Moro reflex, suck).

This can be supported with evidence from amplitude-integrated EEG (aEEG) if available.

8.10 Pulmonary haemorrhage

Answer E: Treatments used in this condition include adrenaline via the ETT and high- frequency oscillatory ventilation

Massive pulmonary haemorrhage (PH) is a potentially life-threatening complication seen most often in the extremely preterm or very-low-birthweight neonate. It characterised by frank blood via the endotracheal tube (ETT) with deterioration in the condition of the infant, and should not be confused with trauma from aspirating from the ETT.

Risk factors for pulmonary haemorrhage

Extreme prematurity:

- Intrauterine growth restriction
- Surfactant therapy
- Patent ductus arteriosus (PDA) due to high flow left-to-right shunt and high pulmonary blood flow.

Pulmonary haemorrhage is uncommon in babies with haemorrhagic disease of the newborn, thrombocytopenia or haemophilia. It is, however, common to have secondary disseminated vascular coagulation (DIC) after PH.

Clinical presentation:

- Commonly days 2–4 of life
- Sudden deterioration of infant's condition: pallor, desaturation, bradycardia and/or apnoea together with frank blood or pink frothy fluid seen in the mouth, up the ETT or between the cords at intubation
- Signs of underlying cardiovascular instability are common:
  - tachycardia
  - PDA murmur
- Widespread crepitations with reduced air entry throughout the chest.

Radiological appearances of massive PH characteristically show 'white-out' with air bronchograms.

Treatment

Resuscitation:

- Airway management: suction relatively contraindicated unless clot is obstructing the airway
- Breathing: intubation and ventilation if not already done
- Circulation: bolus of colloid (fresh frozen plasma [FFP]/blood/platelets).

Ventilation strategies:

- ETT adrenaline
- High-frequency oscillatory ventilation (HFOV)
- Aim not to change ETT unless clearly blocked/displaced
- May need high PIP >30 cmH_2O
- High PEEP (positive end-expiratory pressure) 6–7 cmH_2O
- Long inspiratory time (0.4–0.5s)
- Suction with caution
- A single dose of surfactant once stabilised may improve oxygenation.

Circulation:

- Treatment of underlying heart failure, including ionotropes and diuretics. Management of resulting coagulopathy/anaemia.

Complications:

- Air leaks and later chronic lung disease
- Often associated with intraventricular haemorrhage so cranial ultrasonography is indicated in all cases
- High mortality rate of approximately 30-40%.

8.11 Retinopathy of prematurity

Answer A: retinal detachment is a potentially sight-threatening consequence of the neovascularisation occurring in retinopathy of prematurity

Retinopathy of prematurity (ROP) is a vasoproliferative disorder that affects preterm infants. Predisposing factors include:

- Severity of associated illness (respiratory distress syndrome [RDS], bronchopulmonary dysplasia [BPD], intraventricular haemorrhage [IVH], patent ductus arteriosus [PDA], pulmonary haemorrhage and sepsis) – this appears to be the main predictor of severe disease
- Extreme low birthweight particularly (<1000 g)
- Small for gestational age (<10th percentile for gestational age)
- Young gestational age- (<27 weeks)
- African ethnicity appears to be protective.

It is a disorder in which normal development of retinal vessels is interrupted. Retinal vasculature begins to develop around 16 weeks' gestation; retinal vasculogenesis starts at the optic nerve and grows circumferentially into the retina throughout fetal life and becomes fully mature by term. Preterm infants are born with avascular peripheral retina.

ROP is described by severity, location, extent and the presence or absence of disease.

- Stage 1: demarcation line
- Stage 2: ridge
- Stage 3: ridge with extraretinal fibrovascular proliferation
- Stage 4: partial retinal detachment
- Stage 5: → total retinal detachment.

Approximately 50–70% of all infants born weighing <1250 g display some changes consistent with ROP; however, severe disease is relatively infrequent. The median age of onset of ROP was 35 weeks corrected gestational age. Screening for ROP should include all infants <32 weeks' gestation or ≤1500 g at birth.

Screening for babies <27 weeks should start at 30–31 weeks post-menstrual age. Other babies who meet screening criteria are first screened at 4–5 weeks. Screening continues until complete retinal vascularisation is achieved. This is usually around term or, in the presence of ROP, when there is evidence that progression has stopped and regression has commenced. Laser therapy is currently the treatment of choice.

ROP may regress (as is the case in over 90%) or lead to scarring, retinal detachment and blindness. Other sequelae include the following:

- Visual impairment
- Myopia
- Astigmatism
- Strabismus
- Amblyopia
- Glaucoma
- Cataract.

8.12 Meconium aspiration syndrome

Answer B: Meconium aspiration is associated with the deactivation of endogenous surfactant

Meconium aspiration syndrome (MAS) is defined as respiratory distress with antenatal passage of meconium and characteristic radiology appearances (hyperinflation and patchy interstitial shadowing), without an alternative reason for respiratory distress.

- The incidence of MAS requiring ventilation is between 0.43 and 2.1 in 1000 live births.
- Mortality rates of 3–5% are reported.
- Mostly affects term/post-term infants.
- Induction of labour at <41 weeks has been shown to reduce the incidence of MAS.

- More than 10% of deliveries at >37 weeks have antenatal meconium, most of which have no consequences.

The passage of meconium can be in response to hypoxic/ischaemic stress *in utero* which can lead to reflex gasping and aspiration into the fetal airways. The pulmonary characteristics of MAS are as follows:

- Chemical pneumonitis
- Surfactant inhibition
- Failure of pulmonary vascular relaxation and perinatal adaptation
- Mechanical airway obstruction (uncommon).

Typically a neonate will present with tachypnoea, respiratory distress, cyanosis and chest hyperinflation immediately after birth or more rarely with increasing symptoms over the first few hours of life.

Management

Tracheal suctioning:

- Intrapartum suctioning of the oropharynx is no longer recommended.
- Tracheal suctioning in a vigorous neonate (heart rate >100 beats/min) after delivery is no longer recommended.
- Tracheal suctioning in a floppy, apnoeic neonate before starting timely positive pressure resuscitation is accepted practice but not evidence based.

Ventilation strategies:

- Conventional ventilation
- HFOV commonly used
- Increase fractional inspired oxygen (FiO_2) to keep well saturated and minimize pulmonary hypertension
- Nasal-continuous positive airway pressure (NCPAP) controversial due to concerns about increased risk of pneumothorax in this population
- Consider surfactant replacement or lavage (with multiple doses)
- Nitric oxide.

Cardiovascular:

- Maintain blood pressure to minimise right-to-left shunting
- Exclude structural cardiac disease.

Supportive measures:

- Intravenous fluids (often fluid restriction as risk of syndrome of inappropriate ADH section [SIADH] and poor renal function), nil by mouth, monitor and treat glucose, calcium and magnesium levels
- Intravenous antibiotics (most culture negative)
- Treat metabolic acidosis
- Maintain adequate sedation; muscle relaxants often beneficial.

Finally:

- Monitor oxygenation index {([MAP × FiO_2]/PaO_2 in mmHg) × 100} and discuss with extracorporeal membrane oxygenation (ECMO) centre early if severe or deteriorating (MAP = mean arterial pressure).

There is an association with MAS and perinatal hypoxic ischaemic insult and as such there is a risk of long-term adverse neurological outcome in this population. If significant concerns in a muscle-relaxed baby an EEG can be helpful. Good pulmonary recovery is usual; however, severe cases can have a prolonged oxygen requirement.

8.13 Immunisation in preterm infants

Answer D: Influenza vaccine is recommended for all preterm infants with chronic lung disease once they have reached 6 months of age

It is known that preterm infants especially <28–32 weeks' gestation are relatively immunodeficient. This is due to immaturity of the innate immune system combined with a lack of maternal immunoglobulins which are actively transported across the placenta predominantly in the latter half of the third trimester.

It is recognised that, despite the vulnerability of preterm and low-birthweight infants to preventable diseases, there is often some delay in their immunisation due to parental concern/physician misinformation.

Immunisation should occur on time, as per the routine schedule according to chronological NOT corrected gestational age. Additional protection should be considered:

- Protection against RSV (respiratory syncytial virus) with the humanised monoclonal antibody palivizumab for all children considered high risk due to their prematurity, age at the start of RSV season and underlying chronic health problems, including chronic lung disease and haemodynamically significant congenital heart disease (for details consult the Department of Health's *Green Book of Immunisations*). Passive immunity is conveyed by monthly injections over the RSV season.
- Influenza vaccine is recommended for infants with chronic disease including chronic lung disease. It can be given once to those aged >6 months (immunisation during pregnancy conveys some protection to neonates).

Some retrospective studies have shown an increased rate of apnoea and bradycardia in preterm infants after immunisation; this is not a universal finding. As with all infants, the risk and benefits should be discussed with the parents and, if adverse events do occur, further doses should be considered under supervision rather than omitted. The *Green Book* states that very preterm infants (born <28 weeks) who are in hospital at the time of their immunisations should have 48–72 hours of respiratory monitoring after immunisation and, if the child displays apnoea, desaturation or bradycardia, the next immunisations should be given in hospital with 48–72 hours of respiratory monitoring.

8.14 Persistent fetal circulation

Answer E: Treatment with minimal handling, paralysis, sedation and nitric oxide is useful in this population

Persistent fetal circulation (persistent pulmonary hypertension of the newborn, PPHN) is characterised by hypoxia that is out of proportion to the severity of lung disease, a structurally normal heart and evidence of right-to-left shunting either at the ductus arteriosus or through the foramen ovale. It affects 0.1–0.2% of all births each year and is associated with a mortality rate of 10–20%. Echocardiography is the investigation of choice to confirm the diagnosis and exclude structural cardiac disease. Risk factors include perinatal compromise, group B streptococcal sepsis, pulmonary hypoplasia (diaphragmatic hernia, oligohydramnios and pleural effusion), MAS, RDS, maternal indometacin, congenital pneumonia and post-date delivery. Despite this, in many cases a definite cause cannot be identified. Management includes ventilation, minimal handling, sedation and paralysis, maintenance of a suprasystemic arterial blood pressure (often needing ionotropic support), normalisation of acid–base status, close attention to electrolytes and broad-spectrum antibiotics.

Ventilation strategies that maximise oxygenation and minimise lung trauma are preferred and high-frequency oscillation may be employed often together with inhaled nitric oxide to act as a pulmonary vasodilator. Historically, hyperventilation with resulting alkalosis was used to try to increase pulmonary vasodilatation but this practice is no longer employed due to concerns about reduced cerebral perfusion with hypocapnia. Nitric oxide has been shown to improve the outcome in near term hypoxaemic infants and decreases the need for ECMO; however, mortality rates for both treatments are similar. Thirty per cent of children will fail to respond to nitric oxide treatment. Other pulmonary vasodilators used to treat PPHN include magnesium sulphate, tolazoline, prostacyclin and sildenafil. Survivors of PPHN can experience significant morbidity associated with chronic lung disease, seizures and neurodevelopmental abnormalities.

Extracorporeal membrane oxygenation

ECMO is a form of cardiopulmonary bypass that allows gas exchange outside the body and increases systemic perfusion. The morbidity and mortality of ECMO are influenced by delay in institution of treatment, so early transfer is imperative.

8.15 Air leak syndrome in the newborn

Answer E: Surfactant use decreases the risk of developing an air leak in a preterm baby

Pulmonary air leaks include pneumothorax, pulmonary interstitial emphysema (PIE), pneumomediastinum and pneumopericardium. A pneumothorax is present in approximately 1% of all newborns and may be asymptomatic. Rates are higher in preterm babies; however, the administration of exogenous surfactant administration appears protective. Air leaks in the first 24 hours of life in low-birthweight (<1500 g) infants are associated with increased rates of BPD, IVH and death. Pneumothoraces are usually a complication of mechanical ventilation but can occur spontaneously. Risk factors associated with air leaks in neonates include causes of uneven lung compliance, leading to alveolar over-distension and rupture:

- Respiratory distress syndrome
- Meconium aspiration

- Congenital lung abnormality
- Pulmonary hypoplasia.

Direct trauma from suctioning and introducers through an ETT and central venous catheter placement can also lead to air leaks.

Risk factors in ventilated babies:

- High peak pressure and mean airway pressure
- High PEEP
- Poor patient synchronisation with the ventilator
- Prolonged inspiratory time.

High rates of ventilation (>60 beats/min) may prove protective in conventional ventilation.

Asymptomatic or minimally symptomatic pneumothoraces in term babies can be treated with increased oxygen concentration (relatively contraindicated in preterm population because high concentrations of oxygen associated with increased risk of retinopathy) to hasten absorption. Insertion of a chest drain with underwater seal is indicated in all infants with moderate/severe symptoms and in virtually all ventilated babies with a pneumothorax. Acutely unstable infants with suspected tension pneumothorax should be managed with needle thoracocentesis. Optimising ventilation indices and strategies in all patients is essential. PIE may cause slow progressive deterioration of blood gases and increased requirement for ventilatory support. All air leaks can result in an acute deterioration in the clinical state of a ventilated baby and a pneumopericardium may cause cardiac tamponade.

8.16 Small-for-gestational-age neonates

Answer D: Growth hormone is licensed for the treatment of continued short stature (>4 years) in children born small for gestational age

A neonate is considered small for gestational age if its birth weight is ≤10th centile. About 40% of this population will have failed to meet their genetic potential for growth *in utero*; most of the remainder will be constitutionally small and therefore will not be at risk of the consequences detailed below. There are also babies born above the 10th percentile who have not grown to their genetic potential, and are therefore growth restricted, but will not meet the definition of small for gestational age. Small-for-gestational-age neonates can be symmetrically or asymmetrically growth restricted (head growth spared), the latter being more common.

Intrauterine growth restriction occurs when gas exchange and/or nutrition delivered to the fetus are not sufficient to allow it to thrive *in utero*.

Causes of infants being born small for gestational age

Maternal:

- Physiological: maternal height, age <20 or >35, multiparity
- Pathological: placental insufficiency – toxaemia, hypertension, smoking, alcoholism, malnutrition, chronic disease, drug misuse.

Fetal:

- Physiological: genetic potential, multiple pregnancy
- Pathological: chromosomal, malformation, infection, syndromal.

Placental:

- Infarction, tumour, abruption, twin-to-twin transfusion.

Problems associated with growth restriction

- Late fetal death/stillbirth (↑ 10 ×)
- Prematurity
- Perinatal compromise
- Hypothermia
- Hypoglycaemia
- Polycythaemia
- Thrombocytopenia
- Neutropenia
- Meconium aspiration syndrome
- Persistent fetal circulation
- Pulmonary haemorrhage
- Necrotising enterocolitis
- Renal failure
- Increased risk of infection.

Longer-term complications also occur including:

- Short stature in later life (70–80% catch-up in the first few years of life; growth hormone is licensed for those children born small for gestation who remain small at ≥4 years)
- Metabolic syndrome in adulthood (obesity, hypertension, hypercholesterolaemia, cardiovascular disease and type 2 diabetes)
- Increased risk of neurodevelopmental problems.

8.17 Steroid therapy in the neonate

Answer C: There is clear evidence that postnatal administration of corticosteroids produces acute improvement in respiratory mechanics and therefore facilitates extubation

Corticosteroids were frequently used in the past to prevent and treat chronic lung disease in preterm infants, particularly those who were ventilator dependent. Studies, mostly using dexamethasone, showed acute improvement in lung function, shorter time to extubation and decreased rate of BPD.

Later evidence from individual trials and meta-analyses performed in the 1990s has shown an association between the use of postnatal steroids and adverse long-term neurodevelopmental outcome. The effect appears to be most significant if steroids are used early (<96 h) compared with those used after age 3 weeks – in which combined rates of death and cerebral palsy appeared similar (more cerebral palsy, fewer deaths in treated group). There were limited data on the neurological outcomes of neonates treated with corticosteroid between 7 and 14 days, but there appeared to be no increase in adverse neurological outcome. Higher rates of neurodisability were seen in children given prolonged courses at high dose, and in early short courses using lower doses, demonstrating both total dose-dependent and timing-dependent toxicity effects. Animal studies have suggested that corticosteroids other than dexamethasone may have less neurotoxic effects; however, one trial using early hydrocortisone was stopped prematurely due to an increased incidence of gastrointestinal perforation in the treatment arm.

Corticosteroids are still cautiously used in neonates with severe BPD after assessment of risks versus benefit. The following are the proposed mechanisms of action:

- Stabilisation of membranes
- Reduction in pulmonary oedema
- Increased surfactant synthesis
- Reduction of airway inflammation
- Relief of bronchospasm.

Side effects of steroids in neonates:

- Hypertension
- Gastrointestinal bleeding
- Gastric perforation
- Hyperglycaemia
- Sepsis
- Cataracts
- Cardiomyopathy
- Leukocytosis
- Candidiasis
- Poor growth
- Concerns about neurodevelopment as detailed above.

8.18 Necrotising enterocolitis

Answer D: Breast milk and to a lesser extent donor breast milk decrease the probability of developing NEC in high-risk neonates when compared with formula-fed control infants

Necrotising enterocolitis (NEC) is a condition of unknown aetiology that occurs most commonly in infants <1500 g and is characterised by transmural intestinal necrosis. Presentation is with abdominal distension and tenderness, with increasing bile-stained aspirates, blood in stools, apnoea and acidosis. The characteristic finding on plain abdominal radiograph is intramural gas (pneumatosis); this may be accompanied by portal gas, persistently dilated, fixed loops of bowel and pneumoperitoneum. Predisposing factors are:

- Prematurity

- Intrauterine growth retardation (IUGR), abnormal Doppler scans
- Hypoxia
- Hypotension
- Perinatal compromise
- Sepsis
- Hypothermia
- Exchange transfusion/umbilical catheterisation
- Anaemia
- Polycythaemia
- Formula feeding/hyperosmolar feeds
- Cardiac causes with impaired gut perfusion including PDA, coarctation, left ventricular outflow tract obstruction, transposition of the great arteries.

NEC has been reported after a blood transfusion.

Preventive strategies include:

- Standardised feeding regimens within units
- Maternal breast milk
- Donor breast milk
- In growth-restricted infants with abnormal Doppler scans parenteral nutrition with minimal enteral feeding for the first week was commonly practised; however, recent data (ADEPT 2010) shows no significant difference in NEC between early and late fed infants.
- A possible role for pre- and probiotics (emerging evidence, ongoing trials).

NEC can occur in outbreaks but in <50% of cases an organism is found. Organisms isolated include *Escherichia coli*, *Staphylococcus epidermidis*, rotavirus and *Clostridium perfringens*. Term neonates who develop NEC usually have a predisposing factor such as perinatal hypoxia–ischaemia or congenital heart disease. Medical treatment consists of stopping enteral feeds with nasogastric decompression, total parenteral nutrition and intravenous broad-spectrum antibiotics. Ventilatory and circulatory support are often required and analgesia should be provided. Patients require regular monitoring (clinical, haematological, biochemical and radiological). Babies with NEC who fail to respond to medical therapy need to be assessed by a paediatric surgeon. Indications for surgery include perforation of the bowel, persistent bowel obstruction, presence of a fixed mass and continued deterioration despite medical therapy. Surgery may involve laparotomy or, in very sick infants too unstable for laparotomy, primary peritoneal drainage can be used. This may avoid the need for subsequent laparotomy in up to a third of cases.

Late complications of necrotising enterocolitis:

- Stricture formation
- Short bowel syndrome
- Anastomotic leak
- Blind loop syndrome
- Cholestasis

- Fistula formation
- Neurodevelopmental sequelae.

8.19 Birth injuries

Answer E: the clavicle is the most common bone to fracture during labour and delivery

Fractures

- One per cent of infants sustain fractures at the time of their birth, clavicular fractures being the most common (usually obvious on radiograph). Risk factors include shoulder dystocia, macrosomia and breech delivery.
- Injury to the cervical spine is rare but can occur (with or without radiological changes). Excessive rotation during cephalic deliveries results in injury at the C1–2 level whereas breech deliveries with excessive traction result in damage at C6–T1. Hypotonia, hyporeflexia and hypoventilation ensue. Magnetic resonance imaging (MRI) is useful for diagnosis. Permanent quadriplegia is likely after this injury.

Brachial plexus injuries

These usually result from traction associated with shoulder dystocia; 97% are from cephalic deliveries, 1–2% from breech deliveries and 1% from caesarean sections.

- Upper brachial plexus, Erb–Duchenne paralysis (C5–6): affected arm is held in the waiter's tip position. Biceps and supinator reflexes are absent. Hand grasp is preserved. Associated diaphragmatic (phrenic nerve) palsy represents a severe injury and may require surgical treatment.
- Lower brachial plexus injury, Klumpke paralysis (C8–T1), claw hand deformity, absent triceps jerk and palmar grasp with occasional ipsilateral Horner syndrome (eyelid ptosis and papillary miosis).
- Total brachial plexus injury, Erb–Duchenne–Klumpke palsy: combines features of both.

Depending on the severity of the injury recovery may take up to 3 months, but is incomplete in about a third of cases. Surgery may be indicated if recovery is not evident by this time.

The scalp

Caput succedaneum	Cephalohaematoma
Oedema of presenting part	Haematoma between the skull and periosteum
Diffuse, ecchymotic, oedematous overlying skin	Normal overlying skin
Present at birth	Not present until a few hours after birth
Disappears over days	Reabsorbed over 2 weeks to 3 months
	Can calcify
May extend over suture lines	Limited by suture lines
No treatment needed	May require phototherapy

8.20 Recurrent apnoea in preterm infants

Answer E: Nasal CPAP is an effective treatment for recurrent apnoeas in preterm neonates that do not respond to medical treatment

Apnoea defined as a pause in breathing of more than 20 seconds, or shorter when associated with desaturation, bradycardia, pallor or reduced tone. It is a common symptom in preterm babies, especially those less than 30 weeks' gestation and can be primary or secondary to other phenomena. Recurrent apnoeas are recorded in 10% of babies born at 34–35 weeks' gestation increasing to 50% of babies at 30–31 weeks' gestation. Apnoea can be further classified as central, obstructive or mixed.

Causes of secondary apnoea:

- Infection (bacterial, fungal or viral)
- Gastrointestinal: NEC, GORD (gastro-oesophageal reflux disease), abdominal distension, overfeeding, passage of stool
- Metabolic: hypoglycaemia, hypernatraemia, hyponatraemia, hypocalcaemia, hypothyroidism
- Cardiovascular: hypotension, fluid overload, cardiac failure
- Respiratory: hypoxia, pneumonia, RDS, aspiration
- Nervous system: haemorrhage, hypoxia–ischaemia, seizures, congenital malformations
- Drugs (infant and maternal): opiates, magnesium, prostaglandin, phenobarbital, benzodiazapines
- Pain
- Haematological: anaemia
- Mechanical: airway malformation, head position, obstruction (reduced tone, secretions)
- Vasovagal: suctioning, siting nasogastric tubes.

Apnoea with no underlying cause in an otherwise healthy infant is apnoea of prematurity and is a diagnosis of exclusion. This usually presents in preterm infants within a few days of birth and disappears by about 34 weeks' gestation. Many factors are thought to have a role in pathogenesis including immaturity of the respiratory centre, upper airway collapse, environmental temperature and sleep state. Apnoea of prematurity is usually treated with a respiratory stimulant such as caffeine. Initial studies into the long-term outcomes of infants with apnoea treated with caffeine show a reduction in death and survival with neurological disability and a reduced incidence of cerebral palsy and cognitive delay at 18–21 months. An ongoing trial due to report in 2016 will further define the long-term effects of the use of caffeine (CAP trial). Respiratory support measures are often used. High-flow oxygen via nasal cannula, nasal CPAP and non-invasive positive pressure ventilation all appear to be effective in reducing apnoea.

8.21 Respiratory distress syndrome

Answer A: Radiant heat sources and the use of occlusive plastic bags to decrease the incidence of hypothermia are advantageous strategies to help to prevent/reduce the severity of RDS

RDS is caused by immaturity of the lungs, in particular the surfactant system (type 2 alveolar cells).

Surfactant deficiency results in high surface tension and atelectasis, which decreases lung compliance resulting in a failure to establish a functional residual capacity. This leads to poor gas exchange and high pulmonary arterial pressures. Alveolar epithelial necrosis (hyaline membrane formation) occurs within hours, further decreasing gas exchange.

The incidence is related to gestation:

- 60–80% born at 26–28 weeks
- 15–30% at 32–36 weeks.

Predisposing factors for RDS:

- Prematurity
- Male sex
- Maternal diabetes
- White ethnicity
- Pulmonary infection/haemorrhage
- Twin pregnancy (second twin at greater risk)
- Pre-labour caesarean section
- Hypothermia
- Perinatal compromise
- Familial predisposition.

Treatment/Prevention:

- Antenatal steroids administered to the mother 48–72 hours before delivery reduce the incidence of RDS and decrease the incidence of neonatal death, IVH and NEC. Antenatal steroids accelerate lung growth and increase surfactant production. Repeated doses may affect the final numbers of alveoli and somatic growth.
- Exogenous surfactant can decrease the severity and mortality of RDS. There is some evidence that CPAP without elective intubation and surfactant administration may be an acceptable alternative to elective intubation in spontaneously breathing neonates as young as 25/40 (COIN trial). However, if intubation is needed in neonates born <30 weeks surfactant therapy should be considered.
- Oxygen in high concentrations is potentially toxic to the respiratory epithelium. Resuscitation in all infants should start with air, with increasing oxygen concentration as required.
- Prevention of hypothermia improves endogenous surfactant production; radiant heat sources and occlusive plastic bags are beneficial for small preterm babies.

8.22 Phototherapy

Answer D: Clinical detection of jaundice can be difficult in children, especially those with increased skin pigmentation, so a low threshold for measuring serum bilirubin is essential

Phototherapy reduces serum unconjugated bilirubin levels. It uses light at a wavelength of 420–550 nm and causes bilirubin to become water soluble; this allows excretion without conjugation. It is indicated for the treatment of infants with pathological levels of unconjugated hyperbilirubinaemia for the prevention of kernicterus. It reduces the need for exchange transfusion in infants with hyperbilirubinaemia, but when indications for exchange exist it is not a substitute.

There are National Institute for Health and Clinical Excellence (NICE) guidelines (2010) that specify how and when to start and stop phototherapy, and the indications for exchange transfusion. These guidelines include threshold graphs individualised for each week of gestation from 26 to ≥38 weeks. Parents should be fully informed about the need for eye protection and the likelihood of rebound hyperbilirubinaemia after stopping phototherapy. Complications of phototherapy include loose stools, rashes, dehydration, temperature instability and the potential risks of reduced mother–infant bonding and interference with lactation. There are some data that show that phototherapy may have DNA-damaging effects but the long-term significance of this is not clear. There is no evidence that there is an increased risk of malignant melanoma.

If single phototherapy is indicated, short breaks for feeding, changing and cuddles may be allowed, and feeding and lactation should be encouraged. Additional fluids or feeds should not be used routinely in this group, but hydration should be monitored with daily weights and assessment of nappies and electrolytes. If continuous multiple phototherapy is indicated it should not be interrupted for feeding. Intravenous fluids/enteral feeding should be started and lactation supported as maternal breast milk is the feed of choice.

The colour of the skin does not alter phototherapy's efficacy, but skin colour is an inaccurate method of assessing the bilirubin level in a jaundiced baby. Clinical assessment of level of jaundice may be difficult, particularly in infants with dark skin tones and, so once detected a serum measurement of bilirubin should be recorded.

8.23 Neonatal polycythaemia

Answer B: Trisomy 21 is a predisposing factor for developing polycythaemia

Polycythaemia refers to a raised haematocrit (packed cell volume). Neonatal polycythaemia is usually said to be present if the venous packed cell volume is >65%. The viscosity of blood increases exponentially above a haematocrit of 65%. Haematocrit increases after birth and peaks at 2–12 hours of age; only 40% of children who have a haematocrit >64% at 2 hours still have polycythaemia after 12 hours of age. Predisposing factors are:

- Post-maturity
- Small for gestational age/IUGR/placental insufficiency
- Delayed cord clamping (maternal–fetal transfusion)
- Twin-to-twin transfusion

- Infant of a diabetic mother
- Trisomies 13, 18 and 21
- Beckwith–Wiedemann syndrome
- Hyperthyroidism.

Clinical features/complications are as follows:

- Respiratory: tachypnoea, respiratory distress, apnoea
- Cardiovascular: cardiac failure, acrocyanosis, central cyanosis, persistent fetal circulation, priapism in boys
- Gastrointestinal: feeding problems, vomiting, NEC
- Renal: renal vein thrombosis
- Nervous system: lethargy, hypotonia, seizures, irritability, jitteriness, tremor, stroke
- Skin: plethora
- Haematological: thrombocytopenia
- Biochemical: hypoglycaemia, hypocalcaemia, hyperbilirubinaemia.

Treatment of polycythaemia includes ensuring an adequate fluid intake, attention to predisposing factors and exclusion of alternative aetiology for symptoms. Symptomatic infants may require a partial exchange transfusion with 0.9% saline to achieve a haematocrit of 50–55%. FFP and 4.5% human albumin are alternative exchange fluids but should be used with caution. The indications for dilution are controversial because evidence of long-term benefit is limited. Consideration of exchange should be in those infants who are symptomatic with a packed cell volume >65% or those who have a packed cell volume >70%. Late neurological sequelae are seen in some infants with symptomatic polycythaemia. NEC is associated with umbilical partial exchange transfusion, especially if colloid is used.

8.24 Hypoxic ischaemic encephalopathy

Answer D: Persistent fetal circulation is a recognised complication of HIE

Perinatal asphyxia occurs in 4–9/1000 live births. It is defined as impaired maternal–fetal gas exchange resulting in hypoxaemia, plus development of combined respiratory and metabolic acidosis. Although the insult is global. brain injury depends on the extent and length of time of the insult. Injury occurs as a direct consequence of hypoxia–ischaemia and also due to reperfusion injury.

Risk factors and causes:

- Maternal: diabetes, smoking, hypotension, hypoxia
- Cord: prolapse, occlusion
- Placenta: insufficiency, abruption
- Fetal: multiple pregnancy, growth restriction, congenital abnormality.

Hypoxic–ischaemic injury can cause multiorgan dysfunction:

- Respiratory: PPHN, pulmonary haemorrhage, surfactant deficiency, meconium aspiration

- Cardiovascular: myocardial dysfunction (and rarely infarction), hypotension
- Central nervous system: encephalopathy, seizures, cerebral oedema, bleeding/infarction/stroke
- Renal: acute tubular necrosis, adrenal haemorrhage
- Gastrointestinal: feed intolerance, perforation, NEC
- Metabolic: hyponatraemia (SIADH and renal impairment), hypoglycaemia, hypocalcaemia, deranged liver function, lactic acidosis
- Haematological: disseminated intravascular coagulation, haemorrhage, thrombocytopenia.

The severity of HIE is related to neurodevelopmental outcome, development of cerebral palsy and cognitive disability later in life. It is graded as follows:

- Grade I: irritability, mild hypotonia, poor suck, no seizures (good outcome)
- Grade II: lethargy, abnormal tone, requirement for tube feeds, seizures (20% disability)
- Grade III: comatose, severe hypotonia, failure to maintain respiration without respiratory support, prolonged seizures (pre-cooling 50% died; all had disability)
- Less than 10% of cerebral palsy is as a consequence of perinatal asphyxia (but medicolegal costs are high)
- Cerebral palsy secondary to severe HIE is most commonly quadriplegic ± dystonic features
- Cognitive delay is seen in addition to cerebral palsy but is rarely isolated
- Of survivors of grade III HIE 5–10% are deaf and blind
- Of survivors of grade III HIE 5–10% have ongoing seizures.

Trials have shown that the use of moderate hypothermia within 6 hours of moderate HIE can improve neurodevelopmental outcome in this population, as covered earlier in this chapter.

8.25 Bile-stained vomiting

Answer A: Most cases of duodenal atresia occur as isolated abnormalities

Duodenal atresia

This accounts for 25–40% of all intestinal atresias, but is rare, occurring in approximately 1 child per 10 000 births. Most cases of duodenal atresia will be isolated abnormalities but associated abnormalities do occur; 20–30% of cases are associated with Down syndrome. Other associations include malrotation, oesophageal atresia, anorectal malformations and congenital heart disease. Fifty per cent will be diagnosed *in utero* during antenatal scanning. Early onset of bilious vomiting within hours of birth is the norm for postnatal presentation. Fifteen per cent of babies with duodenal atresia will not have bile-stained vomiting due to the atresia being proximal to the ampulla of Vater. Classical radiological appearance is of the 'double bubble'. Treatment is surgical.

Pyloric stenosis

This has multifactorial inheritance. There is projectile non-bilious vomiting, with onset most commonly between age 3 weeks and 5 months. The baby presents hungry and with weight loss. Firstborn boys are more commonly affected. Palpable pyloric tumour and visible gastric peristalsis are present. Mild unconjugated hyperbilirubinaemia and hypochloraemic/hypokalaemic metabolic alkalosis also occur. Ultrasonography confirms the diagnosis. Treatment is by pyloromyotomy (Ramstedt procedure) after correction of electrolyte and acid–base disturbance.

Malrotation

This refers to incomplete rotation of the midgut during fetal development, resulting in the small bowel occupying the right side of the abdomen and the large bowel the left. The caecum is often subhepatic. The mesentery along with the superior mesenteric artery is attached by a narrow stalk, which can twist around itself producing a midgut volvulus. Infants can present with bile-stained vomiting with or without abdominal distension in the first few weeks of life, or later with episodes of abdominal colic and vomiting. Diagnosis is by upper GI contrast; barium enema may show a malpositioned caecum but is less reliable. Meconium can still be passed with obstruction of the upper small bowel. Bilious vomiting in a neonate is a surgical emergency until proven otherwise.

Other causes of intestinal obstruction in the neonatal period include Hirschsprung disease, meconium ileus and imperforate anus. Distal obstructions may present with abdominal distension, delayed passage of meconium and absence of transitional stools, rather than bilious vomiting.

8.26 Neonatal haematology

Answer D: There is no clear evidence that using a restrictive red blood cell (RBC) transfusion policy to manage neonates on the NICU leads to an increased length of admission to NICU or an increase in rates of intraventricular haemorrhage, NEC or chronic lung disease

Cord haemoglobin levels in term infants range from 16 g/dl to 20 g/dl, rising in the first 24 hours then falling slowly to as low as 9.5 g/l by the ninth week of life. The levels in preterm infants are lower because they show an increased rate of fall of haemoglobin even in the absence of iatrogenic sampling. Over the first few months a physiological anaemia occurs, due at least in part to reduced red cell survival, low erythropoietin levels and increasing blood volume caused by increasing weight. Anaemia at birth is commonly due to immune haemolysis or acute blood loss. Anaemia due to reduced red cell production is not usually noticed till 3–4 weeks of age. Fetal haemoglobin constitutes 70% of the haemoglobin at birth. It contains two α and two γ chains. α Thalassaemia may present in the neonatal period; β thalassaemia does not usually present until the latter half of the first year of life when the γ-chain production is switched off. Fetal haemoglobin is resistant to alkaline denaturation, unlike adult haemoglobin; this is the basis of the Apt test used to differentiate fetal blood from swallowed maternal blood in the gut (eg on a gastric aspirate). The direct Coombs test is positive in patients with immune-mediated haemolysis.

Transfusion in the neonatal period is controversial, but there has been a trend towards a decreased rate of transfusion in neonates over the last 15 years. Observational studies conducted over this time have not shown any increase in need for respiratory support, increase in faltering growth, increase in length of hospital stay, or increase in the rate of IVH, NEC or chronic lung disease in neonates managed with a restrictive RBC transfusion policy.

Causes of anaemia in the neonate include the following.

Blood loss

- Internal fetal haemorrhage:
  - intraventricular haemorrhage
  - cephalohaematoma, subgaleal bleed
  - pulmonary haemorrhage
  - retroperitoneal bleed
  - ruptured liver or spleen
- Obstetric accidents:
  - placental abruption
  - placenta praevia
  - rupture of placenta or umbilical cord
- Occult haemorrhage before delivery:
  - fetofetal haemorrhage
  - fetomaternal bleed
- Iatrogenic: frequent sampling.

Haemolysis

- Immune:
  - ABO incompatibility
  - rhesus disease
  - other antibody (Kell, etc.)
- Hereditary:
  - hereditary spherocytosis
  - glucose-6-phosphate dehydrogenase deficiency
  - α and γ thalassaemia
  - galactosaemia
- Macro-/Microangiopathic:
  - cavernous haemangioma
  - large vessel thrombosis
  - renal artery stenosis.

Impaired production

- Pure red cell aplasia – Diamond–Blackfan syndrome.
- Acquired bacterial/viral infection
- Congenital infection, eg CMV/rubella/parvovirus.

8.27 Neonatal seizures

Answer E: There is evidence that anticonvulsive medication commonly used to control neonatal seizures may have detrimental effects on developmental outcome when used in neonates; however, the balance of risks is still in favour of treating seizures to try to get the best outcome possible for the patient

Convulsions are the most common neurological sign seen in the newborn; they are four times more common in the preterm neonate (although more commonly unrecognised) than the term neonate, and overall rates are around 2.6/1000 live births. Seizure types can be diverse, subtle and difficult to detect, and can vary within the same patient over a short period of time. Subtle manifestations of neonatal seizures can include lip smacking, tongue thrusting, mouthing, cycling movements of the lower limbs and swimming movements of the upper limbs. Apnoea can be a common manifestation of subtle seizures, particularly in the preterm population.

Causes of neonatal seizures:

- Hypoxic ischaemic encephalopathy (38–40%)
- Cerebral infarction (20%)
  - MCA (middle cerebral artery) infarction
  - sagittal sinus thrombosis
- Intraventricular haemorrhage (12–20%)
- Congenital malformation (5–10%)
- Infection (3–20%)
- Hypoglycaemia/hypocalcaemia (3–19%)
- Hyponatraemia
- Hypernatraemia
- Inborn error of metabolism (1%)
- Kernicterus
- Benign familial neonatal convulsions
- Benign sleep myoclonus
- Fifth day fits
- Drug withdrawal
- Idiopathic.

Not all clinical manifestations of seizure activity in the neonate correspond to abnormal EEG findings; conversely, not all electrical seizure activity on EEG corresponds to overt abnormal movements (electroconvulsive dissociation). Anticonvulsants commonly used to control neonatal seizures have relatively low rates of EEG seizure control 43–62%. Data suggest that the antiepileptic drugs (AEDs) commonly used to control seizures in the neonatal period may in themselves lead to neuronal death as a result of apoptosis, with lasting effects on development. These effects appear to be additive with the use of more than one AED. However, there is also evidence that frequent seizures cause additional damage to the developing brain and so, in refractory seizures, a balance needs to be struck between treatment side effects and the risks of ongoing or recurrent seizure activity.

Prognosis of neonatal seizures reported in one study of term babies was relatively good, with a reported favourable outcome in 72%; however, this decreases to 50% if seizures secondary to HIE are considered separately.

8.28 Congenital dislocation of the hip

Answer C: If a Pavlik harness can be fitted before 6 weeks of age, the treatment will be successful in approx. 90% of patients

Congenital dislocation or developmental dysplasia of the hip is a common disorder present in 15–20/1000 live births, with frank dislocation in 1–2/1000 births. It is either present at birth or develops over the first 3 months of life as a consequence of the femoral head being partially or fully displaced from the acetabulum.

Risk factors for congenital dislocation of the hip:

- Family history (positive in 20%)
- Female sex (female:male 6:1)
- Breech presentation (factor in 30%)
- Spina bifida
- Being firstborn
- Oligohydramnios.

The left hip is more likely to be dislocated than the right. Ultrasonography is the best test for diagnosis. The clinical tests of hip instability are the Ortolani (relocation) and Barlow (dislocation) tests.

The management of this condition varies according to the time of diagnosis. The earlier the diagnosis, the better the prognosis. Currently all neonates are screened at birth and at 6–8 weeks by clinical examination. Prognosis is better for those picked up on screening (<3 months) than those children presenting later (>3 months). Delayed diagnosis beyond 3 months almost always requires surgical intervention but the timing of surgery is debatable. Surgery is sometimes delayed to try to decrease the complication of avascular necrosis of the femoral head. Treatment using the Pavlik harness has good prognosis if started early, <6 weeks, with 90% successful outcome. It should be fitted as early as possible and kept *in situ* for 6 weeks with weaning over the next 6 weeks. The hips should be monitored closely and treatment discontinued if there is no response due to the increased risk of avascular necrosis of the cartilaginous femoral head.

8.29 Prolonged neonatal jaundice

Answer E: Conjugated and unconjuugated bilirubin

Prolonged jaundice is defined as jaundice lasting more than 14 days in term babies and 21 days in preterm babies. It is common and affects 15–40% of term breastfed infants. It is imperative to have full assessment of all children with prolonged jaundice to exclude the rare but potentially catastrophic missed cause of this common condition, biliary atresia (jaundice is not a symptom, it is a clinical sign).

THE NICE guidelines (2010) for management of prolonged jaundice state the following:

- **Visual inspection for pale chalky stools and/or dark urine is obligatory.**
- **Measure conjugated bilirubin, FBC (full blood count), blood group and direct antiglobulin test (DAT), and culture urine.**
- **Ensure that routine metabolic screening had been performed (Guthrie/neonatal blood spot test).**
- **Conjugated bilirubin levels >25 μmol/l should be referred for expert advice because they may indicate underlying serious liver disease.**

This baby is most likely to have physiological breast milk jaundice. Breastfeeding should not be stopped.

The Guthrie/neonatal blood spot card currently screens for congenital hypothyroidism, phenylketonuria, sickle cell disease, cystic fibrosis and medium-chain acyl-CoA dehydrogenase deficiency (MCADD).

8.30 Oxygen transfer from the placenta to fetus

Answer A: Oxygen transfer from the placenta to fetus is possible because of relative left shift of the oxygen dissociation curve in haemoglobin F

The left shift of the dissociation curve enables haemoglobin F (HbF) to pick up oxygen transplacentally. None of the other factors is true or has any bearing on this. HbF is composed of α_2- γ_2-globin chains whereas adult Hb is mainly α_2 β_2. HbF has reduced 2,3-diphosphoglycerate (2,3-DPG), causing a left shift in the oxygen dissociation curve – in other words for a given PO_2 the saturation increases. HbF therefore has a high affinity for oxygen, which helps transplacental transfer. This does mean, however, that unloading of oxygen into the tissues is slower. 2,3-DPG levels rise rapidly in the first few days to cope with metabolic demand.

Other causes of a left shift in the curve:

- Alkalosis
- Hypocapnia
- Hypothermia.

8.31 Presentation of floppy neonate

Answer E: Genetic testing for deletion on chromosome 5q

This is the picture of congenital/severe spinal muscular atrophy (SMA) type 1, also called (eponymously) Werdnig–Hoffman disease. It is an autosomal recessive disorder affecting 1 in 10 000 live births. Cases present any time from birth to 6 months of age, with 95% having symptoms before age 3 months and 60% being floppy at birth, and 30% reporting decreased movement *in utero*. Affected infants show progressive muscle weakness and hypotonia with absent reflexes, leading to problems with sucking, swallowing and respiratory function. Patients have intact extraocular muscles and facial weakness is minimal or absent. Babies often appear alert and there is no evidence of cerebral involvement.

Examination reveals diffuse muscle weakness and hypotonia greater in the proximal than the distal muscles. Deep tendon reflexes are absent; tongue fasciculations are usually present but may be confused with the normal random movements unless atrophy is present. Arthrogryphosis can be present at birth as a consequence of *in utero* hypotonia. Creatine kinase (CK) is typically normal in SMA type 1 and only mildly raised/normal in the other types. Cerebrospinal fluid (CSF) findings are normal. Prenatal and postnatal genetic testing are now available to identify this condition; 95% of cases of SMA involve a homozygous deletion of the *SMN1* gene on the long arm of chromosome 5 (5q). Muscle biopsy may be needed if genetic testing is not definitive.

Neonatal nerve conduction studies are difficult to interpret and may be delayed until 6 months of age. There is no curative treatment and, even with supportive measures, the median survival is 7 months with a 95% mortality rate by 18 months, with respiratory infection leading to death in most cases.

8.32 Systolic murmur

Answer A: Four limb saturations

The prevalence of murmurs in the neonatal period varies widely. Many types of congenital heart disease can be associated with an asymptomatic murmur. Non-pathological' murmurs in the neonate are generally related to blood flow through the ductus arteriosus or turbulent flow through the pulmonary arteries. In one study of 50 infants with murmurs, 60% had PDA – all closed by 6 weeks; 50% had pulmonary branch stenosis – all resolved by 6 months

Management:

- Careful clinical examination of the whole cardiovascular system is essential and this should be repeated daily if the infant remains in hospital.
- Four limb blood pressure is variable and not reliable in identifying duct-dependent heart disease.
- Chest radiograph is unlikely to be helpful.
- ECG can be helpful, particularly if abnormal axis or consistent with LVH – indicating cardiac disease.
- Pulse oximetry should be performed in all neonates with clinical murmurs. It may detect subtle or evolving hypoxaemia and difference between pre- and post-ductal saturation may reveal a duct-dependent lesion, saturations <95% being regarded as abnormal.
- Refer any child with significant symptoms or signs (other than the murmur), those who have dysmorphic features or other congenital abnormality or a harsh/loud murmur, or who show hypoxaemia on pulse oximetry.
- Departments vary but in one large audit all children who were well with low intensity murmurs (10% of neonates) and normal pulse oximetry were discharged with written advice about significant symptoms and reviewed weekly and, if the murmur was still present at 2 weeks, a referral to cardiology was made. A third of referrals were found to have a structural heart defect. Only 6% of infants fitting these criteria discharged in the latest 4 years of audit had a structural heart defect, none of which was life threatening.

EMQ Answers

8.33–8.35 Theme: The differential diagnosis of shock presenting in the neonatal period

8.33

Answer F: Duct-dependent cardiac lesion

Moderate-to-severe congenital heart defects occur in around 5–8/1000 live births. Despite major advances in diagnosis and management over the last 10 years, these defects still account for 3% of all infant deaths and 40% of deaths from congenital malformations.

Duct-dependent defects include:

- Critical coarctation of the aorta
- Hypoplastic left heart
- Interrupted aortic arch
- Critical aortic valve stenosis
- Transposition of the great arteries
- Pulmonary atresia.

Presentation of duct-dependent lesions:

- Within the first few weeks of life (usually <6 weeks)
- Dramatic: often asymptomatic until duct closure, then present in shock with circulatory compromise and metabolic acidosis; in its most severe form may present as acute collapse and sudden death
- Insidious: poor feeding, lethargy, breathlessness, respiratory distress, hypothermia, cyanotic episodes
- Poor pulses, significant pre- or post-ductal saturation difference, decreased lower limb blood pressure
- Cardiac failure
- Heart murmur
- Dysmorphic features or other congenital malformations
- Arrhythmias.

Differential diagnosis includes sepsis and metabolic disorders:

- Chest radiograph can be useful but pulmonary vasculature may be more helpful than cardiac shadows.
- Pulse oximetry can be used as a screening tool for detection of aortic arch abnormalities and cyanotic congenital heart disease (saturations <95% or a difference of >3% between pre- and post-ductal saturations is significant).

Management:

- **Resuscitation and stabilisation with correction of metabolic acidosis**

- Start prostaglandin E_1 infusion to keep arterial duct open at a dose of 5 ng/kg per min, doubled after 20 min if no improvement. If duct already closed, doses of up to 100 ng/kg per min may be required. This can be life saving and should be commenced while waiting to confirm the diagnosis.

8.34

Answer A: Group B streptococcal sepsis

Sepsis must be part of the differential for any severely unwell neonate. The two most common pathogens in early (<48 h) neonatal sepsis are Group B streptococci and *E. coli*. Risk factors for neonatal sepsis include prematurity, prolonged rupture of the membranes and maternal infection/pyrexia. GBS is a normal vaginal commensal found in about 30% of healthy women but can cause devastating infection in the neonatal period, either early (<5 days), often with septicaemia and pneumonia, or later in infancy up to 3 months post-delivery, when meningitis and septicaemia are common. Treatment is with resuscitation, oxygen, supportive measures and antibiotics. Antibiotic prophylaxis in labour for known carriers of GBS is known to reduce the incidence of early onset GBS infection but has no effect on the incidence of late-onset disease.

The hyperoxia test can sometimes be useful in helping to differentiate cyanosis due to primary pulmonary disease from that of cardiac disease with the presence of a right-to-left shunt. In cyanotic heart disease no amount of oxygen in the pulmonary circulation will alter the desaturating effect of the shunt. If the cyanosis is secondary to a respiratory cause, it is likely to correct, or at least improve, with an increased concentration of inspired oxygen. Any neonate with an oxygen saturation of <85% in both air and 100% oxygen is likely to have an intracardiac shunt; however, this test is not reliable and any unwell baby with suspected cardiac disease should have formal echocardiography. You should be aware of the theoretical risk of closure of the duct on exposure to 100% inspired oxygen.

8.35

Answer I: Congenital adrenal hyperplasia

This is a group of disorders inherited in an autosomal recessive pattern, the most common being 21-hydroxylase (21OH) deficiency, which accounts for 95% of cases. Congenital adrenal hyperplasia (CAH) is due to enzyme deficiencies in the adrenal cortex, where the metabolism of cholesterol to cortisol and aldosterone is interrupted and excess androgenic steroids accumulate as a byproduct of the process. CAH phenotype can vary greatly depending on the specific enzyme involved and the severity of its functional mutation. Severe forms of CAH can be fatal and present as described in the clinical case with severe cortisol and aldosterone deficiencies, leading to salt wasting, hyponatraemia, hyperkalaemia, dehydration and shock. Girls with 21OH deficiency often present with virilisation or ambiguous genitalia at birth, whereas boys may present from 5 days of age with a salt-losing crisis preceded by a history of poor feeding, vomiting and weight loss.

Patients with less severe 21OH deficiencies can present later in childhood with early pubic hair growth and phallic enlargement, accelerated linear growth and skeletal maturation. Diagnosis of 21OH deficiency is confirmed with increased 17OH-progesterone in serum – usually >100 nmol/l; a urinary steroid profile and specific genetic analysis can further define the exact point of disruption on the metabolic pathway. Management of a salt-losing crisis in the neonatal period includes primary resuscitation of the child with 0.9% saline to correct dehydration and 10% dextrose to correct hypoglycaemia. Replacement hydrocortisone is given 6 hourly intravenously, initially to correct the cortisol deficiency. Once the baby is more stable replacement sodium, hydrocortisone and fludrocortisone can be given orally. Parents should be warned about the potential dangers of decompensation during intercurrent illness, and the need for increased (doubled) doses of replacement hydrocortisone in these circumstances.

8.36–8.38 Theme: Syndromes associated with congenital heart disease

8.36 Down syndrome

Answer J: AVSD

This is the most common chromosomal disorder occurring in approximately 1 in 800 live births. It is due to trisomy 21 in 95% of cases (other cases being due to mosaicism or translocation) and is associated with multiple congenital malformations. Congenital heart disease (CHD) is a major cause of morbidity and mortality in children with Down syndrome, and affects 40–50% of infants.

Cardiac problems:

- Atrioventricular septal defect (AVSD) – 45%
- Ventricular septal defect (VSD) – 35%
- Secundum atrial septal defect (ASD) 8%
- PDA 7%
- Tetralogy of Fallot 4%
- Mixed lesions 1%
- In addition further cardiovascular abnormalities can develop in adolescence, including mitral valve prolapse (46%) and aortic regurgitation (17%).

It is important to note that examination alone cannot diagnose CHD in all children with Down syndrome. In one study 34% of children with Down syndrome remained undiagnosed with CHD at 6 weeks of age and 24% for up to 12 weeks. This is due in part to the propensity for children with Down syndrome to have pulmonary arterial hypertension. Thus, in a neonate with a large VSD or a complete AVSD, the normal fall in pulmonary vascular resistance that occurs over the first 6 weeks of life may be postponed, indefinitely in some cases. This consistently high pulmonary vascular resistance will mean that, despite these major lesions, pulmonary blood flow does not increase and so the usual presentations of cardiac murmur and breathlessness do not occur or occur late.

It is vital that echocardiography be performed in the first few weeks of life in babies with Down syndrome to reliably identify those who have CHD.

8.37 Noonan syndrome

Answer G: Pulmonary valve stenosis

This is a genetic disorder inherited in an autosomal dominant fashion or occurring sporadically. It is associated with gene mutations but a normal karyotype distinguishing it from Turner syndrome, with which it was previously confused. It occurs in between 1 in 1000 and 1 in 2500 live births and has equal sex distribution. The cardinal features of Noonan syndrome include typical triangular facial appearances, hypertelorism, downslanting eyes and a webbed neck; these phenotypical features can be difficult to discern in the neonatal period, becoming more classic with increasing age throughout early childhood. Birthweight within the normal range is common but short stature is present in 80% of affected children; 25% of children will have learning difficulties, and a bleeding diathesis is present in 50%. CHD occurs in 50% of cases, the characteristic lesion being a dysplastic/stenotic pulmonary valve, but virtually all types of congenital heart defects have been described in patients with Noonan syndrome. Hypertrophic cardiomyopathy (obstructive and non-obstructive types) is present in as many as 30% of patients.

8.38 Edward syndrome

Answer A: VSD

This is the most common autosomal trisomy after trisomy 21. It occurs in 1 in 6000–8000 live births but is a common cause of spontaneous abortion. Survival rates are low, with the mean survival time being 14.5 days; 38.6% survive to 1 month of age and 8.4% to 1 year. Severe psychomotor and growth retardation are present in all those who survive. Live-born cases of Edward syndrome are more commonly girls (3:1), representing a higher *in utero* death rate in affected males. Apnoeic episodes and poor feeding with failure to thrive are common.

Characteristic features:

- Microcephaly
- Prominent occiput
- Micrognathia
- Cleft lip and palate
- Low set ears
- Overlapping fingers
- Rocker-bottom feet
- Renal abnormalities
- Apnoea, which is a very common cause of death.

Cardiac defects are present in over 90% of infants born with trisomy 18. The most common abnormalities are VSDs (94%) in combination with polyvalvular heart disease (pulmonary and aortic valves). Many other lesions may occur including ASD (68%), PDA (77%), overriding aorta, coarctation of the aorta, hypoplastic left heart syndrome, tetralogy of Fallot and transposition of the great arteries.

Treatment on the whole is supportive and palliative. including enteral feeding, antibiotics for infection management of any distress and medical management of cardiac problems. However, there is an increasing trend towards surgical management of cardiac conditions and full supportive care.

8.39–8.41 Theme: Conjugated hyperbilirubinaemia

Causes of conjugated hyperbilirubinaemia in the neonatal period include the following:

- Infectious: hepatitis A, B and C, cytomegalovirus, rubella, herpes simplex virus
- Metabolic: cystic fibrosis, tyrosinaemia, galactosaemia, fructosaemia
- Intrahepatic: Alagille syndrome, congenital hepatic fibrosis
- Extrahepatic: biliary atresia, choledochal cyst, inspissated bile syndrome
- Toxic: total parenteral nutrition related, sepsis, urinary tract infection, drugs
- Endocrine: hypopituitarism, hypothyroidism
- Miscellaneous: intestinal obstruction.

8.39

Answer J: Congenital CMV (cCMV)

This is the most common congenital infection in the developed world with an incidence of 0.18–6.2% of all births. Defined as isolation of CMV within 3 weeks of birth, it can be asymptomatic (but not without long-term sequelae) in the vast majority of patients. The risk of placental transfer and symptomatic cCMV is much higher with primary maternal CMV infection (10–25%) versus secondary reactivation (around 2%). Postnatally acquired infection does not seem to be associated with the same long-term sequelae as congenital infection. Positive serology (IgM) is present in 70% of cases of cCMV. PCR (polymerase chain reaction) from saliva and urine can identify viral shedding which can be prolonged – lasting up to 2 years in 98% of cases of cCMV.

Clinical features of cCMV:

- IUGR
- Microcephaly
- Hepatosplenomegaly
- Petechiae (thrombocytopenia)/blueberry muffin rash
- Pneumonitis
- Jaundice
- Chorioretinitis
- Seizures
- Dental enamel defects
- Other neurological abnormalities, eg tone and posture/focal neurological signs.

Investigation abnormalities in cCMV:

- Thrombocytopenia
- Anaemia
- Coagulopathy
- ↑ AST/ALT aspartate and alanine aminotransferases)
- Conjugated hyperbilirubinaemia
- CSF abnormalities
- Abnormal cranial ultrasonography/CT/MRI (lissencephaly, polymicrogyria, dilated ventricles, periventricular calcification).

Mortality rates for symptomatic cCMV are quoted between 10 and 30%. Long-term sequelae include sensorineural hearing loss, chorioretinitis and neurodevelopmental delay. Those who are symptomatic at birth have a 40–58% risk of long-term sequelae compared with 13.5% in those who had no symptoms at birth. The neurological outcome is worse in children who have evidence of CNS involvement (including chorioretinitis) in the neonatal period. Hearing loss appears to be progressive in 50% of cases and can be late onset, with some patients presenting over 6 years after the original congenital infection.

Management:

- Supportive treatment including correction of coagulopathy and vitamin K for hepatitis
- Intravenous ganciclovir (may be associated with improved outcomes; also current research into effectiveness of oral valganciclovir)
- Ophthalmological follow-up to monitor and identify retinal disease that may be delayed in onset and progressive
- Hearing should be tested every 3–6 months in year 1, every 6–9 months in years 2 and 3 and yearly from 4 to 6
- Neurodevelopmental follow-up.

8.40

Answer A: Biliary atresia

This is a sclerosing cholangitis that can start *in utero*, around the time of birth or early in postnatal life. There are three major patterns of disease:

1. Type 1: atresia confined to the common bile duct (8%)
2. Type 2: atresia of the common hepatic duct with residual patency of the right and left hepatic ducts (2%)
3. Type 3: atresia of the whole of the extrahepatic duct system (90%).

Aetiology: unknown:

- 10–20% associated with cardiovascular system/gastrointestinal/genitourinary anomalies
- 10% abnormalities of biliary tree can be seen on antenatal ultrasonography.

Management:

- Untreated → progressive hepatosplenomegaly, portal hypertension, jaundice and ascites. Failing liver and malabsorption lead to progressive emaciation, growth failure, rickets, pruritis and hypersplenism. Death at 2 years from systemic/respiratory infection, GI bleeding or liver failure.
- Surgical correction (Kasai procedure – portoenterostomy):
  –<60 days – 90% will drain bile and 70% will lose their jaundice
  – >13 weeks 20% drainage and loss of jaundice
  – postsurgical predisposition to recurrent episodes of bacterial cholangitis (recurrent episodes are associated with progressive cirrhosis)
  – 30–40% overall will survive >10 years with native liver; most still have evidence of cirrhosis
  – biliary atresia is the most frequent indication for liver transplantation in infancy and childhood.

Differential diagnosis includes choledochal cyst, spontaneous perforation of the common bile duct, gallstones and inspissated bile syndrome. These conditions are rare but cannot be easily differentiated on clinical grounds.

8.41

Answer G: Alagille syndrome

This is an autosomal dominant disorder with variable expression; 15–50% occur as spontaneous mutations. Incidence is 1 in 100 000 live births.

Clinical features:

- Characteristic facial features (broad forehead, deep-set eyes and pointed chin) which become more obvious as the child grows older
- Poor linear growth
- Ophthalmological:
  – 75% have posterior embryotoxon (a thin line seen at the edge of the iris)
  – Axenfeld anomaly (iris attachment to the Descemet membrane), retinitis pigmentosa, papillary abnormalities and abnormalities of the optic disc.
- Cardiovascular:
  – most commonly peripheral pulmonary artery stenosis
  – ASD, VSD, tetralogy of Fallot, PDA and pulmonary atresia are also associated and represent an increased mortality risk for those in whom they are present
  – a subset of patients also have Wolff–Parkinson–White syndrome.
- Hepatic:
  – hypoplasia of the intralobular ducts leads to cholestatic jaundice, pruritis from ↑ serum bile acids and hypercholesterolaemia (xanthomas)
  – hepatosplenomegaly is common
  – fat-soluble vitamin deficiencies and their consequences are common (vitamins A, D, E and K).

- Skeletal: anomalies of the vertebrae (butterfly hemivertebrae), ribs and hands are seen.
- Neurological: mild developmental delay and learning difficulties are reported in some children.
- Renal: hypertension may be caused by occult renal artery stenosis, lipoid nephrosis or glomerulosclerosis.
- Vascular: anomalies occur in around 6% of cases and include basilar artery aneurysms, internal carotid artery anomalies, middle cerebral artery aneurysms, moya-moya disease and aortic aneurysms, coarctation of the aorta and renal artery stenosis.

Treatment of fat-soluble vitamin deficiencies is vital, along with treatment of pruritis which can be severe and disabling. Liver transplantation may be indicated in patients with progressive hepatic dysfunction, severe portal hypertension, resistant failure to thrive, intractable pruritis and osteodystrophy.

8.42–8.44 Theme: Neonatal meningitis

Neonatal bacterial meningitis is a significant cause of morbidity and mortality. Of all age groups the neonatal period has the highest incidence of meningitis due to the relative immaturity of the immune system. In the UK there are approximately 0.22 cases per 1000 births. The overall mortality rate is 10%, with 50% of cases developing some form of disability and 24% being classified as serious. These long-term disabilities include cerebral palsy (8.1%), learning difficulties (7.5%), seizures (7.3%) and hearing problems (25%). More subtle long-term problems include behavioural and educational difficulties which may not be immediately apparent.

Aetiology of neonatal bacterial meningitis in the UK:

- Group B streptococcus (up to 50%)
- *Escherichia coli* (18–26%)
- Other Gram-negative enteric bacteria (8–12%):
  - *Klebsiella* spp.
  - *Enterobacter* spp.
  - *Citrobacter* spp.
  - *Serratia* spp.
  - *Listeria monocytogenes* (5–7%).

Streptococcus pneumoniae, Haemophilus influenzae and *Nesseria meningitidis*, although among the leading causes of childhood meningitis, are rare under the age of 2 months.

Neonatal meningitis is closely associated with sepsis, which is five times more common. Risk factors for both sepsis and meningitis in the neonatal period include:

- Prematurity
- Low birthweight (<1500 g)
- Maternal colonisation with GBS
- Premature rupture of membranes
- Low socioeconomic status

- Male gender
- Invasive monitoring/need for resuscitation
- Fetal hypoxia
- Maternal peripartum infection including chorioamnionitis.

Symptoms and signs of neonatal bacterial meningitis include:

- Fever/hypothermia, poor feeding, apnoea, lethargy, vomiting, respiratory distress (>50%)
- Seizure (40%)
- Irritability (32%)
- Full/bulging fontanelle (28%).

Note that nuchal rigidity occurs in <25% of affected neonates.

Early onset meningitis is usually associated with features of systemic illness rather than neurological signs. Respiratory distress can be prominent within hours of birth in GBS, *E. coli* and listeria meningitis. Late onset (>48 h) is more likely to be associated with focal neurological signs.

A lumbar puncture should be performed in all cases of suspected meningitis because blood cultures may be negative. A normal CSF (cells, protein and glucose) does not exclude meningitis because 13% may go on to yield organisms. Antibiotics vary but generally cefotaxime and amoxicillin should be used in community-acquired neonatal meningitis. and an aminoglycoside should be added for patients on or recently discharged from a neonatal unit (local advice is vital). Current advice is not to use corticosteroids to treat meningitis in children aged <3 months.

8.42

Answer E: Listeria monocytogenes

Listeria monocytogenes is a Gram-positive rod with a number of animal vectors. Transmission outside the neonatal period is often by a food-borne route (soft cheeses, uncooked meats, etc.). In pregnant women, infection gives a 'flu-like' illness, but may be asymptomatic. Transplacental infection, ascending infection after rupture of membranes or acquisition during vaginal delivery are all possible routes of vertical transmission. Infection can precipitate preterm delivery and passage of meconium, which is unusual because prematurity tends to be associated with delayed passage of meconium due to neuromuscular immaturity. Early onset neonatal listeria infection mostly presents as septicaemia and disseminated disease ± meningitis; late-onset disease (mean 14 days) usually presents with meningitis. Respiratory difficulty is common, including cyanosis, tachypnoea and grunting. Treatment is with amoxicillin in addition to broad-spectrum cover with gentamicin or cefotaxime until diagnosis is established (depending on local policy).

8.43

Answer J: HSV meningitis

The incidence of neonatal herpes simplex virus (HSV) meningitis is 0.02 cases per 1000 births; mortality rate runs at approximately 15% and long-term morbidity is seen in up to 50% of cases. Vertical transmission is the most likely cause (90%), although many women are unaware of having had herpes as a primary infection and recurrences may be subclinical. Instrumental delivery and fetal scalp electrodes can increase vertical transmission. Caesarean section decreases but does not exclude vertical transmission.

Late-onset meningitis/encephalitis, presenting with seizures, lethargy, temperature instability and/or poor feeding in the second week, is most common. Disseminated HSV infection typically presents in the first week of life with non-specific signs suggestive of sepsis, including temperature instability, apnoea, hypoxia, poor feeding and irritability. Some of these patients will go on to develop respiratory distress secondary to pneumonitis or seizures if there is CNS spread, hepatic dysfunction and disseminated intravascular coagulation (DIC). Vesicular rash should be looked for but is absent in 70% of cases with CNS involvement. CSF examination typically shows a haemorrhagic lymphocytosis with normal glucose and slightly increased protein. Raised aminotransferases and thrombocytopenia with or without DIC are associated with systemic spread. Neuroimaging commonly shows inflammation in the temporoparietal region, and this may correspond to characteristic EEG changes. Treatment is with a prolonged course (21 days) of intravenous aciclovir, which should be initiated early.

8.44

Answer F: GBS

Group B streptococcus colonises the genital and GI tracts of 15–45% of women. Vertical transmission rate is approximately 50% but only 1–2% of infants develop invasive disease. GBS is the most common cause of neonatal sepsis but it is uncommon in itself with an incidence of 0.5/1000 births. Neonatal group B streptococcal infection can be divided into early disease, which is usually seen within 24 hours of birth but can present up to 7 days of life; septicaemia and pneumonia are common, meningitis less common, and late-onset disease defined as that presenting >1 week or <3 months, more commonly associated with bacteraemia and meningitis. There are guidelines issued by The Royal College of Obstetricians and Gynaecologists for the prevention of early onset group B streptococcal disease using antibiotic prophylaxis in labour in known carriers, but this does not affect the incidence of late-onset disease.

8.45–8.47 Theme: Neonatal presentation of congenital abnormalities

8.45

Answer D: Turner syndrome

Turner syndrome is caused by the absence of one set of genes on the short arm of one X chromosome. This may be due to an XO karyotype or as a consequence of a more limited deletion of one of the X chromosomes. Clinical features include:

- Short stature (<50th centile <11 years and absent adolescent growth spurt) – an indication for growth hormone
- Ovarian failure (no breast development by age 12, no menses by 14 years)
- Normal pubic hair
- Hypoplastic/Hyperconvex nails
- Webbed neck
- Increased carrying angle of the arm
- Shield chest
- Lymphoedema of hands and feet
- GI bleeding (increased vascular abnormalities/increased ulcerative colitis and Crohn disease)
- Hip dislocation
- Scoliosis
- Hypertension (even in the absence of coarctation and renal abnormalities)
- Hypothyroidism
- Neonatal lymphoedema of hands and feet
- Coarctation (about 20%)/hypoplastic left heart/bicuspid aortic valve
- Infertility
- Normal or near normal intelligence.

Prenatal signs:

- Nuchal cystic hygroma, pedal oedema
- Horseshoe kidney
- Left-sided cardiac abnormalities (may not be apparent before ductal closure)
- Non-immune fetal hydrops.

8.46

Answer C: Prader–Willi syndrome

Prader–Willi syndrome is the first syndrome attributed to the loss of genetic material differentially expressed due to its parental origin (genomic imprinting). Deletion of material from the15q11–13 locus from the paternally inherited gene results in Prader–Willi syndrome (70%) and deletion from the same locus on the maternally inherited gene results in Angelman syndrome. Twenty-eight per cent of cases of Prader–Willi syndrome result from maternal uniparental disomy of chromosome 15 (no paternal 15q).

Infants with Prader–Willi syndrome often present with neonatal hypotonia (hallmark), poor suck, weak cry, genital hypoplasia (cryptorchidism/clitoral hypoplasia) and failure to thrive. Other features include:

- Delayed motor development (toddlers)
- 1–6 years: development of hyperphagia
- Progressive obesity
- Short stature
- Sleep disturbances (narcolepsy, obstructive sleep apnoea)
- Behavioural issues (obsessive–compulsive disorder, temper tantrums, psychosis, food seeking/binging)
- Decreased IQ.

8.47

Answer H: VATER association

An association is defined as a group of congenital abnormalities that are associated in a non-random fashion but the grouping and aetiology are not strongly defined enough to be termed a syndrome. VATER/VACTERL is an example of an association.

This baby has abnormalities of at least two systems: renal and (clinically) oesophageal. The picture is typical of an oesophageal atresia, and can be confirmed by failure of passage of a nasogastric tube into the stomach. Often there is an associated tracheo-oesophageal fistula. Features of VATER include:

- V = vertebral, eg bifid vertebrae
- A = anorectal, eg atresia
- T = tracheo-oesophageal fistula
- E = oesophageal atresia
- R = renal (eg horseshoe kidney).

The additional findings of cardiac abnormalities and limb defects (predominantly radial defects), in association with the above, has led to some preferring to call this the VACTERL association.

8.48–8.50 Theme: Neonatal thrombocytopenia

Neonatal thrombocytopenia (platelets $<150 \times 10^9$/l) occurs in 5–10% of newborn infants, with severe thrombocytopenia (platelets $<50 \times 10^9$/l) occurring in 0.1–0.5% The occurrence is higher in sick babies, with 8% of preterm babies and 6% of all babies in NICU having severe ($<50 \times 10^9$/l) thrombocytopenia at some point during their stay.

Classification is as follows.

Fetal

- Alloimmune (NAIT)
- Congenital infection (CMV, toxoplasmosis, rubella)

- Chromosomal abnormalities/aneuploidy (trisomies 13, 18 and 21)
- Maternal autoimmune (ITP [idiopathic thrombocytopenic purpura], SLE [systemic lupus erythematosus])
- Severe rhesus disease.

Early onset neonatal (<72 h)

- Placental insufficiency (pre-eclampsia, IUGR, maternal diabetes)
- Perinatal asphyxia
- Sepsis ± DIC, low-grade bacteraemia from indwelling catheters
- Congenital infection
- Thrombosis (renal vein, aorta)
- Alloimmune (NAIT)
- Maternal autoimmune (ITP, SLE)
- Severe rhesus disease
- Aneuploidy.

Late-onset neonatal (>72 h)

- Late-onset sepsis
- NEC
- Congenital infection
- Maternal autoimmune (ITP, SLE).

Rare congenital/inherited conditions causing thrombocytopenia also occur (Wiskott–Aldrich syndrome, Kasabach–Merritt syndrome, thrombocytopenia, absent radius syndrome).

8.48

Answer A: Neonatal alloimmune thrombocytopenia

NAIT occurs due to sensitisation of a HPA (human platelet antigen)-negative mother to a HPA-positive baby (HPA-positive father) with transplacental transfer of IgG, in much the same way as rhesus sensitisation occurs. In 80% of cases these are anti-HPA1a antibodies. It is frequently severe and, unlike rhesus disease of the newborn, occurs during the first pregnancy in up to 50% of cases. Intracranial haemorrhage occurs in about 10–15% of cases and can be detected antenatally. Approximately 20% of survivors are left with significant long-term neurodevelopmental sequelae. Affected neonates may present with signs of intracranial haemorrhage such as seizures and irritability, or may be asymptomatic and present with petechiae or an incidentally noted thrombocytopenia. Diagnosis is made by demonstrating platelet antigen incompatibility between maternal and neonatal platelets. Treatment of severely affected infants (eg those with bleeding or platelet counts $<30 \times 10^9$/l) is by transfusion of HPA-matched platelets with intravenous immunoglobulin (IVIG) in refractory cases. Prenatal management in future pregnancies may involve fetal blood sampling with platelet typing and transfusion of compatible platelets if required, or a less invasive approach of maternal IVIG therapy.

8.49

Answer C: TORCH infection

This baby has features of intrauterine infection. The lens opacities and low platelets with IUGR are classic for congenital rubella, but there is overlap with the other TORCH infections (*Toxoplasma*, **O**ther, **R**ubella, **C**MV, **H**erpes). Features of congenital TORCH infections include:

- microcephaly
- cataracts
- deafness
- congenital heart disease
- IUGR
- hepatosplenomegaly
- petechiae/purpura.

In congenital toxoplasmosis the following triad is classic:

- Hydrocephalus
- Intracranial calcification
- Chorioretinitis.

8.50

Answer H: Maternal systemic lupus erythematosus

Congenital heart block suggested by a well baby with a profound bradycardia and low platelets strongly suggests maternal SLE. Mothers of patients with neonatal lupus erythematosus may be asymptomatic but often develop autoimmune disease including SLE and Sjögren syndrome. Maternal IgG anti SS-A/Ro and anti-SS-B/La antibodies are almost always found in cases of neonatal SLE; the IgG antibodies cross the placenta and account for the clinical syndrome. Most effects are self-limiting and resolve. Cardiac pacing may be necessary as heart block is permanent. Platelet transfusion is indicated if the platelet count drops $<20 \times 10^9$/l and thrombocytopenia may be accompanied by neutropenia and haemolytic anaemia. Other features of neonatal SLE include cutaneous changes that can be urticarial and desquamative in nature and rarely hepatobiliary disease (fulminant liver failure, conjugated hyperbilirubinaemia or isolated raised aminotransferases).

CHAPTER 9

Nephrology Answers

MTF Answers

9.1 Renin–angiotensin system

Answer: C

Intravascular depletion causes a reduction in renal perfusion and release of renin from the juxtaglomerular apparatus where it is synthesised and stored. Renin acts on angiotensinogen (in plasma and the kidneys) and converts it to angiotensin I. Angiotensin I is converted by angiotensin-converting enzyme (ACE) to angiotensin II in the plasma, vascular endothelial cells, kidney, lungs and many other tissues.

Angiotensin II has multiple actions:

- It causes arteriolar vasoconstriction especially potent in the blood vessels of the kidney, mesenteric plexus and the skin.
- Renal actions:
  – stimulates Na^+ reabsorption in the tubules
  – lowers the glomerular filtration rate (GFR)
- Increases synthesis and release of aldosterone from the adrenal cortex.
- Stimulates Na^+ and water absorption from the gastrointestinal (GI) tract (especially the small bowel).

Aldosterone promotes sodium and chloride reabsorption in the distal tubules and collecting ducts, with excretion of potassium and hydrogen ions. It also acts to increase sodium and water absorption from the large bowel.

9.2 Inappropriate ADH secretion

Answers: A B C

Antidiuretic hormone (ADH) is synthesised by the supraoptic and paraventricular neurons in the hypothalamus and then transported along the nerve axons to be released in the posterior pituitary. The release is stimulated by increased plasma osmolality or reduced plasma volume. It acts on the distal tubules and collecting ducts to increase water reabsorption. In inappropriate ADH secretion there is water retention with hypo-osmolality and hyponatraemia. The urine osmolality is inappropriately high. There is no volume depletion. Investigation is with paired plasma and urinary electrolytes and osmolality.

Causes of inappropriate ADH secretion include:

- Birth asphyxia
- Hyaline membrane disease
- Intraventricular haemorrhage
- Meningitis (particularly pneumococcal)
- Encephalitis
- Other infections, eg pneumonia
- Trauma, eg head injury
- Tumours
- Surgery
- Iatrogenic
- Drugs, eg vincristine, nicotine, barbiturates, carbamazepine, oxytocin.

Phenytoin inhibits ADH secretion. The management is with fluid restriction to 30–50% maintenance and treatment of the underlying cause.

9.3 Hyperkalaemia

Answers: B C

The following are useful in the emergency treatment of acute hyperkalaemia:

- Intravenous calcium gluconate, which antagonises the effects of potassium on the heart by stabilising the myocardium. It does not lower the serum potassium. It should be used if either an arrhythmia or electrocardiogram (ECG) changes of hyperkalaemia are present. Dose is 0.5 ml/kg of 10% calcium gluconate (maximum 20 ml).
- Salbutamol either intravenously or nebulised: nebulised dose is 2.5–10 mg, intravenous dose 4 μg/kg. Salbutamol results in potassium entry into the cell.
- Intravenous sodium bicarbonate: dose is 2.5 mmol/kg. Give if pH <7.3. Sodium bicarbonate promotes the uptake of potassium into cells. In addition, acidosis will impair myocardial function and needs to be corrected. Need to check calcium because, if patient is hypocalcaemic, bicarbonate may lower the ionised calcium, precipitating tetany, convulsions, hypotension or arrhythmias.
- Glucose insulin infusion: dose of dextrose is 0.5 g/kg per h and insulin is 0.05 U/kg per h i.v. Promotes the uptake of potassium into cells.
- Ion exchange resin, such as calcium resonium, which facilitates Na^+/K^+ exchange in the gut and can be given orally or by enema. Dose 1 g/kg initially and then 1 g/kg per day.
- Dialysis/haemofiltration.

Hydrocortisone is not useful.

Adenosine is used to control supraventricular tachycardia.

ECG changes of hyperkalaemia:

- Prolongation of the PR interval
- Peaked T waves

- Widening of the QRS complex
- ST depression
- Ventricular fibrillation.

9.4 Renal osteodystrophy

Answers: A B

Renal osteodystrophy is a potentially life-threatening complication of chronic renal failure. A reduction in GFR causes a reduction in the excretion of inorganic phosphate. The decline in renal function reduces the production of 1,25-dihydroxy-vitamin D from 25-hydroxy-vitamin D, thus decreasing calcium absorption from the gut. Hyperphosphataemia and low serum calcium stimulate parathyroid hormone (PTH) secretion (secondary hyperparathyroidism).

PTH:

- **Increases calcium reabsorption in the distal tubule**
- **Decreases phosphate reabsorption in the proximal tubule**
- **Stimulates the synthesis of 1,25-dihydroxy-vitamin D in the proximal tubule**
- **Promotes osteoclastic bone resorption.**

Biochemical features of renal osteodystrophy include:

- **Normal or low serum calcium**
- **Increased plasma phosphate**
- **Increased plasma alkaline phosphatase**
- **Markedly increased parathyroid hormone level**
- **Normal or reduced 25-hydroxy vitamin D**
- **Reduced 1,25-dihydroxy vitamin D.**

The management is dietary phosphate restriction, use of a phosphate binder (such as calcium carbonate, aluminium hydroxide) and 1α-hydroxycholecalciferol or 1,25-dihydroxycholecalciferol.

Vitamin D

Sources of vitamin D are the diet and ultraviolet radiation. Vitamin D is hydroxylated to 25-hydroxy-vitamin D in the liver. 25-Hydroxy-vitamin D is further hydroxylated to 1,25-dihydroxy-vitamin D in the kidney, which promotes:

- Calcium resorption from bone
- Calcium and phosphate reabsorption from the kidney
- Calcium and phosphate absorption from the gut
- Cell growth and differentiation.

	Vitamin D deficiency	Hypophosphataemic rickets	Renal osteodystophy
Calcium	Reduced	Normal	Normal
Phosphate	Reduced or normal	Reduced	Increased
Alkaline Phosphatase	Increased	Increased	Increased
PTH	Increased	Normal	Markedly increased

9.5 Metabolic acidosis

Answers: D E

Pyloric stenosis results in hypochloraemic metabolic alkalosis due to chloride and hydrogen ion loss through vomiting.

Cystinuria

Defect in the intestinal absorption and renal tubular reabsorption of the dibasic amino acids cystine, lysine, arginine and ornithine. The consequence is the formation of renal calculi, which can lead on to repeated urinary tract infections (UTIs), haematuria, obstructive nephropathy and ultimately renal failure. Treatment is to alkalinise the urine with bicarbonate/citrate. It is inherited in an autosomal recessive pattern.

Bartter syndrome

The basic defect of Bartter syndrome is impaired tubular chloride reabsorption. The biochemical features are of hypokalaemia, hypochloraemia, hyponatraemia, metabolic alkalosis, hyperreninaemia and hyperaldosteronism associated with a normal blood pressure, and high urinary losses of potassium and chloride. Clinically patients display failure to thrive, polyuria, polydipsia, muscle weakness, constipation, salt craving and tetany (alkalosis leads to ↓ ionised Ca^{2+}). Treatment is with potassium and sodium supplements, diuretic supplementation and indometacin.

Cystinosis

This is a disorder of transport of cysteine out of lysosomes causing malfunction of the Na^+/K^+ pump. The biochemical features are those of Fanconi syndrome, with metabolic acidosis associated with a high plasma chloride and a low potassium and phosphate. Presentation may include failure to thrive, polyuria, polydipsia and hypophosphataemic rickets. Renal failure ensues by the end of the first decade. Treatment is by the use of cysteamine, which combines with intralysosomal cystine to slow elimination by an alternative pathway.

Pseudohypoaldosteronism

Pseudohypoaldosteronism is characterised by unresponsiveness of the distal tubule to aldosterone (genetic mutation in the gene encoding the aldosterone receptor (autosomal dominant and autosomal recessive inheritance). It presents with vomiting, faltering growth and dehydration with hyponatraemia and hyperkalaemia. Metabolic acidosis can occur (type IV renal tubular acidosis). Plasma renin and aldosterone levels are raised.

9.6 Proteinuria

Answers: A B C

A positive dipstick for protein in the urine of children or adolescents is not always indicative of renal disease. In most cases it is transient and induced by factors such as fever, exercise or upright posture. Repeated dipsticks of first void urines at weekly intervals over 4 weeks in children who are well and found to have proteinuria will show a decreased prevalence, from 11% who have one positive test to 0.1% who have four positive tests. Values of 3+ or 4+ of protein in a first voided urine is almost always pathological; trace and negative results usually exclude significant proteinuria. It is now well recognised that the quantification of protein in a first voided urine specimen expressed as a ratio to urinary creatinine correlates well with a timed overnight urine protein collection, whereas a protein:creatinine ratio in a random urine sample correlates with a 24-hour urine collection – these single void collections being much more practical for children.

Orthostatic

Of adolescents 2–5% will have orthostatic proteinuria that becomes increasingly uncommon over the age of 30 years. This aetiology is responsible for the vast majority of proteinuria detected in childhood and adolescence (60% and 75%, respectively). Orthostatic proteinuria is characterised by an increased protein in the urine in the upright posture, but normal excretion of protein when lying flat. Proteinuria is variable but can be large. It is a benign condition. Renal function is normal and family history negative.

9.7 Chloride

Answers: C D E

Chloride is the major anion of extracellular fluid. The reabsorption of tubular fluid must be isoelectric. Sodium and potassium transfer with chloride and bicarbonate. Chloride is actively transported in the ascending limb of the loop of Henle and in the gut. Chloride and bicarbonate act such that, if extracellular chloride is reduced, bicarbonate reabsorption is increased (hypochloraemic metabolic alkalosis) and, if bicarbonate is reduced in the extracellular fluid, chloride reabsorption is increased (hyperchloraemic metabolic acidosis).

Hypochloraemia (<95 mmol/l)

Loss of hydrochloric acid from the stomach results in a metabolic alkalosis and volume depletion. This activates the renin–angiotensin system and promotes sodium reabsorption (with bicarbonate and chloride depletion) in the proximal tubule, and sodium exchange for potassium and hydrogen ions in the distal tubule.

Hyperchloraemia

There are three settings:

1. Excessive intake
2. Increased absorption from the gastrointestinal tract
3. Renal tubular acidosis.

Excessive chloride in the extracellular fluid will suppress bicarbonate reabsorption and lead to the development of a metabolic acidosis. Renal tubular acidosis manifest by a bicarbonate leak will increase chloride reabsorption.

9.8 Membranous glomerulonephritis

Answers: A C E

Males predominate in this condition which represents less than 1% of childhood nephrotic syndrome but 20–40% of adult nephrotic syndrome. It can present with full-blown nephrotic syndrome or mild proteinuria and haematuria. It can be idiopathic or secondary to other diseases such as systemic lupus erythematosus and hepatitis B. The C3 is initially low in membranous glomerulonephritis due to either of these conditions. Steroids are beneficial in the adult but rarely so in childhood. Definitive diagnosis is made on renal biopsy. Progression to renal failure is rare; the outcome depends on the renal function at diagnosis and the amount of proteinuria present. Possible outcomes range from spontaneous remission without treatment to progressive end-stage renal disease. Identification and treatment of secondary underlying causes of membranous nephropathy may be curative; secondary causes include:

- Hepatitis B
- Malaria
- Schistosomiasis
- Ankylosing spondylitis
- Leprosy
- Systemic lupus erythematosus (SLE)
- Mercury
- Gold
- Sickle cell disease
- Rheumatoid arthritis.

Other types of glomerulonephritis which present as nephrotic syndrome include:

- Focal segmental glomerulosclerosis
- Mesangiocapillary (membranoproliferative) glomerulonephritis
- Mesangial proliferative glomerulonephritis.

BOF Answers

9.9 Chronic kidney disease

Answer D: Early recognition and treatment of chronic kidney disease can delay progression of the disease and improve long-term outcome

Chronic kidney disease (CKD) is classified into five stages by GFR.

Causes include:

- Congenital dysplasia ± obstruction
- Reflux nephropathy
- Chronic glomerulonephritis
- Genetically inherited, eg Alport syndrome, polycystic kidney disease
- Systemic disease: HSP (Henoch–Schönlein purpura), SLE

Principles of management of CKD:

1. Evaluation and management of reversible causes of renal dysfunction
2. Decrease progression:

   – control BP with ACE inhibitors or angiotensin receptor blockers; drugs can ↓ GFR further!

   – low-protein diet slows progression of kidney disease in adults (no paediatric evidence) but over-restriction may limit growth.
3. Treat complications:

   (a) anaemia (NICE guidelines 2011): iron and folate supplementation + erythropoiesis-stimulating agent (ESA). Hyperparathyroidism should be treated to avoid worsening anaemia and blood transfusion should be avoided due to risk of sensitisation before transplantation

   (b) dietary sodium and fluid restriction ± diuretics until dialysis is indicated (note that some CKD may conversely lead to polyuria and hyponatraemia)

   (c) hyperkalaemia: low potassium diet, loop diuretics and correction of metabolic acidosis may help but renal dialysis may be indicated.

   (d) metabolic acidosis: sodium bicarbonate is the first-line treatment but again dialysis may be indicated.

   (e) bone disease:

   – secondary hyperparathyroidism: ↓ calcitriol secondary to ↓ renal mass → ↑ PTH and ↓ Ca^{2+}. PO_4^{3-} retention secondary to ↓ GFR will also lead to ↑ PTH; this combination leads to bone disease and in addition calcification of vessels and muscles may occur; treat with low phosphate diet, phosphate binders and vitamin D_3 analogues

   – dynamic bone disease: mainly affects those on dialysis and is caused by ↓ PTH and ↑ Ca^{2+}

   (f) hyperlipidaemia

(g) malnutrition is multifactorial and common

(h) growth failure is common – growth hormone indicated

4. Renal replacement – GFR <15 ml/min per 1.73 m^2

(a) haemodialysis

(b) peritoneal dialysis (often preferred in children)

5. Pre-emptive renal transplantation with a live related donor is optimal.

9.10 Acute scrotal pain

Answer C: If torsion of the testis cannot be excluded clinically exploration of the scrotum is the only safe management of an acutely inflamed scrotum

The acute scrotum is defined as the sudden onset of testicular pain; there are many causes.

Testicular torsion (25%)

- Torsion can occur at any time during childhood but peaks in the neonatal and peripubertal periods.
- Testis is acutely very tender.
- Testis lies high in the scrotum accompanied by scrotal redness and oedema.
- It is indefensible if in doubt not to explore the testis if torsion is suspected.
- Infarction occurs within 10 h from onset of symptoms.
- Spermatogenesis is decreased post-torsion in a viable testis.
- Loss of testis may be managed cosmetically with a prosthesis.

Torted hydatid of Morgagni

- Pedunculated small cystic remnant of the müllerian ducts usually attached to the upper pole of the testis.
- Torsion of the appendage presents with acute scrotal swelling, localised tenderness ± hydrocele.
- Transillumination reveals a blue/black spot lying at the superior pole of the testis.
- If diagnosis is clear there is no indication for surgery.
- Natural history of spontaneous resolution of symptoms within 48 h.

Orchitis, epididymo-orchitis

- Orchitis is now rare in childhood post-MMR.
- Epididymo-orchitis: most cases are viral, if urine culture positive then 7 days of oral antibiotics are indicated.
- Due to differential scrotal exploration is needed to exclude torsion of the testis if the diagnosis is not certain.
- Prognosis is good but recurrence should raise suspicion of abnormal urinary anatomy.

Idiopathic scrotal oedema

- Inflamed scrotum/hemi scrotum in young boys that may spread up the shaft of the penis or onto the perineum
- Unknown aetiology
- Self-limiting, resolves within 1–4 days
- Treatment – analgesia
- If superinfection occurs (rare) antibiotic cover with flucloxacillin is indicated.

Further differential diagnoses of an acutely painful testis include an incarcerated inguinal hernia or a tense hydrocele. Painless swelling of the scrotum can occur due to a number of different causes including HSP, hydrocele and generalised causes of oedema such as nephrotic syndrome.

9.11 Cranial diabetes insipidus

Answer B: Irritability, growth retardation, hyperthermia and weight loss may be the presenting features of the disorder in infancy

This is a failure of ADH secretion. It can be familial or sporadic (autosomal dominant and X-linked dominant families have been described). It can be idiopathic or secondary due to:

- Tumours, eg craniopharyngioma
- Infiltration, eg histiocytosis X
- Granulomatous disease, eg tuberculosis
- Trauma, eg head injury, pituitary surgery (most common cause).

The clinical features include the following:

- Polyuria
- Polydipsia
- Nocturia
- Severe dehydration, hypernatraemia, cardiovascular collapse and death can occur in children due to their decreased ability to search out water
- In infants, crying, irritability, growth retardation, hyperthermia and weight loss may be the presenting features of the disorder.

Differential diagnosis:

- Nephrogenic diabetes insipidus
- Psychogenic polydipsia
- Diabetes mellitus
- Urinary tract infection.

Investigation by the water deprivation test:

- Continue to deprive child of water for a maximum of 6–8 hours
- Urine osmolality, child's weight, pulse rate and BP are measured hourly
- Plasma sodium levels and osmolality are measures 2 hourly
- Terminated if:

  - >5% of body weight lost
  - serum osmolality >295 mosmol/kg in the face of urine osmolality <300 mosmol/kg
  - patient becomes unwell or clinically dehydrated
- Diabetes insipidus (DI) diagnosed if:
  - plasma osmolality >290 mosmol/kg (plus inappropriately low urine osmolality)
  - urine osmolality of > 800 mosmol/kg is normal.
- DDAVP (desmopressin) is given at the end of the test to distinguish cranial from nephrogenic DI:
  - a rise in urine concentration confirms cranial DI
  - if no response to DDAVP the diagnosis is nephrogenic DI.
- If the water deprivation test is normal in a child with polydipsia and polyuria, for which other causes such as diabetes mellitus have been excluded, then the diagnosis is psychogenic polydipsia.

Nephrogenic diabetes insipidus can be observed in chronic renal insufficiency, lithium toxicity, tubulointerstitial disease, and hypercalcaemia and hypokalaemia.

9.12 Nocturnal enuresis

Answer C: Increasing day-time fluid intake can be an effective intervention in helping to decrease the symptom of nocturnal enuresis in some children

Definition: wetting the bed three to more nights per month or one night per week:

- 8–10% of 5–6 year olds
- 5–7% of 7–10 year olds
- 1–3% by adulthood
- Enuresis can be monosymptomatic (two-thirds) or non-monosymptomatic (a third), in combination with lower urinary tract symptoms/bladder dysfunction including daytime urgency, frequency and small daytime voiding volumes
- The male:female ratio is 2:1
- The incidence doubles with a positive parental history
- 70% incidence if both parents suffered
- About 20–30% are secondary (after >6 months of night-time dryness).

Enuresis mechanisms

- An inability to wake during sleep in response to need to void
- Nocturnal polyuria (two-thirds respond to DDAVP)
- Reduced bladder capacity (small size ± overactive bladder)

Management

General

- Simple advice on fluid intake (may need to increase during the day, nil <1 hr before bed)

- Regular toileting during the day (more than four but less than seven times)
- Avoid anger/blame from parents
- Advice on reward system to use alone or together with other therapies (star charts for compliance with treatment – not dry nights)
- Suggest a trial without nappies for all dry by day for >6 months
- Avoid lifting
- Treat co-morbidities (constipation, obstructive sleep apnoea, recurrent UTIs)
- Consider alternative diagnoses: diabetes mellitus, maltreatment, learning difficulties/ attention deficit hyperactivity disorder)
- Under age 5 years – reassurance.

Specific

- Enuresis alarm: 35% learn to wake, 65% sleep through (65% success, 42% relapse)
- Desmopressin: >50% ↓ in wet nights in 60–70%); break for 1 week every 3 months to assess progress
- Anticholinergics, eg oxybutynin: ↓ detrusor overactivity; can be used in combination with desmopressin.

An adequate (not excessive) fluid intake must be maintained when on DDAVP and the medication should be stopped if vomiting occurs in order to prevent severe hyponatraemia.

9.13 Berger disease (idiopathic IgA nephropathy)

Answer D: Overall 20-30% of patients diagnosed with IgA nephropathy will develop end-stage renal failure 15-20 ears after the onset of the disease

Berger disease presents with incidental finding of microscopic haematuria or macroscopic haematuria post-upper respiratory tract infection (URTI). It is the most common cause of primary glomerulonephritis throughout the developed world:

- 85% present aged 16–35 years, rare <10 years
- Histological diagnosis: granular deposition of IgA and C3 in the mesangium of the glomerulus in the absence of systemic disease, eg systemic lupus erythematosus or abnormal plasma immunoglobulins or complement levels
- Male:female ratio is 2:1. ↑
- ↑ Asian and white individuals; rare in African individuals.

Presentation:

- 60–80%: macroscopic haematuria concurrent with an URTI may be recurrent
- 25%: incidental finding of microscopic haematuria ± mild proteinuria ± ↑ BP ± ↓ creatinine clearance
- 12% acute nephritic presentation: heavy proteinuria ± ↑ BP ± ↓ creatinine clearance
- 10% present with nephrotic syndrome
- Overall 40–50% of cases are proteinuria associated.

Investigation:

- Serum IgA increased in 8–16% of children affected
- Serum C3 normal.

HSP and IgA nephropathy share identical histological changes on renal biopsy but are distinct clinical entities. It is important to keep patients with both conditions normotensive and there is good evidence that angiotensin-converting enzyme (ACE) inhibitors decrease proteinuria and decrease progression towards renal failure.

The prognosis for most children is good, although 20–30% will develop end-stage renal failure 15–20 years after onset of the disease

Poor prognostic features at presentation include advanced age, heavy proteinuria, hypertension and impaired renal function, in addition to proliferative lesions on renal biopsy.

Berger disease commonly recurs in transplanted kidneys (with 30–60% graft failure rate) and resolves if kidneys with IgA deposits are transplanted into recipients without IgA nephropathy.

9.14 Renal failure

Answer B: Urinary sodium 10 mmol/l

In prerenal failure there is a reduction in the intravascular volume which results in a reduced GFR. This activates the renin–angiotensin system and results in the secretion of aldosterone, which promotes sodium reabsorption and potassium excretion in the distal tubule. Intravascular depletion results in a more concentrated urine being passed. This urine is characterised by a high osmolality (>500 mosmol/l) and low sodium (<20 mmol/l). The urine:plasma creatinine ratio is high (>40).

The fractional excretion of sodium is calculated as follows:

$$[(\text{Urine Na}^+ \times \text{Plasma Cr})/(\text{Urine Cr} \times \text{Plasma Na}^+)]$$

where urine Na^+ = urinary sodium, urine Cr = urinary creatinine, plasma Na^+ = plasma sodium, plasma Cr = plasma creatinine.

The fractional excretion of sodium is <1% in prerenal failure and >1% in renal failure.

In neonates, sodium reabsorption is less efficient and the fractional excretion of sodium is closer to <2.5% in prerenal failure and >2.5% in renal failure.

This approach is not helpful if either mannitol or diuretics have been given, which will interfere with the urinary electrolytes.

Diarrhoea can precede prerenal failure (gastroenteritis) or renal failure (haemolytic uraemic syndrome).

9.15 Henoch–Schönlein purpura

Answer A: Renal involvement in HSP occurs in 20-50% of cases

HSP is the most common vasculitis in children. Diagnosis is based on finding a palpable, purpuric rash predominantly affecting the lower limbs and buttocks. It may often follow a

URTI and is associated with seasonal variation. At presentation 85% will have joint involvement, 48% will have abdominal pain and over the course of the disease 20–50% will have renal involvement. This is usually mild with microscopic haematuria and proteinuria although a nephrotic or nephritic picture may occur. Up to 2% develop long-term renal problems.

The underlying pathophysiology is deposition of IgA in the affected tissue, causing an inflammatory reaction and tissue damage. The renal manifestations are usually present within the first month but can present later and almost always present (97%) within 6 months. Careful follow-up of blood pressure, urine microscopy and plasma creatinine is required in patients with renal involvement until the manifestations disappear. Pregnancy is a time of particular vulnerability for women with a previous history of HSP nephritis with hypertension and pre-eclamptic toxaemia increasing to 70% from a background of 5–10%.

Renal biopsy should be considered if:

- There is significant and persistent proteinuria:
  - urine protein:creatinine ratio of >200 mg/mmol for 2 weeks
  - >100 mg/mmol for 4 weeks
  - serum albumin <25 g/l at any time
- There is evidence of renal insufficiency: creatinine persists >100 µmol/l.

  High-dose immunosuppression is given to those with severe renal involvement. ACE inhibitors may be of benefit for proteinuria.

The differential diagnosis includes:

- Systemic lupus erythematosus
- Post-streptococcal glomerulonephritis
- Haemolytic uraemic syndrome.

The prognosis of Henoch–Schönlein nephritis depends on the extent of glomerular lesions. Poor prognostic factors include:

- Clinical evidence of renal insufficiency
- Clinical evidence of nephrotic syndrome
- Glomerular sclerosis
- Glomerular necrosis
- Extensive crescent formation.

9.16 Renal syndromes

Answer B: Alport syndrome is inherited in an x-linked dominant pattern

Nephrogenic diabetes insipidus

X-linked recessive:

- Characterised by resistance of the kidney to ADH
- The symptoms: polyuria, polydipsia, dehydration, failure to thrive and learning disability

- Biochemistry is characteristic:
  - hypernatraemia,
  - hyperchloraemia
  - hyperosmolality.
- Diagnosis is by a water deprivation test: failure to concentrate the urine despite exogenous ADH
- Treatment:
  - low-salt diet
  - hydrochlorothiazide and indometacin.

Alport syndrome

X-linked dominant (occasional families demonstrate autosomal dominant inheritance):

- Characterised by haematuria, progressive impairment of renal function, deafness, ocular manifestations and a characteristic appearance on renal biopsy.
- Males are more severely affected than females.
- Progression:
  - silent in childhood
  - presents in adolescence with microscopic haematuria and proteinuria.

Hartnup disease

Autosomal recessive:

- Characterised by a tubular and intestinal defect in the reabsorption and absorption of cyclic and neutral amino acids.
- Clinical features (secondary to tryptophan malabsorption): photosensitive rash and cerebellar ataxia.
- Diagnosed by characteristic aminoaciduria.
- Treatment with nicotinamide corrects the clinical features.

Vitamin D-resistant rickets

X-linked dominant:

- Present between 12 and 18 months
- Biochemistry:
  - normal plasma calcium
  - ↓ low phosphate
  - ↑ alkaline phosphatase
  - normal parathyroid hormone level
  - normal vitamin D level.
- Treatment is with phosphate and vitamin D.

Cystinosis

Autosomal recessive:

- Accumulation of cysteine in lysosomal membranes → severe renal Fanconi syndrome.
- Presentation in infancy is with failure to thrive, rickets, recurrent vomiting and dehydration.
- Presentation in second decade of the less severe juvenile cystinosis.
- Biochemistry is of a:
  - metabolic acidosis
  - ↓ plasma potassium
  - ↓ plasma phosphate.
- Diagnosis: measurement of the white cell cystine.
- Treatment is with potassium, bicarbonate and cysteamine, and can delay renal failure.

9.17 Minimal change nephrotic syndrome

Answer C: Minimal change nephritic syndrome has a male predominance

Nephrotic syndrome (NS) is a disease of the glomerulus of the kidney characterised by significant proteinuria (early morning protein:creatinine ratio of >200 mg/mmol) leading to hypoalbuminaemia (<25 g/l) and oedema. NS may be congenital (rare) or acquired. Acquired NS can be primary (idiopathic – common) or secondary (rare).

Primary NS is classified according to clinical response to steroids as steroid-sensitive NS or steroid-resistant disease. Primary glomerular disease may be further divided on histology into three distinct groups:

1. Minimal change disease
2. Focal segmental glomerulosclerosis
3. Membranoproliferative glomerulonephrosis

Causes of secondary NS:

- Infection: hepatitis B, HIV/AIDS, malaria, syphilis, toxoplasmosis
- Systemic disease: SLE, HSP, sickle cell disease, IgA nephropathy, post-infectious glomerulonephritis
- Drugs: penicillamine, gold, non-steroidal anti-inflammatory drugs (NSAIDs), pamidronate, interferon, mercury, heroin, lithium
- Immune/allergic disease: Castleman syndrome (non-cancerous proliferation of B cells), bee stings
- Malignancy: lymphoma, leukaemia.

Idiopathic steroid-sensitive NS is the most common subtype of acquired NS in childhood. It has a male predominance. Peak incidence is in the age range 2–5 years. It is rare in the first year of life but can occur in adult life. It is often preceded by a history of a URTI. In the UK the incidence is approximately 2/100 000 children and is four to six times more common in the UK Asian population. Haematuria is usually absent. The presence of haematuria implies that a more serious form of glomerulonephritis should be considered, as does the presence of hypertension or abnormal renal function tests. Complement levels are normal.

Complications of nephrotic syndrome are:

- Hypovolaemia
- Hypertension
- Hypothyroidism – secondary to loss of thyroid-binding globulin.
- Infection (primary peritonitis or septicaemia)
- Thrombosis
- Hyperlipidaemia (↑ cholesterol and triglycerides)
- Acute renal failure.

9.18 Urinary tract infection

Answer B: Treatment with a 3-day course of oral antibiotics is appropriate in a 2-year-old child with proven UTI and symptoms of a lower UTI

- Ten per cent of girls and 3% of boys have had a UTI by 16 years.
- Vesicoureteric reflux (VUR) is present in approximately a third of children with a UTI.
- Children aged <3 years should have microscopy not dipstick.
- *E. coli* accounts for 70–90% of community-acquired UTIs.
- Non-*E. coli* UTIs are associated with increased underlying obstructive structural abnormalities

The National Institute for Health and Clinical Excellence (NICE) guidance (2007) recommends assessing for signs of severe underlying pathology, and defines atypical UTIs as:

- Poor urine flow
- Previous UTIs
- Recurrent pyrexia of unknown origin
- Antenatal diagnosis of renal abnormality
- Family history of VUR or renal disease
- Constipation
- Dysfunctional voiding
- Enlarged bladder
- Abdominal mass
- Evidence of spinal lesion
- Poor growth
- Hypertension
- Seriously ill child/septicaemia
- ↑ serum creatinine
- Failure to respond to treatment in 48 hours

- Infection with non-*E. coli* organisms.

Although UTIs do predispose to scarring, the degree of damage is unpredictable and evidence has swung against intensive investigation. NICE guidelines detail imaging needed for follow-up stratified by age group at diagnosis, response to treatment by 48 hours, and recurrent and atypical presentations.

Treatment depends on age and severity of symptoms and ability to tolerate oral antibiotics.

- <3 months intravenous antibiotics.
- >3 months with upper tract signs:
  - oral antibiotics for 7–10 days,
  - unable to tolerate oral antibiotics: 48 h of intravenous antibiotics followed by 8 days of oral
- Lower tract signs – 3 days of oral antibiotics
- Prophylaxis should be considered in recurrent UTIs
- Treatment should be with a different antibiotic if infection occurs on prophylaxis.

Follow-up long term is indicated for all with bilateral renal abnormalities, impaired renal function, hypertension and/or proteinuria:

9.19 Haemolytic uraemic syndrome

Answer E: Pneumococcal pneumonia and meningitis are implicated in the development of HUS

HUS is characterised by haemolytic anaemia, thrombocytopenia and acute renal failure in the absence of disseminated intravascular coagulation (DIC). It usually follows a diarrhoeal illness (D + HUS in 90–95%) and most commonly is associated with verotoxin-producing *Escherichia coli* (VTEC) of the O157 serotype. There are three major routes of transmission: person-to-person contact, contact with animals (cattle), and contaminated food and water sources. Peak incidence occurs during the summer months.

Non-diarrhoeal-associated HUS (D– HUS) accounts for approximately 5% of childhood HUS:

- Forty per cent of these cases are associated with pneumococcal sepsis.
- Rarely there is a family history of D– HUS representing a genetic basis for the syndrome. Multiple mutations in the gene encoding factor H, a factor vital in the regulation of the complement pathway, have been identified in families with a predisposition to develop HUS.

Typical clinical course:

- Watery diarrhoea
- Fever is low grade or absent
- Bloody diarrhoea develops over 2–3 days
- Rectal prolapse, intussusception, toxic dilatation of colon ± perforation rarely occur
- Anaemia and thrombocytopenia precede oliguria
- Oliguria between 1 and 14 days after diarrhoea onset
- Oedema (25%)

- Dehydration (25%)
- Hypertension (20–30%)
- Other rarer extrarenal manifestations: CNS involvement (20%) with seizures, altered consciousness, hemiparesis and brain-stem dysfunction; cardiomyopathy, liver dysfunction, pancreatitis and diabetes
- Resolution (85%) is usually heralded by a rise in platelet count.

Management:

- Antibiotics and anti-diarrhoeals – ↑ risk of HUS
- Infection control!
- Careful fluid and electrolyte management
- Blood transfusion
- Platelets for active bleeding
- Dialysis may be needed in >50%
- BP treatment usually straightforward (difficult in D– HUS)
- Plasma exchange (associated with decreased mortality).

Outcome:

- Mortality rate (acute) 2–12%, ↑ to 20% in D– HUS
- Long-term impaired renal function, proteinuria and hypertension occur in 25% over 10 years
- 50% of D– HUS cases develop end-stage renal failure
- Extrarenal involvement may lead to hemiparesis or diabetes mellitus.

9.20 Hypertension

Answer E: The vast majority of children are asymptomatic but hypertensive encephalopathy presenting as severe hypertension with headache, vomiting, hyperreflexia and seizures is a medical emergency requiring admission to hospital for a controlled gradual decrease in BP

- Hypertension in children is rare and usually secondary to renal (80%) or endocrine pathology.
- Primary hypertension in childhood is an increasingly recognised problem.
- Hypertension in childhood is defined as a BP above the 95th centile for age, height and gender.

To measure the blood pressure manually the bladder of the cuff itself should cover at least two-thirds of the circumference of the arm. A small cuff will result in a high reading.

Causes of hypertension in childhood include:

- Renal parenchymal disease:
  - renal scarring/reflux nephropathy
  - acute glomerulonephritis
  - chronic glomerulonephritis
  - chronic renal failure

  - acute renal failure
  - nephrotic syndrome
  - polycystic renal disease
- Vascular disease and renovascular disease:
  - coarctation of the aorta
  - renal artery stenosis
  - renal artery or renal vein thrombosis
- Renal tumours: Wilms tumour
- Catecholamines:
  - phaeochromocytoma
  - neuroblastoma
- Obstructive uropathy
- Corticosteroids:
  - iatrogenic
  - Cushing syndrome
- Neurological causes:
  - raised ICP
  - seizures
  - spinal cord injury
- Drugs:
  - caffeine
  - alcohol
- Essential hypertension.

All children with BPs >25 mmHg above the 95th centile should be admitted for immediate investigation and treatment. Those with less severe hypertension require home ambulatory BP measurements to clarify the diagnosis.

Drug treatment of hypertension includes:

- ACE inhibitors, eg captopril:
  - first line in all renal parenchymal disease (hyperrenninaemia)
  - renal artery stenosis must be excluded first!
- Angiotensin receptor blockage (valsartan, candesartan) useful in primary renal disease
- Diuretics, eg furosemide
- Calcium channel blockers, eg nifedipine
- Vasodilators, eg prazosin, hydralazine, sodium nitroprusside
- β Blockers, eg propranolol
- α and β blockers, eg labetalol.

Complications of hypertension include:

- Nose bleeds and headache
- Left ventricular failure

- Retinopathy
- Hypertensive encephalopathy.

9.21 Acute post-streptococcal glomerulonephritis (APSGN)

Answer C: Hypertensive encephalopathy is a recognised complication

This commonly follows group A β-haemolytic streptococcal infection. The ASOT (anti-streptolysin O titre) is positive in 90%, which is indicative of recent streptococcal infection. The ASOT may not rise after a skin infection whereas anti-DNAse B will rise irrespective of infection site. There are other implicated infectious agents that are less commonly seen. The usual age of presentation is between 3 and 10 years; it is more common in boys. At least two-thirds of patients with laboratory evidence of APSGN are asymptomatic.

Presents 10–14 days post-streptococcal A infection (skin or URTI):

- Macroscopic haematuria (a third) (reddish brown/Coca-Cola coloured)
- Microscopic haematuria in two-thirds
- Oedema (80–90%)often mild and facial
- Nephrotic syndrome – rarer
- Oliguria for first 10 days
- Oedema, ascites and pleural effusions
- Pallor, malaise and anorexia are common
- C3 is low (80-90%) initially and returns to normal within 6–12 weeks
- C4 is less frequently low and if so returns to normal much quicker.

Problems include hypertension, (5% severe with encephalopathy), pulmonary oedema secondary to intravascular fluid overload and renal insufficiency.

Treat fluid overload with fluid restriction and diuretics, and oral penicillin for 10 days to eradicate streptococci (does not influence the time course or severity of the nephritis). Steroids are not indicated without referral to paediatric nephrologist for severe cases. There is an excellent prognosis for recovery but in a small minority of cases renal failure can ensue.

Differential diagnosis of acute nephritis in childhood includes:

- Post-infectious glomerulonephritis
- Henoch–Schönlein nephritis
- IgA nephropathy
- Alport syndrome
- Lupus nephritis.

9.22 Undescended testis (UDT)

Answer C: Early orchidopexy has been shown to reduce infertility in later life

- Of baby boys born at term, 4–5% have either unilateral or bilateral UDT.
- Some 1.5% have UDT by the age of 6 months.

- Spontaneous descent is rare after 6 months.
- Impalpable testes are not necessarily absent and may be intra-abdominal.
- UDT rates ↑ for preterm and low-birthweight babies:
  - 6–10% with a previously affected sibling
  - 70% – undescended testis is on the right
  - 10–25% of cases are bilateral.
- Of cases 10–20% have a completely impalpable testis and in bilateral cases a disorder of sex differentiation must be considered and investigated.
- A small proportion of testes ascend to become permanently impalpable, having been in the scrotum at birth (1.2% at 6 years, 2.2% at 9 years and 1.1% at 13 years).

Important differential diagnoses to consider include:

- Retractile testis (can be 'milked' down into the scrotum)
- Maldescended testis (abnormal route of descent and so will never spontaneously descend)
- Absent testis
- Mixed gonadal dysgenesis (often 45XO/46XY mosaic) associated with hypospadias and UDT
- Disorder of sex differentiation (DSD).

There is an increased risk of infertility and of malignancy in children with undescended testis. In order to minimise these, orchidopexy should be carried out before the end of the second year, increasingly between 6 and 12 months. Early surgical intervention can improve future fertility and may decrease the risk of malignancy. The incidence of testicular tumours in adults is 3/10 000. The risk in males with a history of undescended testis is 4–10 times greater. Sixty per cent of the tumours are seminomas, most of the remainder being teratomas.

Important associations of undescended testis include:

- Spinal muscular atrophy
- Myotonic dystrophy
- X-linked ichthyosis
- Kallmann syndrome
- Prune-belly syndrome.

9.23 Wilms tumour

Answer C: Hemihypertrophy, genitourinary abnormalities and aniridia are all associated with an increased risk of developing Wilms tumours

Wilms tumours are characterised by a malignant proliferation of the metanephric blastema (primitive embryonic renal) cells.

The vast majority of Wilms tumours arise sporadically with no other predisposing malformation syndromes or family history. However, in a small number of cases there is a significant family history of Wilms tumour or one of the following recognised predisposing conditions listed below. In these circumstances regular screening for the development of Wilms tumour with yearly or twice yearly renal ultrasound examinations is advisable:

- Isolated hemihypertrophy
- Beckwith–Wiedemann syndrome
- Neurofibromatosis
- Drash syndrome (Wilms tumour + pseudohermaphroditism + glomerulopathy)
- WAGR syndrome (Wilms tumour + aniridia + genitourinary malformations + learning disability)
- Ambiguous genitalia
- Nephropathy
- Aniridia
- Genitourinary malformations
- Learning disability
- Trisomy 18.

Wilms tumour accounts for 10% of all paediatric tumours; 10% are bilateral. The mean age of diagnosis is 3.5 years. The most common presenting feature is an abdominal mass. Abdominal pain occurs in 30–40% of cases and hypertension, haematuria, anaemia and fever secondary to tumour necrosis may be associated. Ultrasonography is the best investigation to make the diagnosis. Chromosomal analysis and gene mapping are currently available. Treatment is with surgery and chemotherapy, with the addition of radiotherapy for more advanced disease. The overall prognosis is good, with 80–90% 5-year survival rate.

9.24 Hyponatraemia

Answer E: Fluid restriction is appropriate treatment for hyponatraemia when SIADH is suspected to be the cause

Hyponatraemia in hospitalised children is common, with approximately 25% of children in hospital having serum sodium values <134 mmol/l and 1% having values <130 mmol/l. Preterm infants with hyponatraemia have increased morbidity and poor growth and development. Hyponatraemia in adults is also reported to be associated with increased morbidity and mortality.

Causes of hyponatraemia include:

- Inappropriate (hypotonic) intravenous fluid
- Excessive loss in the urine, faeces, vomit or sweat
- Inadequate intake
- Inappropriate ADH secretion (hyponatraemia due to dilution secondary to water retention):
  - CNS disease: meningitis, encephalitis, brain tumour, head injury
  - pulmonary disease: pneumonia, bronchiolitis, asthma
  - cancer
  - nausea, pain, vomiting and anxiety
  - postoperative state
  - cortisol deficiency

- Salt losing state, eg congenital adrenal hyperplasia, Addison disease
- Renal tubular acidosis
- Diuretic therapy.

Interpretation of urinary electrolytes in the context of hyponatraemia:

- Urinary sodium <20 mmol/l suggests non-renal losses (GI), sweat, overhydration with hypotonic fluids
- Urinary sodium >30 mmol/l suggests urinary losses, SIADH, salt-losing endocrine state, diuretics.

Hyponatraemic encephalopathy

This is more common and occurs at higher (less abnormal) sodium concentrations in children than in adults. Mild symptoms should be managed with fluid restriction if the patient is not hypovolaemic; more severe symptoms require immediate treatment with hypertonic (3%) saline.

Clinical features of hyponatraemic encephalopathy include the following.

Early

- Headache
- Nausea and vomiting
- Lethargy
- Weakness
- Confusion
- Agitation
- Altered level of consciousness

Late

- Convulsions
- Coma
- Apnoea
- Pulmonary oedema
- Decorticate posturing
- Pupillary dilatation
- Cardiac arrhythmias
- Central diabetes insipidus.

9.25 Polycystic kidney disease

Answer D: Congenital hepatic fibrosis is strongly associated with autosomal recessive polycystic kidney disease and portal hypertension can be the presenting feature

- Usually presents in the first year of life
- Incidence: 1 in 10 000 to 1 in 40 000
- Characterised by non-obstructive dilatation of the renal collecting ducts.

Presentation:

- **Neonatal respiratory distress (pulmonary hypoplasia) secondary to oligohydramnios**
- **Enlarged kidneys in the neonatal period (may worsen the respiratory compromise)**
- **Patients with ARPCKD always develop congenital hepatic fibrosis (CHF); portal hypertension secondary to CHF can be debilitating with splenomegaly, varices and GI haemorrhage; the hepatic disease can be the dominant clinical presentation**
- **Hypertension and chronic renal failure.**

Death often occurs rapidly from pulmonary complications after delivery, although a number survive and those who do so beyond the first year generally do well but may still develop chronic kidney disease, necessitating renal transplantation; hypertension is often severe.

Antenatal ultrasound appearances include large echo-bright kidneys and oligohydramnios.

Ultrasonography postnatally shows the presence of microcysts with a lack of differentiation between the renal medulla and cortex.

Autosomal dominant polycystic renal disease

- Accounts for 8% of adults in end-stage renal failure.
- Incidence is between 1 in 200 and 1 in 1000.
- The gene is on chromosome 16 in 85% and chromosome 4.
- Cysts can occur anywhere along the nephron and enlarge and increase in numbers throughout life.

Presentation:

- Antenatal ultrasonography – discrete cysts in kidneys
- Microscopic haematuria
- Hypertension
- Renal failure (increases with age; 2% of patients <40 years but 50% of those <70 years)
- Incidental finding of cysts on renal ultrasonography (usually in adult life)
- Rarely: oligohydramnios and pulmonary hypoplasia in the neonatal period.

Cysts in other organs: the liver (30%), pancreas, spleen and lungs; 10–15% have a berry aneurysm in the circle of Willis.

9.26 Vesicoureteric reflux (VUR)

Answer B: The aim of prophylactic antibiotics in childen with vesicoureteric reflux is to minimise the harmful consequences of renal scarring and progression towards renal impairment and subsequent failure

Of children who present to hospital with a confirmed urinary tract infection, 30–40% have VUR (boys > girls). Of those with UTIs, up to 30% develop renal scars. Over 30% of patients who are found to have hydronephrosis on antenatal ultrasound scanning are shown to have VUR on investigations performed postnatally. There is a strong genetic predisposition to the development of VUR, with an occurrence rate of 25–30% in siblings and 66% in children of affected individuals. The diagnosis of VUR is by micturating cystography.

Severity is graded from I to IV, with grade IV implying presence of intrarenal reflux. A MAG-3 indirect cystogram can be used once continence has been achieved; this is both less sensitive and less specific although better tolerated. The object of management is to prevent UTIs and in doing so prevent renal scarring (reflux nephropathy). This is best achieved using low-dose prophylactic antibiotics to prevent infections and appropriate antibiotics if breakthrough infection occurs based on urine culture and sensitivity. Most reflux resolves by the age of 5 years. If not, and recurrent infections occur with progressive renal scarring, ureteric reimplantation is indicated. DMSA is the best investigation to look for renal scars.

Complications of reflux nephropathy include:

- Hypertension
- Impaired renal function (↓ urine concentrating ability and ↓ GFR)
- Renal failure.

9.27 Hypercalciuria

Answer D: Hypercalciuria is an important cause in the differential of any child presenting with haematuria

Hypercalciuria is important as it is a risk factor for the production of renal calculi and can cause other urinary symptoms including polyuria, nocturnal enuresis and dysuria. It is also commonly associated with microscopic haematuria. The gold standard is to measure the 24-hour urinary calcium (upper limit of normal 0.1 mmol/kg per day); the measurement of the urinary calcium creatinine ratio is also useful (upper limit of normal 0.7).

Causes of hypercalciuria can be either normo- or hypercalcaemic.

Normocalcaemic

- Idiopathic (familial)- see below
- Distal renal tubular acidosis }
- Dent disease } reduced renal tubular reabsorption of calcium
- Batter syndrome }
- Furosemide }

Hypercalcaemic

- Increased bone resorption:
  - immobilisation
  - steroids
  - primary hyperparathyroidism
  - McCune–Albright syndrome
  - thyroid disease
  - Cushing disease
- Increased intestinal absorption:
  - calcium
  - vitamin D

- Hypophosphataemia
- Williams syndrome.

Idiopathic hypercalciuria is the most common cause of calcium-containing renal calculi. Children present with gross haematuria, abdominal pain and dysuria.

Thiazide diuretics are currently the mainstay of medical therapy for hypercalciuria. They can reduce the urinary calcium excretion by 30% by stimulating the renal reabsorption of calcium in the distal tubule.

9.28 Congenital nephrotic syndrome

Answer E: Congenital syphilis is a cause of congenital nephritic syndrome

There are multiple causes of congenital nephrotic syndrome which has an onset of symptoms within the first 3 months of life. These include autosomal recessive inherited conditions, congenital syphilis infection and a number of congenital syndromes, including Pierson, Denys–Drash and Frasier syndromes.

The most common congenital nephrotic syndrome is the Finnish type. Incidence is 12/100 000 live births (increased in Finland). It is an autosomal recessive inheritance of mutations in the *NPHS1* gene encoding nephrin, a protein required for normal podocyte function. Babies are often born preterm, small for gestational age and have a large placenta (>25% of mass of the neonate). Proteinuria often occurs *in utero* and the maternal α-fetoprotein is raised in both blood and amniotic fluid secondary to fetal proteinuria. Thirty per cent develop oedema in the first week of life with abdominal distension and ascites. Renal function is normal initially but deteriorates to end-stage renal failure within the first 2 years of life. Renal biopsy is characteristic. There is no available cure. Patients are managed with regular 20% albumin transfusions followed by bilateral nephrectomy, dialysis, high calorie feeding and renal transplantation. There is a recognised risk of recurrence post-transplantation associated with circulating anti-nephrin antibodies.

9.29 Haemolytic uraemic syndrome

Answer D: Admit for investigation and fluid balance

This presentation is typical of haemolytic uraemic syndrome, the most common cause of acute renal failure in children aged <2 years. It classically follows a bloody diarrhoeal illness (*E. coli*, *Shigella* spp.) but there may be non-bloody diarrhoea. Investigations show acute renal failure with thrombocytopenia and anaemia and red cell fragments, and first-line treatment is that generic to acute renal failure, ie fluid management. Transfusion is often required and dialysis for those cases where conservative management fails.

9.30 Posterior urethral valves

Answer B: Urgent renal ultrasonography

This baby has renal failure secondary to posterior urethral valves (PUVs) until proved otherwise and the story is typical.

The diagnosis of PUVs is limited to baby boys and is the most common urological cause of renal failure in childhood. PUVs cause bladder obstruction that can vary in severity ranging from disease so severe that it is incompatible with postnatal life through to disease so minimal that it manifests only in later life. In 70% of cases the diagnosis is suspected on antenatal ultrasonography with findings of a thick-walled, poorly emptying bladder, dilated posterior urethra, bilateral hydronephrosis, echogenic or cystic change in the kidneys ± oligohydramnios. Those cases not diagnosed antenatally can present in infancy with UTI, poor urinary stream, failure to thrive and abdominal mass (palpable bladder or kidneys) ,or later in childhood with persistent day- and night-time wetting or intermittent retention.

The morbidity of PUVs is not just limited to transient urethral obstruction. Obstruction of the urinary tract antenatally at a time of critical organogenesis may result in lifelong dysfunction in both kidney and bladder function.

Ultrasonography at presentation, or in the postnatal period if suspected antenatally, confirms obstruction at the urethral level with ureteric and pelvicalyceal dilatation. The gold standard for diagnosis remains the micturating cystourethrogram. Management includes catheterisation followed by endoscopic resection of valves once the patient is stable. It is important to treat any pulmonary insufficiency secondary to oligohydramnios, exclude UTI, start prophylactic antibiotics, and carefully manage fluid and electrolyte balances to maximise outcome. Approximately a third of patients born with PUVs progress to end-stage renal disease; this represents 10–15% of all children undergoing renal transplantation.

Preauricular tags are common and, though there is an occasional association with renal abnormalities, they do not, as such, warrant further investigation other than a careful history and clinical examination.

9.31 Nephrotic syndrome

Answer A: Start high-dose prednisolone

Nephrotic syndrome usually presents with generalised oedema. Ascites and pleural effusions may develop in more severe cases. There is often a history of URTI that precedes the onset of oedema and children may be lethargic and irritable with poor appetite, and may have diarrhoea and abdominal pain. Blood pressure is usually low or normal. Hypovolaemia is a common finding although difficult to assess. Symptoms and signs associated with hypovolaemia include:

- Cap refill time >2 s
- Toe core temperature gap of >2°C
- Hypotension/hypertension
- Persistent tachycardia
- Abdominal pain
- Urinary sodium <10 mmol/l.

Hypovolaemia should be corrected with fluid resuscitation and cautious use of 4.5% albumin or, more rarely, very cautious 20% albumin.

Treatment is with a course of prednisolone starting at 60 mg/m² daily of prednisolone until remission of the proteinuria (95% in <28 days), followed by 40 mg/m² on alternate days for a further 4 weeks before reduction to stop. Most children have a relapsing–remitting course with 60% having five or more relapses over several years; however, in the long term most show a decline in the rate of relapses and most patients achieve long-term remission by adulthood.

Steroid-sparing agents used in cases found to be steroid dependent or for cases showing frequent relapses include levamisole, cyclophosphamide, ciclosporin and rituximab (CD20 monoclonal antibody). These agents should all be used under the guidance of a paediatric nephrologist.

Referral to a paediatric nephrologist should be considered for the following:

- Age <12 months
- Age >10 years
- Macroscopic or persistent microscopic haematuria
- Impaired renal function not attributable to hypovolaemia
- Persistent hypertension.
- Decreased C3 complement
- Rash or arthropathy
- Failure to induce remission with 28 days of prednisolone at 60 mg/m².

9.32 Urinary frequency

Answer E: Reassure that this is a normal reaction to new siblings and that no investigation is needed

The symptoms are typically non-organic. However, a thorough history should be taken and comprehensive examination, including urinalysis and blood pressure and measuring and plotting of height and weight, should be performed. If there is nothing to note in the history, examination or urinalysis, it is important not to escalate anxiety in this situation; an appropriate next step would be reassurance for the child and the family that there is nothing serious amiss and that she will improve with time as the family dynamics settle down into a new rhythm.

EMQ Answers

9.33–9.35 Theme: Acute kidney injury (previously known as acute renal failure)

9.33

Answer B: Prerenal failure secondary to intravascular depletion

9.34

Answer D: Intrinsic renal failure secondary to haemolytic uraemic syndrome (see question 9.19)

9.35

Answer C: Intrinsic renal failure secondary to Henoch–Schönlein purpura

Acute kidney injury

Acute kidney injury (previously known as acute renal failure) is defined as an abrupt (<48 h) reduction in kidney function, an absolute increase in serum creatinine >26.4 µmol/l (0.3 mg/dl) or an increase of ≥50% or a decrease in urine output (<0.5 ml/kg per h for 6 h).

Common causes of acute kidney injury in children include all of the scenarios listed in the question with the addition of:

- Post-cardiac surgery
- Haematological/oncological and bone marrow transplantation
- Drugs (avoid in renal impairment):
  - NSAID
  - ACE inhibitors
  - aminoglycoside antibiotics
  - radiocontrast agents
  - amphotericin B
  - cisplatin/tacrolimus
  - penicillin and cephalosporins
  - aciclovir.

Pathophysiology:

- Prerenal: after hypotension and hypovolaemia
- Intrinsic: ischaemia and nephrotoxins
- Postrenal (less common): obstruction to urinary flow.

Investigations

Urine

- Dipstick for blood, protein and glucose
- Microscopy:
  - RBCs crenated (scalloped) – glomerulonephritis
  - absent RBCs (+ve dip) – haemoglobinuria (haemolytic process)
  - WBCs – eosinophils are seen in acute tubular nephritis (ATN)
  - multiple WBCs – infection
  - RBC casts – glomerulonephritis
  - WBCs casts – ATN
- Urinary sodium and creatinine:

- Na^+ <10 mmol/l intravascular depletion (prerenal)
- >20 mmol/l – more common with intrinsic acute kidney injury (AKI)
- fractional excretion of sodium, FeNa (percentage of filtered sodium that is excreted) = [(Urine Na^+/Serum Na^+) × (Serum creatinine/Urine creatinine)] × 100:
- FeNa <1% indicative of prerenal AKI
- FeNa 2–3% indicative of intrinsic renal failure.

Blood tests

- Sodium: <135 mmol/l fluid overload secondary to oliguria
- Potassium >6.0 mmol/l common and ↑ with acidaemia; often normal in HUS secondary to increased losses
- Urea: always increased in AKI but proportionally higher than creatinine in prerenal causes: high urea levels are seen with normal renal function in steroid therapy, GI bleed, catabolic states and high protein intake
- Creatinine: indirect assessment of GFR (ml/min per 1.73 m^2) = {(40 × Height (cm)/ Serum creatinine (μmol/l)}:
  - proportional to muscle mass
  - overestimates GFR in chronic renal failure (CRF)
- Acidosis: reduced renal excretion of bicarbonate in AKI
- Phosphate accumulates in AKI secondary to decreased excretion
- FBC:
  - anaemia common, often dilutional
  - microangiopathic anaemia with fragmented RBCs and ↓ platelets in HUS
- Complement :
  - ↓ C3 and normal C4 – postinfective glomerulonephritis
  - ↓ C3 and ↓ C4 SLE
- Autoantibody screen: ANA (antinuclear antibody), DNA ANCA (antineutrophil cytoplasmic antibody), anti-GBM (glomerular basement membrane): positivity suggests autoimmune disease
- Anti-DNAase B and ASOT (positive post-streptococcal infection)
- Lactate dehydrogenase (LDH) ↑ in HUS
- Urine osmolality >500 mosmol/kg – prerenal; <350 mosmol/l intrinsic AKI.

Management of AKI

Fluid management:

- Assessment of fluid status with examination, weight and biochemistry investigations
- If in doubt a cautious fluid challenge of 10–20 ml/kg over 30–60 min
- If no improvement post-bolus and felt to be fluid replete, then intravenous furosemide 2 mg/kg can be given as a one-off dose
- If remains oliguric – millilitre for millilitre replacement for output plus 400 ml/m^2 or 15 ml/kg to cover insensible losses
- Daily weights and strict fluid balance is required.

Hyponatraemia:

- Restrict free water
- If symptomatic correct with 3%.

Hyperkalaemia:

- Treat if >6.0 with ECG changes – see detailed management (answer 9.3)
- ECG manifestations include tall/peaked t waves; prolonged PR interval/flattening of p waves and widening of QRS.

Hypertension:

- Salt and water restriction is sufficient in most patients to control BP.
- Persistent hypertension should be treated with calcium channel blocker or β blocker.
- Hypertensive emergency: with encephalopathy or cardiac symptoms should be admitted to high dependency unit (HDU) and managed in consultation with a paediatric nephrologist.

Drugs:

- Nephrotoxic drugs should be avoided if at all possible
- Drug doses adjusted down if essential, monitoring for levels and toxic effects carefully.

Nutrition:

- Adequate nutrition is essential but a renal diet restricted in fluid volume, potassium, sodium, phosphate and protein should be instigated and managed with the input of an expert dietician.

Indications for dialysis in acute renal injury include:

- Severe or persistent hyperkalaemia
- Fluid overload with hypertension, congestive cardiac failure or pulmonary oedema
- Uraemia with central nervous system (CNS) symptoms, nausea, pericarditis
- Persistent severe acidosis despite bicarbonate therapy
- Severe hypo- or hypernatraemia.

Methods of dialysis:

- Peritoneal dialysis
- Continuous renal replacement therapy
- Haemodialysis.

Prognosis:

- Dependent on the underlying mechanism of injury.
- Factors associated with poor outcome include multiorgan failure, ionotropic support, mechanical ventilation, and the need for dialysis.
- Mortality rates of up to 25% have been reported, with much worse rates (64%) after cardiac surgery.
- Children have a much better prognosis than adults.
- Primary renal disease accounts for the vast majority who progress to chronic renal failure.

9.36–9.38 Theme: Renal biochemistry

9.36

Answer G: Fanconi syndrome

This patient has a background of faltering growth with a period of decompensation before admission. He has features of rickets. He presents with dehydration but not the expected oliguria. His bloods show a metabolic acidosis with a relatively alkaline urine pH. Glycosuria, despite relatively low serum glucose, hypokalaemia, hyponatraemia and proteinuria, suggests a generalised proximal tubular leak.

Proximal renal tubular acidosis (type 2 RTA) occurs as a result of a failure of reabsorption of bicarbonate in the proximal tubule. It is characterised by a high urinary pH, low plasma bicarbonate and metabolic acidosis. Most patients with proximal RTA manifest this tubular abnormality as part of Fanconi syndrome. In patients with proximal RTA, distal tubular acidification (by secretion of H^+) is intact. This means that after an acid load the urinary pH will drop below 5.5.

Fanconi syndrome

This is a generalised transport abnormality in the proximal tubule characterised by excessive urinary losses of amino acids, glucose, bicarbonate, potassium, phosphate, calcium, magnesium and uric acid. It is also characterised by metabolic acidosis, dehydration, hypokalaemia, hypophosphataemia, rickets and growth retardation. There are many causes, both hereditary and acquired (see below):

- Metabolic:
  - cystinosis
  - tyrosinaemia
  - Lowe syndrome
  - galactosaemia
  - Wilson disease
- Heavy metal toxicity: lead, mercury, cadmium
- Idiopathic.

The most common cause in white children is cystinosis, a defect in the transport of cystine out of lysosomes. This leads to Fanconi syndrome, with the addition of photophobia (corneal cystine crystals) and hypothyroidism (thyroid deposition of cystine). Sequentially cystine deposition in other organs can cause diabetes mellitus, male infertility, myopathy and neurological symptoms including dementia.

Treatment

The treatment of proximal RTA is large amounts of alkali as sodium bicarbonate and sodium citrate. Fanconi syndrome requires treatment as appropriate with phosphate, potassium and vitamin D. Specifically, treatment for cystinosis requires mercaptamine (which combines with cystine in the lysosomes, enabling release of the previously trapped cystine); this slows the rate of decline in renal function.

9.37

Answer E: Classic distal renal tubular acidosis (type I)

This patient has metabolic acidosis with relatively alkaline urine pH, with a picture of acquired faltering growth over the 3 months before presentation. He does not currently have a UTI but does have blood and urine results suggestive of RTA without generalised tubular leakage (negative glycosuria and proteinuria).

Distal RTA occurs as a consequence of reduced H^+ secretion in the distal tubule. It is not possible to lower the urinary pH below 5.5 regardless of the acid load.

The condition can be autosomal dominant, sporadic or secondary; causes include:

- Idiopathic
- Familial
- Drugs, eg amphotericin B toxicity, lithium
- Inherited/congenital disease: sickle cell disease, osteopetrosis, Wilson disease, Fabry disease (X-linked lipid storage disease)
- Systemic disease: Sjögren disease, SLE, chronic active hepatitis, amyloidosis
- Diseases causing nephrocalcinosis: hyperparathyroidism, hypercalciuria, vitamin D toxicity, medullary sponge kidney
- Interstitial renal disease: **chronic pyelonephritis**, obstructive nephropathy.

Symptoms and signs:

- Failure to thrive
- Confusion or decreased alertness
- Fatigue
- Muscle weakness
- Tachypnoea
- Tachycardia or dysrhythmia
- Nephrocalcinosis or renal stones
- Rickets, osteomalacia or bone pain
- Muscle cramps
- Polyuria

Investigations:

- Metabolic acidosis on blood gas
- Hypokalaemia
- Hyperchloraemia
- Hypercalciuria
- Low serum bicarbonate
- Urine pH never <5
- Normal anion gap.

The treatment is aiming to restore normal blood pH and electrolyte balance. This will indirectly correct the bone disorders and decrease the calcium deposition as nephrocalcinosis or renal stones. In cases of secondary distal RTA an underlying cause should be sort and treated if appropriate. Alkaline medications such as sodium bicarbonate and potassium citrate act to correct the acidosis and sodium bicarbonate may correct the loss of potassium and calcium. Vitamin D and calcium supplements are not routinely given due to the potential for calcium deposits in the renal tract even after treatment.

9.38

Answer F: Congenital adrenal hyperplasia

This baby presents with vomiting and a hypochloraemic metabolic alkalosis, but the low sodium and high potassium indicate a salt-losing presentation of CAH rather than pyloric stenosis as the most likely underlying aetiology. Of cases of CAH 95% are due to an enzyme abnormality of the 21-hydroxylase deficiency in which progesterone and 17OH-progesterone fail to be converted to deoxycorticosterone and deoxycortisol, respectively, resulting in a failure of production of aldosterone and cortisol with excessive androgen production. The reduced cortisol leads to increased ACTH secretion, which causes the adrenal hyperplasia and excessive precursor and androgen production.
Presentation depends on exact genetic mutation:

- Genital hypertrophy in the male
- Ambiguous genitalia (hypertrophy of the clitoris and labia (which may fuse)) in the female
- Pigmentation of the genital area may occur after several weeks due to the excessive ACTH secretion
- Salt-losing crisis (as in this case): 70% of 21OH deficiency causes salt waste (may occur from days 3–4 until approximately days 21–28):
  - hypotension
  - dehydration
  - vomiting, shock and collapse
  - early increased serum potassium
  - decreased serum sodium
- Hypoglycaemia
- In non -21OH cases presentation may occur later and salt wasting is rare.

Investigations:

- Urine steroid profile
- Genetic analysis
- Raised levels of 17OH-progesterone in the plasma.

Management:

- Treat dehydration with fluid bolus if shocked
- Treat hypoglycaemia
- Intravenous hydrocortisone 6 hourly
- Hyperkalaemia responds well to steroid and fluid administration

- Once stable give oral hydrocortisone and oral fludrocortisone regularly
- Oral sodium supplements are usually given over the first year of life
- Education about the management of double-dose hydrocortisone in intercurrent illness.

9.39–9.41 Theme: Haematuria

Haematuria itself can be macroscopic, intermittent or microscopic. Haematuria needs to be distinguished from other conditions such as excessive beetroot ingestion, rifampicin, haemoglobinuria, myoglobulinuria and inborn errors of metabolism (porphyria), which all produce red urine without haematuria. Urate crystals in the urine of infants may produce a pink stain in nappies, which can be mistaken for haematuria. Positive dipstick results should be verified by microscopy because significant haematuria is defined as more than five RBCs per millilitre; dipsticks are very sensitive and will pick up haemoglobin and myoglobin in tiny amounts; a negative dipstick is, however, good at excluding haematuria. The incidence of macroscopic haematuria in children is very low – <0.2%. Incidental finding of microscopic haematuria is relatively common (0.5–4%) but <30% will have persisting urinary abnormalities 6 months later. It is important to assess whether isolated haematuria in an otherwise well child is either persistent or familial before investigation. If there are two to three early morning urines (EMUs) each week for 6 months report the results in a diary listing any intercurrent illness or episodes of macroscopic haematuria. All first-degree relatives should have three to four EMUs tested over the 6-month period.

The coexistence of proteinuria with haematuria makes a renal parenchymal lesion more likely. Heavy proteinuria suggests glomerular disease. Ultrasonography and plain abdominal radiography are essential to exclude obstruction, calculi or tumours.

9.39

Answer D: Renal calculi in children

- 1–3% present in childhood.
- 30% present with pain and haematuria, but macroscopic haematuria is common
- Renal colic (85%) >8 years
- Diffuse abdominal pain (70%) <8 years
- Other symptoms include dysuria, vomiting or urinary retention
- 20% asymptomatic and identified during investigation for UTIs or unrelated problems.

Investigation

- Radiography and/or ultrasonography
- Urine MC&S
- Metabolic investigations: spot urine for calcium:creatinine ratio, cystine:creatinine ratio, oxalate:creatinine ratio, uric acid:creatinine ratio, serum electrolytes and renal function:
  - 75% have a predisposing condition:

- Infective (30%): can be primary stones leading to stasis or infection leading to stones – proteus infection causes the urease to break down urea into ammonia and CO_2, ↑ pH leading to the formation of struvite (stag-horn calculi) and calcium phosphate stones
- Metabolic (44%) (coexisting infection):
  - often diagnosed late after renal function has deteriorated.
  - red flags include early onset, family history, and recurrent and bilateral stones.

Hypercalciuria (most common):

- Idiopathic (majority)
- Present with gross haematuria, abdominal pain and dysuria.
- Consider secondary causes if there is a family history, failure to thrive, rickets, renal dysfunction, proteinuria, dysmorphic features or poor response to therapy.
- Secondary conditions increase calcium in the urine by (1) decreased renal tubular reabsorption, (2) increased intestinal absorption or (3) imbalance of bone resorption. Nephrocalcinosis, calcium deposition in the kidney parenchyma, is part of the spectrum of calcium-induced renal stones.

Cystinuria (autosomal recessive) responsible for 10% of paediatric stones.

Hyperoxaluria can be primary or secondary to increased oxalate or vitamin C ingestion, pyridoxine deficiency and intestinal malabsorption:

- Structural urinary tract abnormalities – increase urinary stasis leading to increased stone formation and infection
- Idiopathic (26%).

Treatment:

- General measures; ↑ fluid, dietary modifications, treat infection
- Medical (specific to underlying disorder)
- Surgical.

9.40

Answer E: Renal vein thrombosis associated with nephrotic syndrome

This is a recognised complication of nephrotic syndrome. It occurs secondary to the hypercoagulable state associated with nephrotic syndrome, which occurs due to the loss of antithrombin III, a relative excess of fibrinogen and decreased clotting factors. The renal vein is particularly susceptible to clots.

In infants renal vein thrombosis can occur in isolation, associated with dehydration or factor V Leiden mutation. Other associations with renal vein thrombosis include antithrombin III deficiency, protein C or S deficiency, antiphospolipid antibody, postrenal transplantation and steroid administration.

Presentation:

- Asymptomatic (most common)
- Unexplained acute renal failure

- Sudden increase in proteinuria
- Acutely with flank pain and severe macroscopic haematuria.

Investigation:

- Renal ultrasonography – swollen kidneys with prominent echo-poor medullary pyramids. It is often not sensitive enough to make the diagnosis.
- CT with intravenous contrast is currently the investigation of choice, but MRI is emerging as a useful investigation.

Treatment:

- Seek expert advice from paediatric nephrologist
- Control proteinuria in underlying nephrotic syndrome
- Consider anticoagulation especially if pulmonary emboli coexist.

9.41

Answer I: Alport syndrome

This is a group of hereditary syndromes involving the basement membrane of the kidney, cochlea and the eye resulting in hereditary nephritis, sensorineural deafness and anterior lenticonus (conical deformity of the eye). The mode of inheritance varies; 80% are X linked, 15% autosomal recessive and 5% autosomal dominant. The clinical consequences are a result of mutations in type IV collagen genes.

Children with Alport syndrome may present initially with persistent microscopic haematuria with episodic macroscopic haematuria and a family history of haematuria. Auditory and ocular manifestations may appear later in life, deafness arouno 10 years of age, hypertension in mid-teens and eye signs in mid to late teens. End-stage renal failure develops on average around age 21 years, 90% by 40 years of age. Females with X-linked Alport syndrome have persistent microscopic haematuria, with some developing hypertension and end-stage renal failure (40% by 80 years), but this occurs at a later age. Among female patients, the presence of proteinuria and hearing loss increases the risk of development of end-stage renal failure. Ultrasonography is important to exclude alternative causes for haematuria but is usually normal in children with Alport syndrome, but show progressive kidney shrinkage in later stages.

Family history of haematuria, early onset deafness and renal insufficiency is common. If a family history is absent in a patient with typical clinical findings, suspect the rarer autosomal recessive form of the disease which affects male and females equally.

9.42–944 Theme: Blood pressure

9.42

Answer F: Haemolytic uraemic syndrome

This case is a typical picture of haemolytic uraemic syndrome, the most common cause of renal failure in children aged <2 years. It usually follows a diarrhoeal illness and most commonly is associated with verotoxin-producing *E. coli* (VTEC) of the O157 serotype.

Other changes in the FBC and film include RBC fragments and anaemia. Hypertension occurs in 20–30%, often transient around the time of resolution of the oliguria. Management is essentially supportive with strict fluid balance, treatment of hypertension, transfusion and in some cases dialysis. Long-term follow-up is mandatory due to risk of development of renal failure and hypertension. Prognosis is worse in non-diarrhoeal cases.

9.43

Answer I: Vesicoureteric reflux with scarring in infancy

The small kidneys and hypertension strongly suggest chronic pyelonephritis most commonly due to early reflux nephropathy.

VUR is defined as retrograde flow of urine from the bladder to the upper renal tracts. It is associated with infection and many large studies have shown a strong correlation between frequency of UTI and severity of reflux nephropathy in patients with VUR. Scarring of renal parenchyma may result from a single episode of pyelonephritis, especially in very young patients. Over time, when enough renal parenchyma has become scarred, hypertension and renal failure can develop. The incidence of VUR is increased in children diagnosed with a UTI and those who had hydronephrosis on antenatal ultrasonography. There is also a significant increased incidence in children whose siblings and parents have VUR but the specific genetics have not yet been defined.

Currently, under the NICE guidelines for UTI in children, all infants <6 months diagnosed with a UTI should undergo renal ultrasonography within 6 weeks and progress to DMSA and micturating cystourethrogram (MCUG) if they have abnormality on scan or if the UTI is classified as atypical or recurrent. Children between 6 months and 3 years who are diagnosed with a UTI that is classified as atypical or recurrent should undergo renal ultrasonography and progress to a DMSA 4–6 months post-infection. If this is abnormal or if there is a family history of VUR, they should progress to an MCUG, with antibiotic prophylaxis for 3 days before the investigation.

There is controversy about the appropriate management of VUR and the previously widespread practice of reimplantation surgery is now rare due to the long-term follow-up results being similar to those of conservative medical management. A Cochrane review into treatment of VUR reports that there is limited evidence to support the use of prophylactic antibiotics for the prevention of renal parenchymal disease or feverish UTIs, but the studies were small. Endoscopic surgery with the injection of bulking agents at the vesicoureteric junction is currently under review.

9.44

Answer G: Wilms tumour

The vast majority of Wilms tumours arise sporadically; however, there are cases of familial inheritance and strong associations with some syndromes including hemihypertrophy, Beckwith–Wiedemann (2%) and aniridia (1%), which can precede the malignancy by years. Children with hemihypertrophy should have lifelong annual renal ultrasonography.

Wilms tumour is the most common renal tumour of childhood and the fifth most common paediatric malignancy. Six per cent occur bilaterally and the mean age of diagnosis is 3.5 years. The most common presenting feature is an abdominal mass. Other presenting features include abdominal pain, hypertension, haematuria, anaemia and fever caused by tumour necrosis.

Treatment in most cases is a combination of surgery and chemotherapy with radiotherapy being confined to the more advanced stages of disease. The overall prognosis is good with a 90% survival rate, prognosis being worse in bilateral disease.

9.45–9.47 Theme: Investigations

9.45

Answer C: DMSA isotope scan

The DMSA (technetium-99m [or ^{99m}Tc]-labelled dimercaptosuccinic acid) isotope scan is the gold standard investigation for assessing renal parenchymal damage. This particular isotope concentrates well into renal tissue and decreased uptake will indicate areas of scarring (or acute inflammation). DMSA scanning within 6 weeks of a UTI is inadvisable due to false-positive results. The NICE guidelines on the management of children with UTIs state that a DMSA scan should be performed 4–6 months post-infection in all children up to 3 years of age with recurrent or atypical UTIs; it should be performed in all children >3 years with recurrent UTIs. The DMSA scan will also allow visualisation of the collecting system and estimation of the percentage of functioning renal tissue in each kidney.

9.46

Answer J: None of the above

The principal 'investigating' needed at presentation is confirmation of proteinuria. The diagnosis of nephrotic syndrome is based on the triad of proteinuria, peripheral oedema and hypoalbuminaemia, and apart from bloods is clinical.

9.47

Answer E: Renal tract ultrasonography

Ultrasonography is simple and effective and will show perinephric fluid in most cases. Some surgeons prefer an additional CT preoperatively. Percutaneous drainage can be done under ultrasound guidance but open drainage is required for definitive treatment.

9.48–9.50 Theme: The kidney in systemic disease

9.48

Answer I: Amyloidosis

Secondary amyloidosis can result from a number of chronic inflammatory/infective conditions. It is characterised by the extracellular tissue deposition of fibrils that are composed of fragments of serum amyloid A protein. This is a major acute phase protein produced by the liver. Underlying conditions associated with amyloid A deposits include the following.

Infective

- Bronchiectasis
- Osteomyelitis
- Chronic pyelonephritis
- Tuberculosis
- Lung abscess
- Cystic fibrosis.

Inflammatory

- Chronic juvenile arthritis
- Inflammatory bowel disease
- Ankylosing spondylitis
- Familial Mediterranean fever

The most common presentation of amyloid A amyloidosis is renal; it leads to proteinuria or nephrotic syndrome or progresses to renal failure (by deposition). Amyloid can also be deposited in the liver and spleen causing enlargement. Diagnosis is usually by demonstrating deposition of amyloid A in the kidney (renal biopsy) by performing a rectal biopsy.

9.49

Answer A: Systemic lupus erythematosus

Although several of these conditions may have renal impairment after some years only lupus presents with involvement as a glomerulonephritis. Lupus is considered the great mimicker and may present in many ways. Typical presenting features may include:

- Renal disease – often nephritic on urinalysis but can present as nephrotic syndrome
- Polyarthritis
- Malar rash
- General malaise/fatigue and fever.

SLE is defined as an episodic, multisystem, autoimmune disorder characterised by widespread inflammation of blood vessels and connective tissue. Diagnosis is made by autoantibody testing, which shows the presence of ANAs – the gold standard being anti-double-stranded DNA. Diagnosis is only confirmed in the presence of symptoms because ANAs can be seen relatively frequently in children without lupus or any other chronic disease. Lupus is commonly associated with decreased levels of C3 and C4, and almost never associated with raised complement levels. Treatment is often with corticosteroids in the first instance.

9.50

Answer B: Diabetes

The classic 'herald' of renal impairment (nephropathy) in diabetes is asymptomatic microalbuminuria. Microalbuminuria refers to small amounts of albumin in the urine outside the normal range but too low to be detected by normal clinical Albusticks. In adult patients with type 1 diabetes, approximately 30% will develop microalbuminuria by age 20 years; a tenth will spontaneously regress to normoalbuminuria and a third will develop macroalbuminuria or overt nephropathy; thus this is a process that usually occurs in the adolescent age group of patients who have had type 1 diabetes for some years. The risk of progression to permanent microalbuminuria is higher during puberty than during either the pre- or postpubertal periods.

It is known that type 1 diabetes mellitus onset at an early age and metabolic control during the early years can significantly influence the development of persistent microalbuminuria; in addition there appears to be familial factors that can increase the risk of progression to microalbuminuria. Annual urinary screening for the microalbumin:creatinine ratio is recommended. After detection of microalbuminuria tighter glycaemic control can increase the regression rates back to normoalbuminuria, but too tight a control can lead to increased risk of hypoglycaemia and excessive weight gain, so a determined but cautious approach is advised.

CHAPTER 10

Neurology Answers

MTF Answers

10.1 Sudden unexplained death in a person with epilepsy (SUDEP)

Answers: A D E

SUDEP is the sudden unexplained death of a person with epilepsy; it accounts for approximately 500 deaths/year in the UK. Although the exact cause is unknown it is postulated that seizure activity causes changes in a person's breathing and heartbeat that lead to death.

Factors that may increase a person's risk of SUDEP include:

- Having generalised tonic–clonic seizures
- Not taking antiepileptic drugs (AEDs) as prescribed
- Having seizures that are not controlled by AEDs
- Having sudden and frequent changes to AEDs
- Being a young adult (in particular male)
- Having nocturnal seizures
- Having seizures when alone
- Drinking large amounts of alcohol.

10.2 Carpal tunnel syndrome

Answers: A C D E

This results from compression of the median nerve in the carpal tunnel of the wrist. The syndrome progresses slowly resulting in the following:

- Pain, tingling and numbness in the lateral three and a half fingers (the thenar eminence is spared because the branch supplying the skin over this area leaves the median nerve before the carpal tunnel).
- Weakness and wasting of muscles supplied by the median nerve (lateral two lumbricals, abductor pollicis, flexor pollicis brevis, opponens pollicis).

Symptoms are initially worse at night, and are typically relieved by shaking vigorously or immersing in water. Aetiology includes causes of soft-tissue swelling:

- Obesity, pregnancy
- Rheumatoid arthritis

- Hypothyroidism
- Gout
- Amyloidosis
- Acromegaly.

Treatment involves splints, diuretics, topical hydrocortisone injection and surgical decompression.

10.3 Nystagmus

Answers: A D

Nystagmus is involuntary oscillation of the eyes, usually during attempted fixation. It must be sustained for a few seconds to be significant. The direction of the fast or rapid phase describes the direction of the nystagmus. The fast phase is in fact an attempt by the eyes to correct the drift from fixation that has occurred, and it is the slow phase that is pathological.

Nystagmus falls into three categories: jerk, pendular and ataxic.

Jerk nystagmus: distinct fast and slow phases, more obvious on gaze towards the rapid phase. Aetiology includes:

- Vestibular lesions: nerve VIII, inner ear, vestibular pathway; horizontal or rotatory; fast phase away from the side of the lesion; usually transient.
- Central lesions: brain stem, cerebellum; horizontal, rotatory or vertical; fast phase towards the side of the lesion; usually last weeks or longer.
- Positional nystagmus: benign positional vertigo; occurs in one direction only; induced by rapid head movements but delayed; fatigues after short time.

Note that vertical nystagmus originates only from central lesions.

Pendular nystagmus: no fast and slow phases. Aetiology includes:

- Congenital lesions: X-linked or autosomal dominant
- Secondary to poor visual fixation, such as severe visual impairment/blindness, albinism, cataracts, optic atrophy.

Ataxic nystagmus: as in internuclear ophthalmoplegia. A gaze palsy exists – on looking to one side there is nystagmus in the abducting (contralateral to lesion) eye, but no movement in the 'adducting' (ipsilateral to lesion) eye. It is usually due to damage to the medial longitudinal fasciculus (multiple sclerosis). Other causes of nystagmus include drugs – alcohol, barbiturates, phenytoin.

10.4 Cerebral palsy

Answers: D E

Prenatal causes:

- Genetic forms – autosomal recessive and autosomal dominant
- Cerebral malformation

- Alcohol
- Substance abuse
- Infection (TORCH).

Perinatal causes:

- Hypoxic ischaemic encephalopathy
- Ventricular haemorrhage (preterm babies)
- Postnatal causes
- Meningitis
- Encephalitis
- Head injury.

Preterm delivery is a risk factor for, but not a cause of, cerebral palsy.

10.5 Patterns of inheritance

Answers: A E

This is an important question. Patterns of inheritance are often asked in MCQs and should be learnt. The inheritance of the conditions listed are as follows:

- Tuberous sclerosis: autosomal dominant
- Ataxia–telangiectasia: autosomal recessive
- Colour blindness: X-linked recessive
- Haemophilia A: X-linked recessive
- Myotonic dystrophy: autosomal dominant.

Genetic anticipation

Genetic anticipation refers to the situation by which successive generations are more severely affected by a particular disease process and at a younger age.

Examples of this include:

- Fragile X syndrome
- Myotonic dystrophy
- Huntington disease.

10.6 Myoclonus

Answers: A B D

Myoclonus is a simple jerk-like movement that is not coordinated or suppressible. The jerks are usually flexor and occur at an extremity. If the legs are involved a child may be thrown to the ground. In childhood epilepsy myoclonic jerks can either present as the main seizure type (benign myoclonic epilepsy of infancy) or be one of several seizure types seen in an epilepsy syndrome.

West syndrome

- Infantile spasms

- Developmental delay
- Hypsarrhythmia on the EEG.

Lennox–Gastaut syndrome

- Extension of West syndrome occurring between the ages of 1 and 5 years
- Atypical absences, myoclonic, tonic and atonic seizures
- EEG shows slow spike-and-wave discharges
- 90% show moderate-to-severe learning disability.

Landau–Kleffner syndrome

This is rare and is characterised by the almost complete or complete loss of previously acquired language before the onset of seizures, which develop in 70–80%. The EEG is usually abnormal and the outlook poor. Myoclonic jerks are not usually seen.

Juvenile myoclonic epilepsy

JME is characterised by myoclonic episodes with preserved consciousness. The episodes often occur on wakening or after sleep deprivation. EEG abnormalities are usually seen and the response to sodium valproate is good. Prolonged treatment is required.

10.7 Primitive reflexes

Answers: B C

The Moro reflex

This is initiated by sudden movement of the neck and consists of a rapid abduction and extension of the arms with opening of the hands. Eliciting it helps to assess muscle tone. It usually disappears by 3 months. A decrease in it on one side may be an early sign of a hemiparesis.

The startle reflex

This is similar to the Moro reflex, but is elicited by a loud noise. There is no opening of the hands.

The grasp reflex

Stimulation of the palm causes it to close. This reflex usually disappears by 3 months.

The asymmetrical tonic neck reflex

When a baby lies with the head to one side, the arm and leg on that side are extended to the same side, and the arm and leg on the contralateral side are flexed. This appears by 2–3 weeks and disappears by 3 months. Its persistence is suggestive of cerebral palsy

The parachute reflex

This appears between 6 and 9 months and persists. It is elicited by holding the infant in ventral suspension and suddenly lowering him or her. The arms extend as a defence reaction. Asymmetry may be a sign of hemiparesis.

The Babinski (extensor plantar) response is normal up until about 1 year of age.

10.8 Hydrocephalus

Answers: B C D

Macrocephaly is defined as a head circumference larger then two standard deviations (2 SD) from the normal age-corrected mean. Normal/familial large head is the most common cause of macrocephaly. Other causes are hydrocephalus, megalencephaly (large brain) and a thickened skull. Hydrocephalus occurs due to an excess volume of cerebrospinal fluid (CSF) in the skull vault. This can result from either increased production or impaired reabsorption and circulation. CSF is formed in the choroid plexus principally within the lateral ventricle. It flows from the lateral ventricles through the foramen of Munro into the third ventricle and from there via the aqueduct of Sylvius into the fourth ventricle. It exits the fourth ventricle via the foramina of Luschka and Magendie for reabsorption principally through the arachnoid villi.

Hydrocephalus can be either communicating or non-communicating. Non-communicating occurs as a consequence of obstruction at some point in the ventricular system. Megalencephaly is enlargement of the brain substance. Hydrencephaly refers to the replacement of the brain substance by CSF.

Causes of communicating hydrocephalus are:

- Meningitis
- Post-haemorrhagic
- Choroids plexus papilloma
- Meningeal malignancy.

Causes of non-communicating hydrocephalus:

- Aqueduct stenosis
- Arnold–Chiari malformation
- Dandy–Walker syndrome
- Klippel–Feil syndrome
- Mass lesion
- Warburg syndrome.

Causes of megalencephaly:

- Genetic
- Sotos syndrome
- Achondroplasia
- Incontinentia pigmenti
- Neurofibromatosis
- Tuberous sclerosis
- Alexander disease
- Canavan disease
- Galactosaemia
- Mucopolysaccharidosis.

Causes of macrocephaly due to a thickened skull:

- Anaemia
- Rickets
- Renal dwarfism
- Hyperphosphataemia
- Osteogenesis imperfecta.

10.9 Microcephaly

Answer: E

Uncontrolled phenylketonuria in the mother can be neurotoxic antenatally. There are various mechanisms which include disruption of normal metabolism by phenylalanine metabolites, phenylethylamine and phenylpyruvic acid. There may also be associated congenital heart disease and good control (maintaining phenylalanine levels <10 mg/dl) is of great importance. Chickenpox late in pregnancy can cause disseminated disease in the baby if delivery happens <1 week after maternal illness, ie before adequate maternal antibody is passed to the fetus. It does not, however, cause microcephaly at this stage. Dandy–Walker syndrome is fourth ventricular hydrocephalus and associated with a normal or large head. Neither myotonia nor neurofibromatosis is linked to microcephaly.

BOF Answers

10.10 Juvenile myoclonic epilepsy

Answer B: If in the future she wants to become sexually active, discuss the issues around anticonvulsant medication and contraception further as it is important for patients with epilepsy to have pre-pregnancy advice

NICE guidelines on Epilepsy 2004 state that 'Information about contraception, conception, pregnancy, or menopause should be given to girls and women in advance of sexual activity, pregnancy or menopause, and the information should be tailored to their individual needs. This information should also be given, as needed, to people who are closely involved with girls and women with epilepsy. These may include an individual's family and/or carers.'

Information to young people needs to be given at appropriate times but should not be delayed until they have transitioned into adult services. If a child is likely to need ongoing treatment into her childbearing age, such as this case, then it may be worth discussing the risks of any drugs being used and potential risks or benefits of changing medication. Under no circumstances should a patient suddenly stop anticonvulsant treatment because this may precipitate a seizure which in itself could be harmful to a fetus.

10.11 Narcolepsy

Answer B: It is familial

Narcolepsy is characterised by episodes of sudden uncontrollable sleep occurring at any time of the day or night. It involves an abnormal sequence in the stages of sleep – REM sleep occurring within 10 minutes of falling asleep compared with 1–2 hours in normal individuals. It typically commences in adolescence, is familial and up to 90% have cataplexy (sudden loss of tone in the legs, no loss of consciousness). Other associations include psychiatric problems, sleep paralysis and hypnagogic hallucinations (auditory hallucinations while falling asleep). Treatment involves stimulants for narcolepsy, clomipramine for cataplexy and multidisciplinary management of associated problems.

10.12 Raised intracranial pressure

Answer C: Urgent CT Scan

This child needs an urgent scan.

Rising intracranial pressure (ICP) may present in a variety of ways:

- Headaches
- Vomiting
- Alteration in conscious level
- Seizures
- In a trauma setting.

Causes of raised ICP:

- Head injury/trauma (most common)
- Infection (meningitis/encephalitis)
- Intracranial haemorrhage
- Cerebral oedema: of which there are three 'main causes'
- Vasogenic: due to increased capillary permeability
- Cytotoxic: from hypoxia, necrosis
- Interstitial, eg from obstructive hydrocephalus.

After 18 months of age ICP has the potential to rise significantly, as the skull sutures are mostly closed. As this occurs, the raised ICP will 'squash' brain tissue against bone, resulting in two syndromes:

1. Central syndrome: the whole brain is forced towards the foramen magnum through which the cerebellar tonsils herniate (coning).
2. Uncal syndrome: volume increase occurs mainly supratentorially and the uncus herniates through the tentorial opening. This may lead to an ipsilateral dilated pupil due to nerve III compression.

Signs of raised intracranial pressure:

- Abnormal oculocephalic reflexes – doll's eyes movements
- Dilated pupils (ipsilateral then bilateral)

- Altered conscious level progressing to coma
- Abnormal ventilation: rapid/slow/Cheyne–Stokes respiration/apnoea
- Posturing: decorticate progressing to decerebrate
- Papilloedema
- Absence of venous pulsation in retinal vessels
- Cushing triad: often preterminal (bradycardia, high blood pressure, abnormal ventilation).

Treatment is complex and involves the following:

- Adequate analgesia
- Effective nursing
- Raising head end of trolley
- Hyperventilation
- Mannitol
- Neurosurgical referral.

10.13 Gilles de la Tourette

Answer C: Symptoms disappear during sleep

Gilles de la Tourette is a syndrome of involuntary movements. It is a condition in which multiple groups of muscles are affected by tics – spasmodic, repetitive, stereotyped movements, often associated with verbal obscenities, echolalia and echopraxia. The condition is life-long, and may start from as early as 2–3 years of age.

Typical tics:

- Facial grimacing
- Blinking
- Violent, sudden movements
- Progressing to vocalisations:
- Throat clearing
- Coughing
- Sniffing
- Forced utterances
- Swearing.

Associated learning difficulties and compulsive disorders are common. Symptoms are not present during sleep. The condition responds well to dopamine antagonists such as haloperidol and therefore can be induced in normal patients by dopamine receptor agonists such as bromocriptine.

10.14 Head injuries

Answer C: Raised intracranial pressure is less common in infants

Head injuries are the most common cause of death in children, usually as a result of a road traffic accident. Damage to the brain in head injuries occurs as result of:

- primary damage from the injury itself
- secondary damage from the cerebral injury or associated physiological changes.

After 18 months of age, when a child's skull sutures have closed, there is very limited space in which the brain can expand. Hence any space-occupying lesion, such as blood, has the potential to cause the ICP to increase significantly after the failure of early compensatory mechanisms. These include decreased CSF and venous blood volume within the cranium. Before the sutures have closed there is considerable 'give' to allow ICP to remain relatively normal. After initial resuscitation and cervical spine immobilisation, various neurological parameters should be assessed such as conscious level, pupils, fundi and peripheral nervous system examination. For children aged ≥4 years the traditional Glasgow Coma Scale (GCS) is used, but for those aged ≤4 years the modified Children's Coma Scale is essential for accurate scoring. You should be roughly familiar with both of these. A score of ≤8 should prompt intubation and ventilation. Appropriate radiological investigations include skull radiographs, cervical spine radiographs and computed tomography (CT) or MRI if indicated. Referral to a neurosurgical centre may be necessary. Adequate pain control should be given, particularly because there are often other injuries. Poor pain control can lead to a further increase in ICP which will result in a drop in the cerebral perfusion pressure. Intravenous morphine may be appropriate.

10.15 Guillain–Barré syndrome

Answer A: Implicated infectious agents include Coxsackievirus

The pathology of Guillain–Barré syndrome is inflammation with segmental demyelination in peripheral nerves. It is commonly preceded by an upper respiratory tract infection (10–14 days) and can follow gastroenteritis. The implicated infectious agents are:

- Epstein–Barr virus
- Coxsackievirus
- Influenza virus
- Echovirus
- Cytomegalovirus (CMV)
- *Mycoplasma pneumoniae*
- *Campylobacter* spp.

The initial symptoms are of numbness and paraesthesia followed by progressive weakness. This generally starts in the lower limbs and 'ascends' over days or weeks. Weakness is usually symmetrical (90%). Power and tone are reduced with absent or reduced reflexes. About 50% have bulbar involvement. Myalgia may occur early in the disease. Autonomic involvement can occur with flushing and hypotension. Bladder dysfunction may occur early in the disease in about 20%. Fifty per cent have cranial nerve involvement. CSF protein rises with a normal CSF white cell count and glucose. Close monitoring of the vital capacity is essential. Type II respiratory failure can occur secondary to muscle weakness. Recovery is usually complete and treatment largely supportive. Relapses can occur in up to 5% of children. Plasmapheresis, intravenous immunoglobulin, steroids and immunosuppressive drugs are used in patients with rapidly progressive ascending paralysis.

10.16 Spinal muscular atrophy (SMA)

Answer B: The genetic abnormality is localised to chromosome 5

There are three types of anterior horn cell disease:

1. Acute infantile spinal muscular atrophy, SMA type I, Werdnig–Hoffmann disease
2. Intermediate spinal muscular atrophy (late infantile), SMA type II, chronic Werdnig–Hoffmann disease
3. Juvenile spinal muscular atrophy, which is also known as Kugelberg–Welander disease.

All three are usually inherited in an autosomal recessive manner. The gene locus for all three types is on chromosome 5; they are all variants of the same disease. The age of presentation varies with each disorder. SMA type I presents between 0 and 6 months, SMA type II between 3 and 15 years and Kugelberg–Welander disease between 5 and 15 years. Survival of children with SMA type I is rare beyond 3 years.

Clinical features:

- Hypotonia
- Weakness
- Absent reflexes
- Fasciculation of the relaxed tongue
- Normal intelligence.

Diagnosis is by:

- DNA studies
- creatine phosphokinase raised but can be normal
- electromyography (EMG) – fibrillation potentials
- muscle biopsy – characteristic.

Differential diagnosis of Kugelberg–Welander disease:

- Duchenne muscular dystrophy
- Fascioscapulohumeral muscular dystrophy
- Limb-girdle dystrophy
- Inflammatory myopathies.

10.17 Epilepsy

Answer C: Partial seizures begin focally

Simple and complex differentiates between seizures in which consciousness is retained (simple) and those in which consciousness is impaired or lost (complex). Partial seizures begin focally. They can become generalised (secondary generalisation). Symptomatic epilepsy is when the cause is known. Cryptogenic is when there is a likely but unidentified cause and idiopathic is when no cause is known. Most childhood epilepsy is idiopathic. An aura is not necessary for the diagnosis of childhood epilepsy.

10.18 Infantile spasms

Answer E: An urgent EEG

This infant needs an urgent EEG.

Infantile spasms represent 1–5% of childhood epilepsy. The incidence is 1 per 2000–4000 live births. It is more common in boys. Onset is usually between 4 and 9 months, although can occur from birth and appear long into the first decade of life. The spasms are brief and transient but often occur in clusters. A spasm is due to a sudden muscular contraction, which is usually generalised and a mixture of flexion and extension. Clusters of as many as 100 spasms can occur. The EEG is characteristic and shows hypsarrhythmia (high voltage with multifocal spikes, spike-and-wave discharges, chaotic slowing and asynchrony). This is an interictal appearance and may be suppressed during seizure activity. The EEG can be normal, and it is not of prognostic value in individual children.

Aetiology of infantile spasms may be:

- Symptomatic: 70–80%
- Hypoxic ischaemic encephalopathy
- Dysgenesis, eg tuberous sclerosis, Sturge–Weber syndrome
- Infection pre-, peri- or postnatal
- Haemorrhage intraventricular haemorrhage
- Metabolic, eg neonatal hypoglycaemia
- Idiopathic – 20–30%.

Multicentre randomised controlled trials have taken place within the UK and international studies looking at treatment choices are ongoing, but the current standard treatment is with high-dose prednisolone or adrenocorticotrophic hormone (ACTH), to which 70% have a good response. Vigabatrin has also been widely used; its effect is particularly good in seizures secondary to tuberous sclerosis but its side effect of peripheral visual loss although rare is irreversible and difficult to screen for in children.

Other drugs often used:

- Nitrazepam
- Sodium valproate
- Lamotrigine.

The prognosis is worse in the symptomatic group. Early recognition and early treatment of seizures is of benefit:

- 70% have severe developmental delay
- 50–60% develop chronic epilepsy that will be part of a chronic epilepsy syndrome
- 25–30% go on to develop the Lennox–Gastaut syndrome.

10.19 Tuberous sclerosis

Answer B: Adenoma sebaceum is a feature

This shows an autosomal dominant inheritance with a 50% recurrence risk in offspring and 70% are new mutations. The prevalence in children is 1 in 10 000–15 000. The gene is on chromosomes 9 and 11. Seizures are common, often presenting as infantile spasms. All seizure types except petit mal have been described in tuberous sclerosis, and it is a cause of symptomatic epilepsy. The age of seizure onset and the severity of learning difficulties are directly related, with most children in whom seizures develop under the age of 2 years having learning disabilities. Seizures respond well to anticonvulsants but rarely with complete seizure control. Vigabatrin is indicated particularly in seizures associated with hypsarrhythmia on the EEG. Prevalence of significant learning difficulties is 30–50%. Clinical features include the following:

- Skin:
  - hypopigmented macules
  - adenoma sebaceum present in 85% over the age of 5 years
  - periungual fibromas
  - shagreen patches
  - café-au-lait spots
- Teeth: enamel hypoplasia
- Eyes: choroidal hamartomas
- Central nervous system:
  - cerebral astrocytoma
  - malignant glioma
  - hydrocephalus
- Kidney:
  - renal angiomas
  - polycystic kidneys
- Cardiac: rhabdomyomas
- Gastrointestinal: rectal polyp.

Investigations required:

- Echocardiography
- Skull radiograph
- EEG
- CT
- MRI.

Early death may occur due to seizures or tumours affecting the central nervous system, heart or kidney.

Causes of calcification on skull radiograph:

- Arteriovenous malformation
- Tuberous sclerosis

- Sturge–Weber syndrome
- Toxoplasmosis
- CMV infection
- Glioma
- Astrocytoma
- Craniopharyngioma.

10.20 Cerebral palsy

Answer B: Birthweight <1500g is a risk factor

Cerebral palsy is the most common cause of severe neurological disability in childhood. It is a disorder of posture and movement that results from a static injury to the developing brain. Although the injury is static, the manifestations will change as the child develops and diagnosis is not always clear until late infancy.

About 20% have learning difficulties. Prevalence is 2–4 per 1000 live births. Male:female ratio is 1.5:1. It is idiopathic in 75% of cases. Known aetiologies are divided into pre-, peri- or postnatal onset, and include hypoxia, infection, trauma, genetic and cerebral malformation. There is a strong association with low birthweight (51/1000 live births <1500 g will have cerebral palsy), but these account for only a small amount of the total number of children with cerebral palsy. Perinatal asphyxia accounts for no more than 8%. There are several different classifications of cerebral palsy. The Swedish classification is generally used:

- Diplegic
- Quadriplegic
- Hemiplegic
- Dyskinetic (athetoid)
- Ataxic.

10.21 Infantile hypotonia

Answer E: Down syndrome

Hypotonia in the infant can result from neurological abnormality or systemic disease, and the differential diagnosis is wide. The word infants implies age <12 months and the age of presentation needs to be considered when the correct answers are selected. Becker muscular dystrophy presents in late childhood (6–16 years), as does subacute sclerosing panencephalitis. The latter is more likely to manifest with hypertonia.

Neurological causes of hypotonia:

- Cerebral
- Encephalopathy, eg birth asphyxia presenting as hypotonic cerebral palsy
- Abnormal brain structure: trisomy 21, Prader–Willi syndrome, hydrocephalus, agenesis of corpus callosum
- Degenerative disease, eg metachromatic leukodystrophy

- Neurometabolic disease, eg Zellweger syndrome
- Spinal cord transection, eg after complicated breech delivery
- Spina bifida
- Anterior horn cell disease
- Spinal muscular atrophy (Werdnig–Hoffmann disease)
- Type II glycogen storage disease
- Poliomyelitis
- Peripheral nerve disease
- Guillain–Barré syndrome
- Disease of the myoneural junction
- Myasthenia gravis
- Diseases of the muscle
- Congenital muscular dystrophy
- Congenital myotonic dystrophy.

Systemic causes of hypotonia: most acute and chronic childhood illnesses will cause hypotonia.

Particular examples:

- Hypercalcaemia
- Renal tubular acidosis
- Rickets
- Hypothyroidism
- Coeliac disease
- Cystic fibrosis
- Failure to thrive.

10.22 Frontal lobe lesion

Answer B: Impaired memory

Features of a frontal lobe lesion:

- Disinhibition
- Presence of the grasp reflex
- Impaired memory
- Abnormal micturition behaviour.

The prefrontal lobe is concerned with aspects of psychological reactions, the ability to make intelligent anticipation of the future and the emotional consequences of thought.

Features of a precentral gyrus lesion:

- Pyramidal tract lesion (upper motor neuron lesion)
- Contralateral hemiparesis.

Features of a parietal lobe lesion:

- Spatial disorientation
- Apraxia (loss of the ability to perform a pattern of movements although the purpose is known)
- Agnosia (loss of the ability to recognise a pre /iously familiar object)
- Sensory inattention
- Receptive dysphasia
- Contralateral homonymous hemianopia (lower quadrant or both).

Features of an occipital lobe lesion:

- Flashing lights
- Contralateral homonymous hemianopia.

Features of a temporal lobe lesion:

- Visual sensations
- Auditory/gustatory/olfactory hallucinations
- Receptive dysphasia
- Contralateral homonymous hemianopia (upper quadrant).

10.23 Muscular dystrophy

Answer A: Inheritance is X linked

The incidence of Duchenne muscular dystrophy is 1 in 3000 liveborn males. The inheritance is X-linked recessive. The gene locus known and is at Xp21. A third of cases represent a new mutation. Females may be symptomatic as a consequence of the random inactivation of one of the X chromosomes. Cases usually present between age 3 and 5 years with weakness and calf muscle hypertrophy. The reflexes disappear early in the disease, apart from the ankle jerk which disappears late. Creatine phosphokinase is usually raised at birth and high at diagnosis. Diagnosis is made by EMG and muscle biopsy, both of which show typical features. In addition, DNA studies can be done looking for the dystrophin gene. Complications arise from cardiac, respiratory and skeletal muscle involvement.

Becker muscular dystrophy

This presents later than Duchenne muscular dystrophy, but the gene defect is known and is at the same locus as Duchenne muscular dystrophy. Cardiac and respiratory muscle involvement is rare. The creatine phosphokinase is high at diagnosis. EMG and muscle biopsy are helpful in establishing a diagnosis.

McLeod syndrome

This a benign, non-progressive, late-onset myopathy in which the creatine phosphokinase is usually mildly raised. It is X linked. Symptoms are usually mild and splenomegaly is often seen.

10.24 Febrile convulsions

Answer C: Family history of febrile convulsions

Febrile convulsions occur in 3–4% of children. The age range is variably quoted but usually between 6 months and 5 years. Simple (75%) febrile convulsions last less than 15 minutes and are associated with a good prognosis. Complicated (25%) are either focal in origin or prolonged. These have a worse prognosis. Risk factors for recurrent febrile seizures include previous febrile seizures and a positive family history of febrile seizures. The risk factor for siblings of an index case is 10% and the risk if either parent had febrile convulsions is 15%. There is no sex difference. There is no increased risk if there is a family history of epilepsy. A third of children who have a first fit will have a second and a third of these will have a third.

Risk factors for the development of epilepsy:

- Positive family history of epilepsy
- Prolonged or atypical seizure
- Pre-existing neurological problem
- Abnormal neurological examination.

Prophylactic anticonvulsants are not helpful in children with recurrent simple febrile seizures. An interictal EEG is usually normal and the investigation is unhelpful, except in children presenting with atypical febrile seizures.

10.25 Temporal lobe seizures

Answer A: It can present with feelings of déjà vu

Temporal lobe seizures originate in the temporal region; they may be simple partial seizures or complex partial seizures. They can become generalised when consciousness is impaired.

Symptomatology of simple partial include:

- Flushing
- Sweating
- Déjà vu and jamais vu
- Hallucinations
- Feelings of fear and panic.

Symptomatology of complex partial include:

- Semi-purposeful automatisms, eg lip smacking, chewing, swallowing
- Fumbling with clothing
- Staggering and wandering.

The EEG changes are characteristic with focal discharges from the frontotemporal region. There is often a past history of febrile convulsions. Surgery may be helpful in a number of children with resistant seizures.

10.26 Peripheral nerve injuries

Answer E: Palsy causes wrist drop

Peripheral nerve injuries need to be revised as they are often the subject of questions. The small muscles of the hand are supplied by the median and ulnar nerves. The radial nerve (C5–8) supplies two muscle groups:

1. Those that supinate the forearm
2. The extensors of the fingers, wrist and elbow.

The radial nerve also supplies sensation to the back of the hand. Injuries to the radial nerve occur either at the axilla or the elbow. Injury at the axilla will result in an inability to extend the elbow and wrist drop. Involvement at the elbow will result only in wrist drop. Klumpke paralysis results from an injury to the lower part of the brachial plexus (C8–T1). Clinically this manifests as a claw hand with failure of forearm flexion.

10.27 Microcephally

Answer A: Holoprosencephaly

Microcephaly refers to a small head due to a small brain, the head circumference being less than 2 SD below the mean when corrected for age and sex. There are other causes of a small head including craniosynostoses (premature suture fusion). Microcephaly can be primary or secondary. Primary microcephaly refers to the situation whereby there is a genetic or chromosomal abnormality that causes the brain to be small. Secondary microcephaly refers to the situation whereby the brain was initially normal but because of a disease process subsequent growth has been impaired.

Causes of primary microcephaly:

- Familial: autosomal dominant or autosomal recessive
- Chromosomal/syndromes
- Trisomies 13, 18 and 21
- Cri-du-chat syndrome
- Cornelia de Lange syndrome
- Holoprosencephaly.

Causes of secondary microcephaly:

- Intrauterine infection
- Drugs
- Placental insufficiency/alcohol/drugs
- Hypoxic ischaemic encephalopathy
- Meningitis/encephalitis.

10.28 Brain tumours

Answer B: Craniopharyngiomas can present with a visual field defect

Primary brain tumours are the second most common malignancy in childhood after leukaemia. Metastatic tumours are rare in childhood. Between the ages of 2 and 12 years infratentorial (posterior fossa) tumours are the most common. Under the age of 2 years and in adolescence supra- and infratentorial tumours occur with the same frequency. Tumours within the posterior fossa produce symptoms and signs of raised ICP. Supratentorial tumours produce focal signs dependent on the tumour site. Personality changes can occur as a consequence of either. Infratentorial (posterior fossa) tumours include the following:

- Medulloblastoma: most common brain tumour in children under the age of 7 years
- Brain-stem glioma
- Ependymoma
- Astrocytoma.

Supratentorial tumours:

- Craniopharyngioma: common; present with bitemporal visual field defect; treatment is surgical and radiotherapy; residual hypothalamopituitary problems are common
- Optic glioma
- Pineal tumour
- Oligodendroglioma.

10.29 Investigation of first seizure

Answer B: Serum calcium

Blood glucose, full blood count and chemistry are arguably the only essential tests after a first afebrile seizure. Unless the fit is focal or associated with developmental delay or regression, a CT scan is not indicated. EEG is usually carried out after a second fit, although management tends to be clinically based even with a normal EEG, with the latter guiding treatment rather than leading it. Blood and CSF culture are needed if infection/meningitis suspected.

10.30 Horner syndrome

Answer C: Middle-ear infections can be a cause in children

Horner syndrome is a clinical syndrome caused by damage to the sympathetic nervous system.

Features of Horner syndrome:

- Partial ptosis
- Pupil constriction
- Anhidrosis
- Enophthalmia
- Heterochromia iridis
- Normal direct and consensual reflex.

It may be congenital or acquired.

Causes include:

- Neurofibromatosis type 1
- Middle-ear infections
- Goitre
- Klumpke paralysis.

10.31 EEG

Answer C: EEG can help in providing likely prognosis in patients whom an epilepsy syndrome is suspected

EEG (Epilepsy NICE guideline, October 2004)

- This should not be performed in the case of probable syncope because of the possibility of a false-positive result.
- This should not be used to exclude a diagnosis of epilepsy in an individual in whom the clinical presentation supports a diagnosis of a non-epileptic event.
- This should not be used in isolation to make a diagnosis of epilepsy.
- This may be used to help determine seizure type and epilepsy syndrome in individuals in whom epilepsy is suspected. This enables individuals to be given the correct prognosis.

In individuals presenting with a first unprovoked seizure, unequivocal epileptiform activity shown on EEG can be used to assess the risk of seizure recurrence.

For individuals in whom epilepsy is suspected, but who present diagnostic difficulties, specialist investigations should be available.

Repeated standard EEGs may be helpful when the diagnosis of the epilepsy or syndrome is unclear. However, if the diagnosis has been established, repeat EEGs are not likely to be helpful. Repeated standard EEGs should not be used in preference to sleep or sleep-deprived EEGs. When a standard EEG has not contributed to diagnosis or classification, a sleep EEG should be performed, because this is more likely to show abnormalities. In children, a sleep EEG is best achieved through sleep deprivation or the use of melatonin. Long-term video or ambulatory EEG may be used in the assessment of individuals who present diagnostic difficulties after clinical assessment and standard EEG.

10.32 Chorea

Answer D: Sydenham chorea

Chorea is the rapid jerky uncoordinated movements.

Sydenham chorea is a neurological disorder of childhood resulting from infection by group A β-haemolytic streptococci, the bacterium that causes rheumatic fever. Rapid, irregular and aimless involuntary movements of the arms and legs, trunk and facial muscles are characteristic. It affects girls more often than boys and typically occurs between 5 and 15 years of age. Some children will have a sore throat several weeks before the symptoms begin, but the disorder can also occur up to 6 months after the fever or infection has cleared. Symptoms can appear gradually or all at once, and may also include uncoordinated movements, muscular weakness, stumbling and falling, slurred speech, difficulty concentrating and writing, and emotional instability. The symptoms vary widely. The random, writhing movements of chorea are caused by an autoimmune reaction to the bacterium which interferes with the normal function of the basal ganglia.

Treatment:

- Bed rest
- Benzodiazepines
- Penicillin

Other causes of chorea:

- Inherited: Huntington disease, ataxia–telangiectasia, inborn errors of metabolism
- Drugs: L-dopa, amphetamines, carbamazepine
- Endocrine: hyperthyroidism
- Immune: SLE (systemic lupus erythematosus)
- Toxins: carbon monoxide.

10.33 Paediatric stroke

Answer B: Approximately half of children presenting with an arterial ischaemic stroke have a known predisposing condition

Paediatric stroke is thought to have an incidence of 1.3–13 per 100 000 children in the UK. Around a quarter of childhood strokes occur in neonates with the pathology in this group, suggesting an embolic aetiology and a low risk of recurrence. Half of childhood strokes are thought to be haemorrhagic, presenting typically with signs of rising ICP, headache, vomiting and reduced level of consciousness. It is estimated that half of children presenting with arterial ischaemic stroke have a known predisposing condition. Cerebral venous thrombosis may present as stroke but also commonly present as headaches and symptoms of raised ICP.

Predisposing factors for stroke are as follows

Haemorrhagic stroke

- Arteriovenous malformation
- Coagulopathies, eg haemophilia.

Arterial ischaemic stroke

- Sickle cell disease
- Meningitis
- Cardiac disease
- Immunodeficiency
- Neurofibromatosis.

Cerebral venous sinus thrombosis

- Head and neck infections
- Chronic anaemias
- Dehydration
- Nephrotic syndrome
- SLE.

10.34 Craniosynostosis

Answer A: Posterior plagiocephaly

Craniosynostosis is the premature fusion of one or more cranial sutures. Sutures are normally kept open by ongoing brain growth, with skull growth occurring perpendicular to suture lines. Craniosynostosis may be classified as primary (when it is due to an ossification defect – <10% of cases) or secondary (due to failure of brain growth – >90% of cases). If only one suture is affected it is termed 'simple craniosynotosis', whereas compound or complex craniosynostosis affects multiple sutures. It is seen as part of a variety of syndromes including Crouzon and Apert syndromes. In simple primary synostosis, the cosmetic defect is the primary morbidity whereas, in secondary synostosis, the major morbidity is due to the underlying disorder causing failure of brain growth, typically neurodevelopmental delay. Raised ICP can result if multiple sutures fuse while the brain is still increasing in size, but is rare if only one or two sutures are affected. Scaphocephaly is the most common form of craniosynostosis and is caused by premature fusion of the sagittal suture (as seen in preterm infants).

Posterior plagiocephaly is most commonly caused by positional moulding but may also be due to synostosis of the lambdoid suture. The former can be differentiated from the latter by the more anterior position of the ear on the side of the flattening, and frontal bossing seen ipsilateral to the flattening in the positional form. Individuals with craniosynostosis should be followed up developmentally, by monitoring head growth including head circumference, and for symptoms and signs of raised ICP. Surgery is indicated in the presence of elevated ICP and for cosmetic purposes in the more severely affected individual. The best results are obtained in children with syndromic craniosynostosis if surgery is performed early (before 6 months of age). A multidisciplinary approach is required.

10.35 Lumbar puncture

Answer D: Abnormal posturing

Lumbar puncture has diagnostic (meningitis, encephalitis, demyelination, malignancy, benign intracranial hypertension) and therapeutic (intrathecal antibiotics and chemotherapy, and CSF drainage) uses. Complications include headache, bleeding, infection, damage to cord/nerves, cardiorespiratory compromise and cerebral/cerebellar herniation. Lumbar puncture should not be performed in the presence of the following without further evaluation:

- Signs of raised ICP or herniation
- Recent (within 30 min) convulsive seizures
- Prolonged (>30 min) convulsive seizures
- Focal or tonic seizures
- Focal neurological signs including abnormal posturing
- GCS score <13 or deteriorating conscious level
- Cardiovascular or respiratory compromise
- Coagulopathy/thrombocytopenia
- Local superficial infection
- Strong suspicion of meningococcal infection (ie typical purpuric rash).

Even with normal appearances of the brain on imaging, the presence of signs of herniation means that it is not safe to perform a lumbar puncture.

Cellular and biochemical changes persist in CSF for 48–72 hours after treatment, although cultures may be rendered negative by administration of appropriate antibiotics within 2 hours (meningococci), 6 hours (pneumococci), 8 hours (group B streptococci) and 48 hours (coliforms). In cases of suspected meningitis/encephalitis where any of the above contraindications or relative contraindications to lumbar puncture are present, administration of antibiotics or antiviral agents should not be postponed pending further evaluation of the patient.

10.36 Migraine

Answer E: Propranolol and sodium valproate can be used as prophylaxis

Migraine may or may not be associated with aura in childhood – indeed in some cases, headache may not even feature. Variant migraine types include hemiplegic migraine (where neurological deficit can persist for hours or even days and may precede the onset of the headache), abdominal migraine and basilar migraine. The child normally looks pale and ill during an attack – which is typically relieved by sleep. Boys are more commonly affected than girls until the age of 7 years then a female predominance develops in late childhood and on into adulthood. Incidence continues to increase throughout adolescence, but more so in girls. It affects 5–10% of school-age children, but can also affect pre-schoolers. Diagnosis is usually made through history and detailed physical examination – both general and neurological. Neuroimaging and EEG are not required routinely. Treatment involves education about potential triggers (eg caffeine, citrus fruits, chocolate, cheese), plan for treatment during an acute attack and prophylaxis for frequent episodes. None of the prophylactic medications is fully effective in preventing all attacks – drugs that can be tried include pizotifen, amitriptyline, propranolol, topiramate and sodium valproate, but all have potential side effects. Acute attacks can be treated with simple analgesia; if vomiting this may need to be combined with an antiemetic. 5HT (5-hydroxytryptamine or serotonin) receptor agonists can also be used to treat the acute attack.

10.37 Juvenile myoclonic epilepsy (JME)

Answer A: Myoclonic jerks, generalised tonic–clonic seizures and absence seizures

This is an idiopathic generalised epilepsy syndrome accounting for up to 10% of all cases of epilepsy. It is characterised by myoclonic jerks, generalised tonic–clonic seizures and sometimes absence seizures. Jerky movements are typically experienced in the morning – perhaps interfering with breakfast or brushing teeth. It is associated with normal intelligence, onset around adolescence and seizures occurring shortly after wakening. About a third of patients with JME have a positive family history of epilepsy. Precipitating factors for seizures include sleep deprivation, psychological stress, alcohol use, photic stimulation and menses. Neuroimaging is typically normal. Sleep-deprived EEG is the investigation of choice with typical interictal EEG findings of generalised 4–6 Hz spike-and-slow-wave discharges lasting up to 20 seconds. These changes are not, however, pathognomonic of JME. A normal study does not exclude JME. Monotherapy is usually adequate to control seizures, 80% of patients becoming seizure free with sodium valproate. Lamotrigine and topiramate can also be used. Carbamazepine may increase number of myoclonic jerks and also precipitate absences. Withdrawal of anticonvulsants, even after a prolonged seizure-free period, leads to seizure recurrence in >80% of cases – hence life-long treatment is usually required.

10.38 Childhood stroke

Answer B: Screening for sickle cell disease

Risk factors for childhood stroke include the following:

- Sickle cell disease (up to 400 × greater risk of stroke),
- Moyamoya disease (accounts for 10–20% of arterial infarcts)
- Arterial dissection (most commonly secondary to trauma)
- Cardiac disorders account for up to 50% of cases
- Meningitis.

In more than a third of cases, no cause is found. Ischaemic events (due to thromboembolism or angiopathy) are more common than haemorrhagic events, which may be secondary to vascular malformations (most commonly arteriovenous malformations), malignancy, trauma, haemophilia or thrombocytopenia.

Recurrence risk is up to one in three, but depends on cause, the presence of multiple risk factors indicating a worse long-term outcome.

Evaluation of a child with a stroke should include neuroimaging (CT, MRI and MR angiography) as well as investigations to rule out non-vascular causes (haematological and metabolic studies). Cranial ultrasonography is inadequate to identify ischaemic stroke, especially cortical or posterior infarcts. Surgical intervention may be required in some cases, eg embolisation of an arteriovenous malformation. Aspirin at a dose of 5 mg/kg per day can be used for cases of non-haemorrhagic stroke, but not in children with sickle cell disease. No adequate trials have been performed into the use of thrombolytic agents in children, although case reports do exist. Mortality rates are up to 10%, with more than half of survivors developing some degree of neurological or cognitive deficit. Seizures at presentation are associated with a poor outcome.

EMQ Answers

10.39–10.41 Theme: Neurocutaneous syndromes

10.39

Answer A: Sturge–Weber syndrome

Sturge–Weber syndrome is sporadic with an incidence of 1 in 50 000. The condition has two main features:

1. An angiomatous malformation (capillary haemangioma), usually called a port wine stain, present from birth over the skin of one of the branches of the trigeminal nerve, most commonly the first branch. It is usually unilateral.
2. A similar malformation over the occipital area of the ipsilateral cerebral hemisphere which results in cerebral ischaemia, giving rise to atrophy and calcification.

Clinical manifestations:

- Contralateral hemiparesis
- Difficult to control seizures
- Learning difficulties
- Progressive neurological deterioration.

Rail-track calcification on the skull radiograph is characteristic and due to linear calcification lines in the gyri, with the intermittent sulci being spared. The blood supply to the skin and meninges is in common with that of the retina and face; therefore associated anomalies of the eyes such as glaucoma, buphthalmos and retinal defects occur. Treatment involves aggressive treatment of seizures with anticonvulsants, management of disabilities, on occasions occipital lobectomy and rarely hemispherectomy. Pulsed laser has been used for the port wine stain.

10.40

Answer D: Neurofibromatosis type 1

Although many types of neurofibromatosis have been described types 1 and 2 are the most common.

Type 1

- 1 in 4000
- 90% of all cases of neurofibromatosis
- Autosomal dominant inheritance
- 50% new mutations
- Gene locus on chromosome 17.

Diagnosis of type 1 – if two of the following features are present:

- Axillary or inguinal freckling
- Optic gliomas (15%)
- Distinctive osseous lesion, eg kyphoscoliosis, tibial bowing
- Two or more neurofibromas or one plexiform neurofibroma
- Two or more Lisch (iris) nodules (90%, do not occur in type 2)
- Prepubertal child: five or more café-au-lait spots >5 mm diameter
- Postpubertal child: six or more café-au-lait spots >15 mm diameter
- A first-degree relative with neurofibromatosis.

Café-au-lait spots are usually present at birth. Less than 10% of patients have learning difficulties. There are many other clinical manifestations and these should be reviewed. Maternal folate deficiency is a risk factor for spina bifida. There is an increased incidence of the following in type 1 neurofibromatosis:

- Phaeochromocytoma
- Rhabdomyosarcoma
- Leukaemia
- Wilms tumour
- Seizures
- Neurofibrosarcoma
- Schwannoma.

Type 2

- Represents 10% of all cases of neurofibromatosis
- Autosomal dominant inheritance
- Mostly new mutations
- Gene locus on chromosome 22.

Diagnosis of type 2:

- Bilateral acoustic neuromas
- Unilateral acoustic neuroma and first-degree relative with neurofibromatosis type 2
- Two of the following: neurofibroma, meningioma, glioma, schwannoma, juvenile posterior subcapsular lenticular opacities.

10.41

Answer H: Incontinentia pigmenti

Incontinentia pigmenti is an X-linked disorder but occurs more frequently in females and this is thought to be because it can be lethal to the male fetus. It is characterised by skin abnormalities that evolve through life. Infants can be born with linear blistering areas which when healed leave hyperpigmented wart-like lesions. They also have swirl-like hyperpigmented patches that may fade into adulthood. In adulthood hypopigmented lines on the limbs are common. Most people with incontinentia pigmenti have normal intelligence but it may be associated with developmental delay and seizures.

Other associated features:

- Eye abnormalities, eg coloboma, optic atrophy, retinal detachment
- Alopecia
- Dental abnormalities, eg small teeth, failure of primary eruption
- Pitted nails.

10.42–10.44 Theme: Cranial nerve palsies

10.42

Answer A: Nerve III (oculomotor) palsy

Features of a nerve III (oculomotor) lesion:

- Complete ptosis
- Diplopia
- Downward and lateral gaze (unopposed lateral rectus and superior oblique muscles)
- Pupil dilatation
- Failure of the pupil to react to light or to accommodation.

10.43

Answer E: Nerve VII palsy – facial nerve

The most common cause of a facial nerve palsy in both adults and children is a Bell palsy. This is an acute unilateral facial palsy (lower motor neuron lesion). It usually occurs 2 weeks after a viral infection.

Causes:

- Epstein–Barr virus
- Herpesvirus
- Mumps
- Hypertension.

Prognosis is excellent with full recovery in more than 85% and permanent weakness in around 5%. The effectiveness of steroids remains uncertain but they are often prescribed.

Other causes of facial nerve palsy:

- Tumour invasion
- Trauma
- Birth injury.

Other causes of facial weakness:

- Myotonic dystrophy
- Fascioscapulohumeral muscular dystrophy
- Myasthenia gravis.

10.44

Answer B: Nerve VI (abducent) palsy

Features of a nerve VI (abducent) lesion:

- Diplopia
- Failure of lateral gaze.

Causes:

- Neoplasm, eg pontine glioma
- Elevated ICP without tumour, eg venous sinus thrombosis
- Congenital, eg Duane syndrome.

10.45–10.47 Theme: Epilepsy

10.45

Answer D: Benign rolandic epilepsy

This is more common in boys with a peak incidence at age 2–14 years. It represents 15–20% of childhood epilepsy. It is often called benign partial epilepsy with centrotemporal spikes. The fits are often preceded by an aura. The seizures themselves are short-lived (1–2 minutes) and include paraesthesia and unilateral tonic–clonic convulsions involving the face, lips, tongue, and pharyngeal and laryngeal muscles. Consciousness is commonly preserved and seizures usually occur on wakening. Generalised (nocturnal) seizures often occur especially in children under the age of 5 years. There are a proportion of children with this syndrome who only have nocturnal seizures. Interictal EEGs often show centrotemporal spikes. Carbamazepine is the drug of choice and fits are well controlled on it. In some children treatment is not required. Seizures generally disappear around puberty.

10.46

Answer C: Childhood absence epilepsy

This accounts for 5% of childhood epilepsy. The peak age is 3–12 years. It is more common in girls. It shows an abnormal ictal EEG with 3/s spike-and-generalised-wave discharges. The interictal EEG is normal. Hyperventilation will provoke seizures. There is no known aetiology. Clinically, it is characterised by sudden cessation of speech and motor activity, with a blank facial expression and flickering of the eyelids. There is no aura or postictal state. Tone is not lost but the head may fall forward. The drugs of choice are sodium valproate and ethosuximide. The long-term prognosis is good, with most patients becoming seizure free by adolescence although a number do develop generalised seizures.

10.47

Answer E: Panayiotopoulos syndrome

This epilepsy syndrome is thought to be relatively common, affecting about 10% of children with epilepsy, it is also known as early onset benign partial epilepsy with occipital paroxysms. The peak age is pre-school age 3–5 years. The main seizure type is known as 'autonomic'. Children may have a sudden change in behaviour and then they become pale, complain of a feeling of sickness and will usually vomit. The pupils of the eyes often become very large (dilated) and there may be sweating and drooling. They may become unresponsive and their head may turn and become fixed. It may remain turned to the side for many minutes. Very often the seizure will then end by clonic movements down one, or occasionally both, sides of the body. After this the child may become upset then postictal.

Over two-thirds of the seizures will occur in sleep, during the night or during a day-time nap. The seizures are often long-lasting and may last 20, 30 or even 60 minutes.

EEG shows occipital spikes but these may be seen only in sleep EEG. The prognosis is good, with most children going into remission in later childhood, and it is rare for the seizures to continue into adult life. Development is usually normal.

10.48–10.50 Theme: Anticonvulsant treatment

10.48

Answer I: Topiramate

Topiramate has been licensed for use in over 16 year olds for migraine prophylaxis since 2005. It has many mechanisms of action that may contribute to migraine prevention. It inhibits sodium channels and calcium channels and has effects on other neurotransmitters such as enhancing GABA (γ-aminobutyric acid) activity that may contribute, although the exact mechanism for prevention of migraine is unclear. Sodium valporate has been used widely over many years as migraine prophylaxis but remains unlicensed.

10.49

Answer G: Phenobarbital

Phenobarbital is the most commonly used anticonvulsant in the neonatal population. If long-term anticonvulsant treatment is needed this is often switched once the underlying condition has been established.

10.50

Answer A: Carbamazepine

Carbamazepine would be a first-line agent in this case; it is more effective in partial seizures than sodium valporate. Newer drugs could be considered but accepted practice would be, and the NICE guidelines state, that these should only be considered in patients who have not benefited from older AEDs, ie sodium valporate or carbamazepine.

10.51–10.53 Theme: Ataxia

10.51 Friedreich ataxia

Answer C: Genetic analysis of the frataxin gene on chromosome 9

Friedreich ataxia is a progressive ataxia with pyramidal tract dysfunction. Inheritance is usually autosomal recessive. The gene locus is known and is on chromosome 9. It usually presents before the fifteenth birthday with loss of position and vibration sense. Other features include absent tendon reflexes, extensor plantars, nystagmus, pes cavus, kyphoscoliosis, cardiac abnormalities (hypertrophic cardiomyopathy) and an increased risk of diabetes mellitus. Treatment is largely supportive. Death is usually secondary to cardiac complications.

10.52 Ataxia–telangiectasia

Answer A: Genetic studies for ataxia–telangiectasia

Ataxia telangiectasia is an autosomal recessively inherited condition. It occurs in 1 in 40 000 people worldwide.

The ataxia usually presents in early childhood; there is often a history of delayed walking (>18 months) and a history of gait being unsteady for longer than normal. The characteristic telangiectasia may not always be present initially but will usually develop over time.

The gene locus is known and is on chromosome 11; the gene it codes for is important in the control of cell division and involved in DNA repair, explaining in part the increased risk in developing cancer that patients with ataxia–telangiectasia have – a third of these children develop malignancy. There is a 50–100-fold greater chance of developing lymphoreticular malignancy as well as brain tumours. There is an increased risk of recurrent infection with a low IgA and IgG. The α-fetoprotein is usually raised.

10.53 Adrenoleukodystrophy

Answer E: Very-long-chain fatty acids

Adrenoleukodystrophy is caused by an accumulation of very-long-chain fatty acids within the brain due to a dysfunction in the peroxisomes. It is diagnosed by measuring very-long-chain fatty acids within the blood.

Onset is usually in early childhood with behavioural changes such as abnormal withdrawal or aggression, poor memory and poor school performance. Other symptoms include visual loss, learning disabilities, seizures, poorly articulated speech, difficulty swallowing, deafness, disturbances of gait and coordination, fatigue, intermittent vomiting, increased skin pigmentation and progressive dementia.

Up to the point of onset, development is usually normal. After initial neurological symptoms appear, the health of the patients deteriorates rapidly. The average time between the initial symptoms and a vegetative state (where the patient is bedridden) or death is approximately 2 years, although it can range anywhere from 6 months to 20 years.

Treatment options are limited to the use of a mixture of specific oils – 'Lorenzo's oil' has been shown to reduce or delay the appearance of symptoms in some studies.

General comments on ataxia

Clinical features of ataxia:

- Incoordination of voluntary movement
- Abnormal speech – dysarthria
- Ocular incoordination – nystagmus
- Hypotonia
- Intention tremor.

Aetiology of congenital ataxia includes:

- Cerebellar malformation
- Dysgenesis of the cerebellar vermis, eg Joubert syndrome
- Cystic malformation of the posterior fossa, eg Dandy–Walker syndrome
- Perinatally acquired, eg hypoxic ischaemic encephalopathy.

Aetiology of acquired ataxia includes:

- Acute
- Infectious and post-infectious, eg *Mycoplasma* spp., chickenpox, measles
- Structural lesions, eg tumours, hydrocephalus
- Toxic, eg lead, phenytoin
- Metabolic disorders
- Vascular: basilar artery thrombosis
- Intermittent
- Migraine
- Epilepsy
- Inherited recurrent ataxia (eg Hartnup disease)
- Progressive
- Structural, eg tumours
- DNA-repair abnormalities, eg ataxia–telangiectasia, xeroderma pigmentosa
- Metabolic, eg Wilson disease, leukodystrophies, abetalipoproteinaemia
- Spinocerebellar degeneration, Friedreich ataxia.

10.54–10.56 Theme: Hypotonia

10.54

Answer F: Plasma very-long-chain fatty acids

Plasma very-long-chain fatty acids assays are used to diagnose peroxisomal disorders. This child has features of Zellweger syndrome (hypotonia, large anterior fontanelle, hepatomegaly and seizures), which is one of the peroxisomal disorders that include adrenoleukodystrophy, Refsum disease and rhizomelic chondrodysplasia punctata. Functions of peroxisomes include β oxidation of fatty acids longer than C22 (ie very-long-chain fatty acids), the abnormal accumulation of which is the disease hallmark. Other features of Zellweger syndrome include the following:

- High forehead
- Large anterior fontanelle
- Hypoplastic supraorbital ridges
- Epicanthal folds
- Psychomotor retardation
- Hypotonia
- Seizures
- Retinal degeneration
- Impaired hearing
- Hepatomegaly
- Death within first year of life.

10.55

Answer I: Cri-du-chat syndrome

The presence of a distinctive, high-pitched, cat-like cry is suggestive of cri-du-chat. Genetic studies for cri-du-chat syndrome look for a deletion of chromosome 5p.

Other features of this syndrome include growth failure, microcephaly, facial abnormalities and learning difficulties. The child may also have associated cardiac anomalies and cleft lip and palate. The distinctive high-pitched cry in infancy is typically lost by age 2 years. It is more common in girls. Swallowing difficulties and poor suck cause failure to thrive in infancy and may require placement of a gastrostomy. Affected individuals have severe cognitive, speech and motor delays. Behavioural problems include hyperactivity, aggression and tantrums with hypersensitivity to sound.

Females are fertile and therefore have a 50% risk of passing on the condition to their offspring. Males have small testes but spermatogenesis is thought to be normal. Other medical problems encountered include recurrent upper respiratory tract infections, otitis media and severe constipation. Affected children usually attain developmental and social skills consistent with those of a 5 to 6 year old.

10.56

Answer A: Muscle biopsy for congenital myopathy

Congenital myopathies

Reduced muscle bulk in association with generalised hypotonia and hyporeflexia are the typical characteristics of congenital myopathies. These are a group of conditions including nemaline rod myopathy and central core disease. Affected individuals have generalised weakness, often affecting proximal more than distal muscle groups. Typical characteristics include onset in early life with hypotonia, hyporeflexia, reduced muscle bulk and generalised weakness, often affecting proximal more than distal muscle groups. Dysmorphic features may be present secondary to the weakness. They are often relatively non-progressive and hereditary (may be autosomal dominant, recessive or X linked). Both sexes are equally affected. There may be a history of reduced fetal movements or breech presentation. Other features may include poor suck/swallow and respiratory failure.

Arthrogryposis may also be a feature. Creatine kinase levels are either in the reference range or mildly elevated. EMG and nerve conduction studies can also be normal, so muscle biopsy is required for diagnosis.

Treatment is supportive in all cases. The prognosis depends on the type. They can be fatal in the neonatal period or associated with a normal lifespan. Cardiopulmonary insufficiency is the usual cause of death. Duchenne and Becker muscular dystrophies are characterised by elevated creatine kinase levels but do not present in the neonatal period. Features of congenital hypothyroidism are generally not present at birth but develop within the first few weeks of life.

10.57–10.59 Meningitis

10.57

Answer E: Haemophilus influenzae type B

The CSF picture is consistent with a bacterial meningitis. In a baby of this age the presence of Gram-negative rods is most likely to represent infection with *Haemophilus influenzae* (see below).

10.58

Answer C: Pneumococcus

The CSF picture is consistent with partially treated bacterial meningitis (see below). Given the presence of the preceding upper respiratory tract infection and that the child has sickle cell disease, the most likely infecting organism is a pneumococcus.

10.59

Answer B: Listeria monocytogenes

This CSF picture in a neonate is consistent with a bacterial or viral meningitis. However, the presence of Gram-positive rods on Gram staining makes *Listeria* sp. the most likely infective agent.

Meningitis

Neonates

The most common infecting organisms are group B streptococcus, *Escherichia coli*, *Listeria* spp., and herpes simplex and varicella-zoster viruses. Preterm babies are at greatest risk. Symptoms are often non-specific and require a high index of suspicion. Interpretation of CSF findings are complicated by higher levels of glucose and protein normally seen in neonates. Bacterial meningitis typically causes a white cell count >1000/mm³. In cases secondary to *Listeria* spp., this is typically a lymphocytosis. Viral meningitis causes a less dramatic pleocytosis. Results should be interpreted together with any results available from the mother such as swap results, blood culture results, etc. Poor prognostic indicators include low birthweight, significant leukopenia or neutropenia, high CSF protein, coma and seizures lasting more than 72 hours.

Appropriate empirical treatments for neonatal bacterial meningitis include combinations of either an aminoglycoside, or amoxycillin and a third-generation cephalosporin. Treatment should be reviewed in the light of culture results and response to treatment and continued for 10–21 days.

Infants and children

Seventy per cent of cases of bacterial meningitis occur in those under 2 years of age. Most common infecting agents are pneumococci, meningococci and *Haemophilus influenzae* type b, although since the introduction of the immunisation programme against *H. influenzae* type b, its incidence has fallen significantly. In one in two cases of pneumococcal meningitis there is a parameningeal focus or pneumonia is also present. Individuals with sickle cell disease, other haemoglobinopathies or functional or anatomical asplenia are at increased risk. Incidence of penicillin resistance varies from <10% to 60% worldwide. Meningococci cause peaks of incidence in the 6–12 month and adolescent age groups. *H. influenzae* type b primarily affects the unimmunised, with 80–90% of cases occurring between the ages of 1 month and 3 years.

CSF should be obtained in all cases of suspected meningitis, unless performing a lumbar puncture is contraindicated. Opening pressure should be recorded. CSF glucose and protein estimation, total and differential cell counts, Gram stain and culture should always be requested. Also consider agglutination tests or polymerase chain reaction (PCR) evaluation. Patients with early or fulminant disease and those with poor immune response may not show 'normal' CSF changes. Partially treated meningitis may cause culture results for pneumococci and meningococci in particular to be unreliable, but protein, glucose and cell count abnormalities can persist even after treatment with antibiotics. Lymphocytosis may be seen in partially treated patients.

Cefotaxime or ceftriaxone provides coverage against the three most common causes of meningitis – vancomycin should be added in areas where penicillin-resistant pneumococci are prevalent. Duration of treatment varies but is usually continued for a minimum of 7–10 days. Dexamethasone has been shown to be of benefit if given antibiotics in cases of *H. influenzae* type b and pneumococcal meningitis, and now is given routinely in many centres.

CHAPTER 11

Respiratory Answers

MTF Answers

11.1 Oxygen dissociation curve

Answers: B C D

This is a graph of the oxygen saturation of haemoglobin (*y* axis) against the partial pressure of oxygen (*x* axis). It is sigmoid in shape due to the way in which the haem molecule binds each of its four oxygen molecules with increasing affinity. During heavy exercise the oxygen requirements can be delivered to the tissues with a relatively small drops in capillary PO_2 reflecting the steep part of the curve.

There are several factors that can shift the curve and help supply oxygen to more active tissues or increase oxygen take-up in the lungs in times of increased need.

Right shift = decreases in Hb affinity for O_2:

- ↑ PCO_2
- ↑ H^+ concentration
- ↑ temperature
- ↑ 2,3-DPG (2,3-diphosphoglycerate)

Left shift = increased Hb affinity for O_2:

- ↓ PCO_2
- ↓ H^+ concentration
- ↓ temperature
- ↓ 2,3-DPG

The following have an increased affinity for oxygen:

- Carboxyhaemoglobin
- Fetal haemoglobin
- Methaemoglobin.

The Bohr effect describes the shift in the curve caused by changes in the blood PCO_2 and H^+ concentration. As the blood passes through the lung capillaries CO_2 diffuses into the alveoli and thus decreases the PCO_2 and H^+ concentration in the blood. This causes a left shift, allowing greater oxygen uptake and transport to the tissues. In the active tissues where PCO_2 concentrations are high, the opposite occurs, increasing oxygen delivery to the tissues.

2,3-DPG is an organophosphate endproduct of red cell metabolism. It binds to haemoglobin and decreases its affinity for oxygen (right shift). It binds with greater affinity to deoxygenated haemoglobin (in the tissues) than oxygenated haemoglobin (in the lungs), thus increasing oxygen delivery to tissues. Its production is upregulated in states of chronic hypoxia, eg high altitude or chronic lung disease and anaemia.

11.2 Lymphocytic intestinal pneumonitis

Answers: A E

Lymphocytic interstitial pneumonitis (LIP) is a syndrome of fever cough and dyspnoea, with bibasilar pulmonary infiltrates of dense interstitial accumulations of lymphocytes and plasma cells. Nodular formations of polyclonal lymphocytes are commonly seen and can distort the lung architecture.

LIP is an uncommon disease but mostly occurs in association with underlying autoimmune disease or infection with Epstein–Barr virus (EBV) or HIV. LIP occurs in 25–40% of children with vertically acquired HIV and usually presents in the second or third year of life. It is an AIDS-defining diagnosis in children but not adults, where it is much less common.

Its onset is usually insidious, with early symptoms including dry cough and exertional dyspnoea. Long-standing disease is accompanied by finger clubbing and chronic bronchiectasis. In addition physical signs may include hepatosplenomegaly, generalised lymphadenopathy and parotid enlargement. Acute deterioration occurs with bacterial or viral super infection. The differential diagnosis of interstitial infiltrates includes tuberculosis (TB), cytomegalovirus (CMV) infection and infection with *Pneumocystis jiroveci* (formerly *P. carinii* – hence PCP).

Chest radiograph may show bibasilar, interstitial or micronodular infiltrates, and mediastinal and/or hilar enlargement secondary to pulmonary lymphoid hyperplasia. A lung biopsy is occasionally required for diagnosis.

Treatment with corticosteroids may be started empirically for symptomatic HIV-positive children initially at a high dose for 4–12 weeks and then weaned to the lowest maintenance dose that will suppress symptoms. Antibiotics are used to treat secondary infections; oxygen for correction of hypoxia and bronchodilators can be used to treat associated wheezing. There have been reports of improvement with zidovudine alone and highly active antiretroviral therapy (HAART – when three to four HAARTs are taken in specific combinations).

Clinical course is variable over many years; symptoms can be stable over many months and can show spontaneous improvement, but are often recurrent and may occasionally lead to end-stage fibrosis, bronchiectasis or malignant transformation.

11.3 Pulmonary hypoplasia

Answers: B D E

Pulmonary hypoplasia occurs in 1 in 1000 births. It can be unilateral or bilateral. It can be primary but is more commonly secondary, causes of which are summarised below.

Lung compression

- Congenital diaphragmatic hernia
- Congenital cystic adenomatoid malformation
- Pleural effusion
- Asphyxiating thoracic dystrophy
- Thanatophoric dwarfism.

Oligohydramnios:

- Potter syndrome (renal agenesis)
- Prolonged rupture of membranes
- Renal tract abnormalities resulting in markedly decreased urine volume, eg renal obstruction, cystic disease or severe dysplasia.

Decreased fetal breathing

- Congenital myotonic dystrophy
- Spinal muscular atrophy
- Lesions of spinal cord, phrenic nerve and brain stem
- CNS lesions.

Reduced pulmonary vascular perfusion

- Hypoplastic right heart
- Pulmonary artery hypoplasia
- Tracheo-oesophageal fistula
- Tetralogy of Fallot.

Outcome is variable depending on the aetiology but some associations with poor outcome include premature rupture of membranes before 25 weeks, severe oligohydramnios for more than 2 weeks, early delivery and the presence of hydrops fetalis. Babies who are ventilated have a high risk of developing pulmonary interstitial emphysema. Isolated unilateral hypoplasia usually presents late and can be asymptomatic.

11.4 Respiratory failure

Answers: B D E

Respiratory failure refers to inadequate gaseous exchange by the respiratory system and is classified according to the absence or presence of hypercapnia.

Type I respiratory failure

This reflects ventilation–perfusion mismatch causing failure of gaseous exchange. It presents with hypoxia and normal or low PCO_2, as a consequence of hyperventilation. Aetiologies include:

- Pulmonary oedema
- Pneumonia
- Pulmonary embolus

- Acute asthma, before fatigue
- Adult respiratory distress syndrome.

Type II respiratory failure.

This reflects hypoventilation and presents with hypoxia and hypercapnia. Aetiologies include:

- Head injury/encephalitis/meningitis
- Muscle disease
- Drugs
- Kyphoscoliosis
- Severe asthma
- Respiratory obstruction
- Pneumothorax.

Patients with type I respiratory failure can progress to type II when respiratory muscle fatigue occurs or with central nervous system (CNS) depression from hypoxia.

11.5 Bronchoscopy

Answers: A E

Bronchoscopy can be carried out with either a flexible or a rigid endoscope. A rigid endoscope is an open tube and therefore a child can be ventilated through it; it is therefore appropriate for the removal of foreign bodies, large clots and mucus plugs, and in massive haemoptysis. Rigid bronchoscopy requires anaesthetic, and therefore functional assessment of the airway is limited. A flexible endoscope is solid and requires ventilation to occur around it. There is a suction and biopsy channel but large objects cannot be removed through it. It allows inspection of much more of the airway than is possible with a rigid endoscope, including the upper airways. Flexible endoscopy can be performed with sedation and local anaesthetic only, which allows evaluation of the dynamic anatomy of the airway during spontaneous respiration. Bronchoscopy can be therapeutic or diagnostic.

Indications for bronchoscopy are as follows.

Diagnostic

- Congenital stridor
- Evaluation of stridor persisting for >2 weeks
- Suspected foreign body
- Suspected tracheobronchial fistula
- Suspected tracheobronchial stenosis
- Persistent atelectasis or consolidation on radiological investigations
- Evaluation of unexplained persistent cough with concerning history or signs
- Unexplained interstitial disease
- Undiagnosed infection particularly in an immunocompromised host

- Haemoptysis
- Investigation of bronchiectasis
- Evaluation of persistent abnormal cry or hoarseness.

Therapeutic

- Bronchopulmonary lavage
- Removal of clot, mucus plug, foreign body.

Complications of bronchoscopy:

- Hypoxia
- Cardiac arrhythmias
- Bronchospasm (patients with asthma should be premedicated with a bronchodilator)
- Laryngospasm
- Infection (patients should receive prophylactic antibiotics if asplenic, have artificial heart valves or have previously had endocarditis)
- Haemorrhage
- Pneumothorax.

11.6 Sweat test

Answers: B C

The gene responsible for cystic fibrosis (CF) functions as a chloride ion channel and also inhibits the epithelial sodium channel. The CF respiratory epithelium therefore fails to secrete Cl^- (which is absorbed in the sweat gland), hence high sweat levels of electrolytes and hyperabsorbs Na^+ and thus H_2O, dehydrating the airway surface. Secretions are viscid, impairing clearance.

The gold standard investigation for diagnosis of CF remains the sweat test. Traditionally a value of sweat sodium or chloride >60 mmol/l is diagnostic, on a sample weighing >100 mg.

In the general population aged >16 years 10% have sweat sodium > 60 mmol/l. In these patients a fludrocortisone test can be performed to confirm the diagnosis. Fludrocortisone 3 mg/m³ twice daily. for 2 days normalises result in the those who don't have CF but has no effect in patients with CF.

Plasma immunoreactive trypsin (IRT) is now used to screen neonates for CF using the heel-prick blood test on day 5–14.

Causes of raised sweat sodium (false positive):

- Eczema, dermatitis/ectodermal dysplasia
- Malnutrition/anorexia nervosa
- Flucloxacillin therapy
- Untreated hypothyroidism/panhypopituitarism
- Adrenal insufficiency
- Glycogen storage disease/mucopolysaccharidosis

- Glucose-6-phosphate dehydrogenase deficiency
- Fucosidosis
- Nephrogenic diabetes insipidus
- Nephrotic syndrome
- HIV infection.

Causes of false-negative sweat tests:

- Oedema
- Hyponatraemia.

A diagnosis of CF may be further investigated with specific CF genetic testing. Often only the most common genetic mutations are screened for and so >90% of white patients with CF can be confirmed in this way. When a diagnosis of CF is confirmed in a child, it is good practice to investigate all other siblings, even those who have no clinical symptoms of the condition.

11.7 Lung development

Answers: C D

Lung development is divided into four stages according to microscopic appearance:

1. Embryonic (0–7 weeks): lung foundation is laid down. Lung bud develops as a ventral diverticulum of the foregut (endodermal). At the end of this phase the first segments appear in the five lobes of the lung (three right and two left). At this time the pulmonary vessels have formed themselves.
2. Pseudoglandular (7–17 weeks): conducting airways are developed with continuous branching of bronchial buds. Adult numbers of airways proximal to the acini are present by week 16 of gestation. The acinus is a functional unit comprising alveoli, alveolar ducts and respiratory bronchioles. Epithelial lining differentiates. Goblet and serous cells are identifiable by week16. All preacinar vessels are present by week 17.
3. Canalicular (17–26 weeks): this phase sees the maturing of the conducting airways and the development of the terminal respiratory units. There is an increase in size of the proximal airways, with an increase in cartilage, muscular and glandular tissue. By week 22, type I and type II pneumocytes are seen. Type I pneumocytes are responsible for gas exchange in the alveoli and type II for secretion of surfactant.
4. Saccular (27 weeks to term: this period sees the further development of gas exchange units such that, by term, a third to a half of the adult number of alveoli are present. Preacinar airways increase in size and there is a continued increase in the number of goblet cells.

- Alveoli increase in number up until age 4–8 years.

11.8 Peak expiratory flow rate

Answers: D E

The peak expiratory flow rate (PEFR) is the maximal expiratory flow rate following a full inspiration. It is dependent upon the diameter of the airways at the narrowest point and the intrathoracic pressure generated. It is effort dependent. Few children under the age of 5 years can do a peak flow. Normal values are available and relate to height. They can be used for assessing the severity of asthma attacks and the response of the patient to therapy. The British Thoracic Society (BTS) guidelines use PEFR as a guide to good control (>80% predicted PEFR), and also in the assessment of severity of the attack – 33–50% of predicted/best reflecting an acute severe attack and <33% reflecting life-threatening asthma – in appropriate patients. Morning dip in PEFR is a sign of possibly worsening asthma.

Forced expiratory volume in 1 s (FEV_1) is the volume of air that can be forcibly expired in 1 second. It is less effort dependent and more reproducible than the PEFR. The FEV_1:FVC (FVC is forced vital capacity) ratio is used to distinguish a restrictive (normal FEV_1:FVC) from obstructive (considerably reduced FEV_1:FVC) pattern. In asthma the residual volume will increase reducing the FVC and the FEV_1 is considerably reduced compared to the FVC.

BOF Answers

11.9 Parapneumonic effusion (PPE)

Answer B: Ultrasound scan of the chest

Ultrasonography is the most important investigation after initial chest radiograph to guide diagnosis and management of PPE.

PPE is defined as a pleural fluid collection associated with an underlying pneumonia. It encompasses uncomplicated parapneumonic effusions through to thoracic empyema.

The incidence of parapneumonic effusion/empyema has increased in children in developed countries over the past 10 years. The reason for this increase is not currently fully understood.

Presentation of parapneumonic effusion is usually that of a child either with the clinical symptoms and signs of severe pneumonia or who fails to respond to standard therapy for pneumonia.

All children with PPE should be admitted to hospital for management including intravenous antibiotics. The most commonly identified causative organisms include *Streptococcus pneumoniae* in 80% of cases (most serotypes of which are not included in the most commonly administered pneumococcal vaccine), *Staphylococcus aureus, Haemophilus pneumoniae* type b and *Mycoplasma* sp.

Ultrasonography should be used to confirm the presence and nature of a pleural fluid collection and will help to guide interventional procedures; chest CT should not be performed routinely, but can be helpful in cases where there is concern that infection is not the underlying aetiology.

Effusions will respond to conservative management (antibiotics ± simple drainage) in 60–80% of cases but hospital admission may be long, possibly requiring a prolonged stay.

Effusions that are enlarging and/or compromising respiratory function should not be managed conservatively. Consideration should be given to early active treatment including insertion of chest drain and use of intrapleural fibrinolytics if indicated.

Oral antibiotics should be given at discharge for 1–4 weeks; patients should be followed up until symptoms have resolved. A follow-up chest radiography is essential.

11.10 Pneumocystis

Answer B: BAL PCR for Pneumocystis jiroveci pneumonia

BAL (bronchoalveolar lavage) PCR (polymerase chain reaction) for *Pneumocystis jiroveci* pneumonia is positive in up to 98% of cases.

First identified as a protozoan, *P. jiroveci* (PCP – formally *P. carinii*) has been more recently reclassified as a fungus. It is a common opportunistic infection causing pneumonia in patients with severe combined immunodeficiency and vertically acquired HIV, and may be the presenting illness for these underlying conditions. In these circumstances it has a high mortality and often presents in the first 3–6 months. Symptoms include progressive dyspnoea, cough and low-grade fever; signs include hypoxia, tachycardia and tachypnoea but chest auscultation is often unremarkable. Chest radiograph typically reveals bilateral interstitial and alveolar shadowing but may be normal in appearance. Diagnosis often requires BAL and PCR which is positive in up to 98% of cases; occasionally lung biopsy is required. Rarely the organism can be isolated from ordinary respiratory secretions.

Treatment of acute infection is with high-dose co-trimoxazole for a minimum of 3 weeks with the addition of steroids. Surfactant can be of benefit in severe cases requiring ventilation. Prophylaxis is with co-trimoxazole given to all HIV-infected infants for the first 12 months and all HIV-infected patients with previous infection with PCP or low CD4 counts. It is also given to all patients with congenital immunodeficiency and those on immunosuppressive therapy.

Note that anti-HIV IgG is not diagnostic of HIV infection at 4 months because IgG antibodies cross the placenta and may remain in the child's circulation up to age 18 months. Infection with a respiratory virus does not explain the prodrome of faltering growth or profound desaturation with normal chest examination.

11.11 Acute severe asthma

Answer D: Saturations of 90% in air

Pulsus paradoxus describes when there is an exaggeration of the normal drop in systolic blood pressure that occurs on inspiration. Patients with a difference >20 mmHg have severe asthma or cardiac tamponade, hypovolaemic shock or a tension pneumothorax. It is not required to be routinely recorded in every patient presenting with acute asthma following the latest (2009) BTS guidelines, and would be very difficult to elicit in a distressed unwell 2-year-old child.

Any child of 2 years in a stressful environment such as A&E may well appear distressed and confused and this is a better sign of severe attack in an older child.

Most children aged <5 years are unable to perform a peak flow measurement even when well.

Pulse oximetry is a good indicator of the severity of an acute attack of asthma. It is a good predictor of duration of the attack if performed on admission. O_2 saturations <92% are a marker of a severe asthma attack.

BTS guidelines list features of acute severe asthma in children >2 years as:

- SpO_2 (oxygen saturation) <92%
- PEFR 33–50% of predicted or best recorded
- Can't complete sentences in one breath or too breathless to talk or feed
- Pulse >125 beats/min in >5 year olds, >140 beats/min in 2–5 year olds
- Respiratory rate >30/min in >5 year olds, >40/min in 2–5 year olds.

BTS guidelines list features of life-threatening asthma in children >2 years as:

- Hypotension
- Exhaustion
- Confusion
- Coma
- Silent chest
- Cyanosis
- Poor respiratory effort.

11.12 Acute stridor in childhood

Answer D: Oral dexamethasone (no dosage)

The differential diagnosis of acute stridor in childhood includes:

- Acute laryngotracheitis (viral croup)
- Acute spasmodic croup
- Foreign body aspiration
- Bacterial tracheitis
- Acute epiglottitis
- Peritonsillar abscess
- Retropharyngeal abscess
- Laryngeal diphtheria
- Anaphylaxis and hereditary angio-oedema
- Thermal, mechanical (eg post-extubation) or chemical trauma.

Croup

Croup is a frequent cause of stridor in childhood, most commonly affecting children between the ages of 6 months and 3 years. Viral croup is typically associated with a prodrome of 24–48 hours of coryzal symptoms followed by the sudden onset of barking cough, horse voice, stridor and variable amounts of respiratory distress. It is commonly caused by parainfluenza and is associated with a mildly raised temperature.

Spasmodic croup is thought to be a non-infectious variant of viral croup where the presentation may be similar but with less coryzal prodrome and fever; the histology of the subglottic oedema is without the typical inflammatory changes seen in viral croup.

Most presentations of croup occur over night and in the late autumn and winter, but cases are seen throughout the year.

Treatment is with oral dexamethasone which has been shown to reduce the rate of hospital admission and length of stay in emergency departments, the need for nebulised adrenaline and the rate of intubation. Nebulised budesonide is more expensive and probably less effective than oral/intramuscular dexamethasone and so is no longer the first-line treatment.

Nebulised adrenaline is effective in treating severe croup but the effect is temporary, lasting 2–3 hours and close monitoring for recurrence of symptoms is needed after administration.

There is no evidence that humidified air/oxygen is effective in the treatment of croup.

11.13 Bronchiolitis

Answer E: Admit for assessment and commence nasogastric feeding if not tolerating >50% of maintenance requirement during the next feed

Bronchiolitis is a clinical syndrome seen most commonly in the first 6 months of life. Coryzal symptoms are followed by the onset of a harsh cough, tachypnoea, hyperinflation and intercostal recession. Auscultation reveals fine expiratory crepitations and polyphonic wheeze. Improvement is usually seen within 3–4 days after the onset of lower respiratory tract symptoms. Peak incidence occurs between October and March.

Respiratory syncytial virus (RSV) accounts for 50–90% of cases; other causative agents include human metapneumovirus (hMPV), rhinovirus, adenovirus, parainfluenza, influenza, coronavirus, bocavirus and *Mycoplasma pneumoniae*.

Mainly a self-limiting disease, treatment in hospital may be required to correct the main complications of dehydration, hypoxia and apnoea. The guidelines of the Scottish Intercollegiate Guidelines Network (SIGN) for hospital assessment include taking <50% of usual fluid intake in the preceding 24 hours, lethargy, apnoea, respiratory rate >70/min, O_2 sats <92%, respiratory distress and cyanosis.

Treatment is supportive with enteral or parenteral fluid/feed and supplementary oxygen. The syndrome of inappropriate antidiuretic hormone secretion (SIADH) may occur, so parenteral fluids are often restricted to 75% of maintenance. Continuous positive airway pressure (CPAP) and invasive ventilation can be used to correct severe hypoxia and apnoea.

There is no proven therapeutic value for bronchodilators, corticosteroids, antiviral agents, physiotherapy or antibiotics. Nebulised 3% saline administered in combination with a bronchodilator has recently been shown to decrease length of hospital stay.

Palivizumab, an anti-RSV monoclonal antibody, has been shown to significantly decrease risk of hospitalisation, length of stay and need for intensive care in high-risk patients. It is expensive and administered by monthly intramuscular injections throughout the RSV season. It is currently licensed for use in patients at high risk of developing severe bronchiolitis.

Recurrent wheeze after bronchiolitis occurs in 40–50%. Duration of attack, family history of atopy and exposure to cigarette smoke are risk factors.

11.14 Exercise-induced asthma

Answer B: Salbutamol

The BTS guidelines published in June 2009 state that, when you are treating exercise-induced asthma, the first step is to review all regular treatments including inhaled steroids, because exercise-induced symptoms may reflect a generally poor level of control.

The guidelines go on to state that immediately before exercise the drug of choice to alleviate exercised induced symptoms is an inhaled short-acting β_2 agonist.

Treatments to be considered for use in the prophylaxis against symptoms of exercise-induced asthma, in otherwise well-controlled patients, who are already taking inhaled steroids include:

- Leukotriene receptor antagonists
- Long-acting β_2 agonists
- Chromones (eg sodium cromoglicate)
- Oral β_2 agonists
- Theophyllines.

11.15 Cleft lip and palate

Answer D: Mothers with babies born with cleft lip and palate should be offered support and specialist advice to feed their child by their chosen method

The incidence in the UK is 1 in 700 live births; the recurrence rate is 1 in 25. The risk of having an affected child if one parent is affected is 1 in 20. A third of patients have an isolated cleft lip and a quarter have isolated cleft palate. It is an isolated abnormality in 75% but over 300 syndromes are associated with orofacial clefting. Maternal risk factors include antenatal alcohol consumption, periconception smoking, diabetes, nutritional factors (vitamin A, folic acid) and anticonvulsant medication.

Antenatal diagnosis occurs in 25% of cleft lips but isolated cleft palate is more difficult to diagnose antenatally.

Both breastfeeding and bottle feeding are possible in children born with cleft lip and palate, but support is needed. Specialist bottles and teats are available to help. The centralisation of services into nine specialist centres with dedicated multidisciplinary support teams in 2006 has improved the outcomes of children treated in the UK.

Problems associated with cleft lip and palate:

- Feeding difficulties and poor weight gain
- Difficulty with bonding
- Respiratory disease
- Speech delay
- Hypernasal speech
- Glue ear with impaired hearing
- Dental caries
- Problems with secondary dentition
- Cosmetic appearance and psychological adjustment of patient and parents.

Surgical correction is usually undertaken in two main stages. Generally the lip and anterior palate are closed as a primary procedure around 2–3 months of age; the soft palate is closed once the airway is more secure around 4–12 months. Speech and language therapy input at an early stage is vital to aid feeding and help promote best speech development.

11.16 Epiglottitis, croup and bacterial tracheitis

Answer D: Epiglottitis

Epiglottitis is most commonly caused by *Haemophilus influenza* type b and has decreased in prevalence since childhood immunisation was introduced in 1990. Now more common in older children/adults but unimmunised children present more classically at 2–7 years.

Features suggestive of epiglottitis rather than croup:

- Short history/abrupt onset
- High pyrexia with toxaemia
- Absence of cough
- Drooling
- Neck extension.

Treatment includes intubation in the operating room if possible to protect the airway and intravenous antibiotics once the airway is secured.

Viral croup (laryngotracheobronchitis) is usually caused by parainfluenza and presents between 6 months and 3 years.

Factors that suggest croup rather than epiglottitis:

- 1–2 days preceding history of coryzal symptoms
- Low-grade pyrexia without toxaemia
- Barking cough
- Absence of drooling
- Hoarse voice.

Treatment is with oral steroids and nebulised adrenaline for acute symptomatic relief in more severe cases. Intubation is rarely required. Spasmodic croup is a condition in which recurrent attacks of stridor and barking cough occur in the absence of fever and with minimal coryzal symptoms.

Bacterial tracheitis (pseudomembranous croup) runs a more prolonged course. It usually occurs in children aged <3 years. It can occur anew or on the background of viral croup. The most common causative organism is *Staphylococcus aureus*, followed by *Streptococcus pneumoniae*.

Presenting features:

- High fever and toxic
- Rapidly progressing upper airway obstruction
- Unlike epiglottitis, ability to lie flat and control secretions is not impaired.

Treatment is with parenteral antibiotics; intubation is required in up to 80% of cases.

11.17 Inhaler devices for children <5 years

Answer B: Pressurised MDI (metered dose inhaler) plus spacer device

There are the BTS and NICE guidelines that cover the appropriate drug delivery devices for use in children with asthma.

Children <5 years

- Corticosteroid **and** bronchodilator therapy should be delivered by metered dose inhaler and spacer device ± facemask
- **If** this is not effective, depending on the child's condition, nebulised therapy may be considered, and, if >3 years, a dry powder device may be considered.

Children 5–15 years

- Corticosteroid therapy should be routinely delivered by an MDI **and** spacer device.
- Children and carers should be trained to use their chosen device; suitability should be reviewed annually; technique and compliance should be monitored.
- In the case of other inhaled drugs, mainly inhaled bronchodilators, a wider range of delivery devices can be considered due to the greater need for portability and the clear feedback from symptom response.

Devices available include:

- Pressurised MDIs: devices used without spacers may be difficult to coordinate inspiration with actuation and oropharyngeal deposition may be a problem.
- Breath-actuated MDIs: Sound and sensation may be offputting for some children and oropharyngeal deposition may be a problem.
- Dry powder devices: some children (especially younger ones) may not be able to generate inspiratory flows high enough for effective delivery; also delivery may be impaired due to poor inspiration during an acute attack.
- Spacer devices: spacers are prone to attracting electrostatic charge; they should be washed and allowed to drip dry once a month. They are bulky and some children are unhappy to use them due to a perceived stigma. As soon as a child is able to use the mouthpiece, the mask should be removed.

11.18 Primary ciliary dyskinesia

Answer C: Primary ciliary dyskinesia

This is a heterogeneous group of genetic conditions leading to dysfunction in the motility of the cilia in the upper and lower respiratory tracts and fallopian tubes. The stationary or dysfunctionally beating cilia lead to ineffective mucociliary clearance, resulting in mucus retention; this predisposes to recurrent chest infections that can progress to bronchiectasis.

Most are inherited in an autosomal recessive fashion. The incidence is 1 in 15 000 in the UK (↑ in the Asian population due to ↑ consanguinity). Of patients 40% will have Kartagener syndrome: chronic sinusitis, bronchiectasis and visceral situs inversus.

Presentation:

- Infancy to late adulthood, mean age 4 years (0–14 years common)
- Delay is significant; 30% have bronchiectasis at presentation
- Neonatal: unexplained RDS, neonatal chest infection
- Congenital anomalies: situs inversus (35–50%), complex congenital heart disease 12.5%, hydrocephalus, oesophageal atresia, biliary atresia
- Childhood, chronic wet cough, bronchiectasis, atypical treatment-resistant asthma, hearing impairment due to chronic otitis media, rhinosinusitis, learning difficulties
- Adulthood: bronchiectasis, male infertility, female ectopic pregnancy.

Diagnosis:

- Screening saccharine test, (time to taste >60 min is abnormal), or measures of the concentration of exhaled nasal CO_2 (low level <250 ppb – parts per billion) both difficult in those aged <10 years.
- Evaluation of ciliary beat frequency, beat pattern and ultrastructural analysis is the gold standard
- Ciliated epithelial cells are cultured from nasal brushings for analysis of structure and function.

Management:

- Respiratory
  - aggressive antibiotics in exacerbations
  - twice daily physiotherapy + exercise
  - inhaled bronchodilators ± corticosteroids
  - pneumococcal, BCG and annual flu vaccine
  - regular follow-up + spirometry
- Hearing: regular audiology ± hearing aids (avoid grommets)
- Fertility: males and females may require assisted conception
- Psychology: Genetic counselling, support groups, DSS benefits and educational statement.

Prognosis:

A normal lifespan is possible with early diagnosis and aggressive treatment. Delay may cause progressive lung disease requiring lung transplantation.

11.19 Gastrointestinal obstruction in cystic fibrosis

Answer E: Distal intestinal obstruction syndrome

Of children diagnosed with cystic fibrosis 10–15% presented in the neonatal period with meconium ileus, which may be diagnosed antenatally with the presence of 'bright bowel' on antenatal ultrasound scan due to the secondary inspissated meconium. After birth, infants typically present with failure to pass meconium, abdominal distension and bile-vomiting. Microcolon is often seen on contrast enema, and the enema in itself may prove therapeutic by softening the meconium mass to relieve the obstruction. Most cases fail to respond to conservative management and require surgical intervention to remove the impacted meconium and to resect any non-viable gut. Rarely antenatal meconium peritonitis, neonatal volvulus and atresias may occur.

Distal intestinal obstruction syndrome (DIOS) is partial or complete obstruction of the bowel due to viscid mucofaecal material in the terminal ileum, caecum and ascending colon. It can present acutely or subacutely with colicky abdominal pain, and constipation. The diagnosis is often made clinically in a patient with CF presenting as above, with a tender mass in the right iliac fossa. Plain abdominal radiograph typically shows a speckled faecal gas pattern in the right lower quadrant. DIOS often responds to conservative treatment. Adequate hydration is imperative. Treatment involves large-volume bowel lavage with balanced salt solution containing polyethylene glycol taken orally or via nasogastric tube. Mucolytic agents (eg acetyl cysteine) can also be given orally; however, administration of Gastrografin is often more effective – it can be given either orally or per rectum under radiological supervision.

The cause of DIOS is multifactorial but pancreatic insufficiency and poorly controlled steatorrhoea are believed to be the main factors. Children with a history of meconium ileus and those with CF-related liver disease carry an increased risk of developing the syndrome.

11.20 Cystic fibrosis

Answer D: Cystic fibrosis

Cystic fibrosis is inherited in an autosomal recessive fashion. Over 450 mutations of the CF gene are recognised, ΔF508 being most common (70%). The incidence in the UK is 1 per 2000 births. Newborn screening using immunoreactive trypsin (IRT) was introduced in the UK in 2005. In the first week of life the specificity of the raised IRT is low thus genetic testing ± further IRT follows a positive result. Sweat testing isn't possible until 6 weeks. The aim of neonatal screening is to achieve better outcomes with early intervention.

Clinical features

Respiratory

- Wheezing can be persistent in the first 1–2 years.
- Twenty per cent have coexisting atopic asthma.
- Finger clubbing develops in parallel with the progressive suppurative lung disease.
- Ten per cent develop allergic bronchopulmonary aspergillosis (ABPA).

Gastrointestinal

- Meconium ileus
- DIOS
- Malabsorption secondary to pancreatic insufficiency (85%)
- Recurrent rectal prolapse occurs in 10% of undiagnosed CF.

Liver disease

- Prolonged neonatal jaundice
- Fatty infiltration is common in malnourished individuals
- Progressive liver involvement with cirrhosis and portal hypertension occur in the minority; 20% of adolescents with CF develop chronic liver disease
- Children with advanced liver disease may develop acute variceal haemorrhage and haematemesis.

Diabetes

- Endocrine pancreatic insufficiency occurs increasingly for >10 years
- Most patients with CF and diabetes benefit from insulin but should not change to a diabetic diet.

Treatment

Respiratory

- Prevent bacterial infection and colonisation
- Prompt treatment of exacerbations
- Airway clearance, physiotherapy
- Corticosteroids in high dose for treating ABPA
- Mucolytics; hypertonic saline and recombinant human deoxyribonuclease (DNase).

Nutritional support

- Pancreatic enzyme supplementation
- Regular follow-up including nutritional and growth review
- Supportive enteral feeding regimens
- Supplementation of fat-soluble vitamins.

11.21 Bronchiectasis

Answer D: Bronchiectasis

This is defined as persistent dilatation of the bronchi, resulting from inflammatory destruction of its walls, associated with chronic cough with sputum production, which children rarely expectorate. It is characterised by periods of relapse and remission. History suggestive of bronchiectasis includes a chronic wet cough, recurrent chest infections responsive to antibiotics, exertional dyspnoea, symptoms of reactive airway disease and growth failure. Clinical signs include clubbing, chest wall deformity, coarse crackles and wheeze on auscultation. Chest radiograph may show the characteristic appearances of tramlines caused by dilated bronchi in the affected lobe. High-resolution CT is useful for diagnosis.

The BTS guidelines for the assessment and management of cough in children (2008) suggest that all cases of chronic cough (>8 weeks) require investigation. Studies have shown substantial (3–5 years) delays from onset of symptoms to diagnosis in cases of bronchiectasis which leaves the bronchial tree open to ongoing damage.

The most common cause is cystic fibrosis. In a large number of cases an underlying cause cannot be identified.

Known causes of bronchiectasis include:

- Previous infection – measles, pertussis, pneumonia, TB
- Congenital:
  - – structural (congenital lobar emphysema)
  - – other (α_1-anti-trypsin deficiency)
- Congenital immunodeficiency:
  - – hypogammaglobulinaemia
  - – functional antibody deficiency
  - – neutrophil function abnormalities
  - – MCH class 2 deficiency
- Acquired immune deficiency (eg HIV)
- Primary ciliary dyskinesia
- Mechanical:
  - – foreign body aspiration (history can be entirely absent)
  - – extrinsic compression
  - – endobronchial lesion
- Chronic aspiration.

The main stay of the management of bronchiectasis is with physiotherapy and regular and prolonged courses of antibiotics, targeted by clinical symptoms and regular sputum cultures. Surgery is occasionally required if a defined lobe is affected and the patient is unresponsive to medical treatment.

11.22 Obstructive sleep apnoea

Answer E: Referral to respiratory paediatrician for a sleep study

Obstructive sleep apnoea (OSA) is defined as a prolonged upper airway obstruction that disrupts normal ventilation and normal sleep patterns during sleep. The prevalence of OSA in childhood appears to be around 2–3%; the incidence is highest between age 2 and 8 years when tonsillar and adenoidal size are greatest in relation to upper airway calibre.

Factors associated with an increased prevalence of OSA include childhood obesity, family history of OSA, craniofacial abnormalities, Down syndrome, Prader–Willi and Marfan syndromes, and neuromuscular and neurodevelopmental abnormalities.

Symptoms of OSA include both nocturnal symptoms and daytime consequences of the disorder. The most common nocturnal symptoms include snoring, gasping and witnessed apnoeas during sleep, frequent awakenings and continuous movement during sleep, and episodic nocturnal enuresis. Daytime symptoms include mouth breathing, early morning headaches, hyperactivity, inattentiveness, aggressive behaviour and poor school performance. Daytime somnolence appears to be much less of a problem in children with OSA than adults, being present in around 7–10% of cases. Untreated OSA can also lead to right ventricular hypertrophy (RVH), pulmonary hypertension and failure to thrive.

The diagnosis is made by clinical assessment and overnight monitoring. The gold standard is the nocturnal polysomnogram, which includes monitoring of sleep stages, oxygen saturations, and respiratory and body movements. This is not available in all centres due to its complexity and the simplest test for OSA is a sleep study comprising overnight pulse oximetry; however, this does not exclude OSA if negative and carries a specificity and sensitivity of 60% and 70% respectively.

Treatment is mainly surgical, with adenotonsillectomy being curative in 80% of cases. A small proportion of patients experience some recurrence of their symptoms postoperatively; the risk is increased in children with obesity, those with predisposing underlying conditions, such as Down syndrome and those with a family history of OSA.

11.23 *Mycoplasma pneumoniae*

Answer E: Erythromycin and salbutamol

Mycoplasma pneumoniae is a bacterium without a cell wall. It is spread by droplets and humans are the only hosts. The incubation period is 3 weeks. The most common clinical manifestation of infection is atypical pneumonia presenting with cough. Onset of symptoms is usually insidious with fever, malaise, headache and sore throat. The frequency and severity of the cough increase over the first few days. Wheeze is common, especially but not exclusively in those who have asthma. The chest radiograph appearance is usually worse than the symptoms and signs suggest and pleural effusions may be present. The peak incidence is in children aged 5–9 years. Infection is uncommon in the first year of life. Diagnosis is by serology with positive mycoplasma IgM in the acute illness and a convalescent rise in the mycoplasma IgG titre. Culture is difficult. Cold agglutinins will be positive in 50%. White cell count is often normal. Treatment is with azithromycin, bronchodilators and physiotherapy. Tetracyclines can be given in adolescence, but are contraindicated in younger children due to deposition and staining of developing teeth. Prognosis is usually excellent; however, long-term sequelae may be associated with the development of complications. Associations and complications of mycoplasma infection include:

- Skin: erythema multiforme, Stevens–Johnson syndrome
- CNS: meningoencephalitis, aseptic meningitis, cerebellar ataxia, Guillain–Barré syndrome
- Joints: monoarthritis
- Cardiac: myocarditis, pericarditis
- Blood: haemolysis, thrombocytopenia
- Gastrointestinal (GI) tract: hepatitis, pancreatitis, protein-losing enteropathy.

11.24 Acute tonsillitis

Answer A: Give a prescription for phenoxymethylpenicillin and advise the use of the prescription in 48 hours if symptoms continue to increase or there is no sign of settling within this time frame advise to re-present if child looks severely unwell at any time

Acute tonsillitis is rare in infancy, with the peak incidence being around age 5 years. There is a second peak in adolescence. Viral infections are much more common than bacterial infections. The most common viral agent is adenovirus; others include EBV, influenza, parainfluenza and RSV. The most common bacterial cause is group A β-haemolytic streptococci; others include pneumococci, *Haemophilus* sp. and *Mycoplasma* sp.

Patients usually present with fever, sore throat, foul breath, difficult and painful swallowing, and painful cervical lymph node enlargement. Symptoms usually last 3–4 days but can last up to 2 weeks. Tonsillar hypertrophy with exudate does not distinguish between a bacterial and a viral aetiology. The differential diagnosis of tonsillitis includes diphtheria, agranulocytosis and infectious mononucleosis.

Infectious mononucleosis is a clinical syndrome caused by the immunopathological response to infection with EBV in some people. It should be considered in all children with tender cervical, axillary and/or inguinal lymphadenopathy, splenomegaly, severe lethargy and low-grade fever associated with tonsillitis.

The BTS guidelines state that children presenting with three or more Centor criteria (listed below) should have immediate antibiotics as group A β-haemolytic streptococci are the more likely causative agent; those with fewer than three should have delayed antibiotics or no antibiotics provided that they are low risk and systemically well:

- History of fever
- Tonsillar exudates
- Tender anterior cervical lymphadenopathy
- Absence of cough.

The indications for tonsillectomy may include:

- Recurrent tonsillitis + failure to thrive
- Frequent school absence
- Quinsy
- Sleep apnoea
- Exclusion of tonsillar tumour.

11.25 Anaphylaxis

Answer E: Prescription of EpiPen, education re its use and referral to allergist

Anaphylaxis is defined as 'a serious allergic reaction that is rapid in onset and may cause death'; it is a type 1 immediate hypersensitivity reaction that is IgE mediated. The overall rate of anaphylaxis appears to be rising, especially in food-related cases among 0- to 4-year-old children. Anaphylaxis is more prevalent in young children, where food allergy is the most common cause; in adults drugs and insect venom are more common triggers.

Clinical diagnosis is highly likely when there is an acute onset of illness (minutes to several hours) PLUS two or more of the following:

- Respiratory compromise (dyspnoea, wheeze, bronchospasm, stridor, reduced PEFR, hypoxemia)
- Reduced blood pressure or associated end-organ dysfunction (hypotonia, syncope, incontinence)
- Involvement of the skin-mucosal tissue (generalised hives, itch–flush, swollen face, lips, tongue, uvula)
- Persistent GI symptoms (crampy abdominal pain, vomiting, diarrhoea).

Anaphylaxis is potentially life threatening; <2% of cases are fatal. Risk factors for death from food-related anaphylaxis include: active asthma, age 11–30 years, peanut or tree nut allergy, unavailable or delayed use of adrenaline.

Acute management

- Remove allergen, place patient in supine position
- Assess airway, breathing, then circulation and manage as appropriate
- Adrenaline 10 μg/kg i.m., repeat every 15 min as needed
- Hydrocortisone 4 mg/kg i.v.
- Consider colloid 20 ml/kg
- If stridor severe give adrenaline 5 ml 1:1000 nebulised
- If bronchospasm is severe then salbutamol 5 mg nebulised every 15 min
- Observation for 6–8 h to avoid missing biphasic reactions.

Discharge planning

- Trigger avoidance advice
- Education of parents/carers and adolescents (high risk) in the early recognition and treatment of allergic reactions
- Personalised action plans
- EpiPen prescription and training for appropriate cases (previous anaphylaxis, child with food allergy and coexisting persistent asthma)
- Follow-up with allergist
- Management of co-morbidities.

11.26 Pulmonary TB

Answer C: A strongly positive Mantoux test (>15 nn) is suggestive of a diagnosis of TB even if the patient has been immunised with BCG

Mycobacterium tuberculosis is a Gram-positive acid-fast bacillus that is difficult to culture. The reservoir is the mammalian host and spread is by inhalation of infected droplets. Young children are not normally infectious, because they rarely have cavitating disease before age 8–10 years. The clinical features of infection are variable and depend on the balance between bacterial multiplication and host response. Symptoms can either be from a primary complex (Ghon focus) or as a consequence of reactivation, when infection spreads to local lymph nodes, causing invasion or compression of local structures and/or dissemination to more distal sites. The vast majority (>90%) of disease in children follows within 12 months of primary infection. Children aged <3 years and immunocompromised individuals are most at risk of progression to pulmonary or disseminated disease after primary infection.

The diagnosis of TB in childhood is difficult. Sputum is difficult to obtain and rarely positive. Sputum induction should be performed if possible and safe, early morning, gastric aspirates can be used if this is not successful. Pointers include a clinical picture of persistent symptoms, history of contact, suggestive radiology and positive tuberculin test (Mantoux). The Mantoux test is often difficult to interpret. It can be negative in early fulminating disease and in children with HIV infection. False-positive Mantoux tests occur with previous BCG and exposure to environmental mycobacteria. A strongly positive Mantoux test (>15 mm) is suggestive of infection even with previous BCG. Newer interferon-γ immunological tests (QuantiFERON-TB and T-SPOT.TB) are available and these tests should be used as a second line in those patients who have a positive Mantoux test or in whom Mantoux testing may be unreliable.

The BTS guidelines for the treatment of TB (2006) state that the treatment for active respiratory TB in children should be with quadruple therapy: isoniazid, rifampicin (6 months), and pyrazinamide and ethambutol (2 months). BCG immunisation is now targeted and often given in the neonatal period.

11.27 Blood gas analysis

Answer C: Sepsis

The gas shows an uncompensated metabolic acidosis. Key features are a low pH, low HCO_3, negative base excess and lack of respiratory compensation, which would include a low CO_2 and longer term a rise in HCO_3^-. The most likely diagnosis in a child presenting with this gas would be sepsis or shock for other reasons, eg severe gastroenteritis. Other causes include congenital heart disease, inborn metabolic errors and ingestion of toxins (in older children). Diabetic ketoacidosis (DKA) causes a metabolic acidosis but you would expect a more markedly raised blood sugar than seen in this case; the mild hyperglycaemia is much more likely to reflect the systemic stress of sepsis than the hyperglycaemia associated with the total lack of insulin predisposing to DKA.

The management of a child presenting in this way comprises providing adequate oxygenation and circulating volume, and treating the underlying cause.

11.28 Congenital lobar emphysema

Answer B: If symptomatic, wil usually present with tachypnoea and signs of respiratory distress in the neonatal period

Congenital lobar emphysema is a rare congenital lung abnormality caused by overexpansion of one or more pulmonary lobes, with resulting compression of the remaining ipsilateral and sometimes contralateral lung. Intrinsic cartilaginous deficiencies or external bronchial compression may be the cause (eg large pulmonary artery). The left upper lobe is the most likely to be affected. Approximately 10% have associated abnormalities, the most common being cardiac. Antenatal diagnostic accuracy is almost 100%. Congenital lobar emphysema, if symptomatic, will usually present in the neonatal period with increasing respiratory difficulty. However, many patients experience no symptoms and so it may be an incidental finding in an older child. The chest radiograph findings are typically those of overinflation and/or hyperlucency of the affected segment.

The differential diagnosis includes the following:

- Pneumothorax
- Bronchial mucus plug with associated hyperinflation
- Agenesis/hypoplasia of the contralateral lung
- Congenital cystic adenomatoid malformation.

The diagnosis should be confirmed with further imaging such as CT or MRI. Those with significant symptoms should be considered for surgery (lobectomy), but conservative management is appropriate for those who are asymptomatic or have only mild symptoms.

11.29 Palivizumab

Answer A: Reduces admission rates to hospital and ICU in infants with BPD when compared with placebo

Palivizumab is a humanised monoclonal immunoglobulin G1 that prevents entry of RSV into the cells lining the respiratory tract.

The IMpact study was a placebo-controlled study of intramuscular palivizumab every 30 days in over 1500 high-risk infants. It showed that palivizumab significantly decreased the risk of hospitalisation, duration of hospital stay and need for intensive care.

Palivizumab is currently licensed in the UK for the prevention of RSV infection in:

- Children born at less than 35 weeks' gestation who are 6 months old at the start of the RSV season.
- Children <2 years old who have received treatment for BPD within the last 6 months.
- Children <2 years with haemodynamically significant congenital heart disease.

It is given as monthly intramuscular injections during the RSV season (half-life given intramuscularly is 18–20 days). Cost is prohibitive with a course of five injections costing upwards of £2500 per patient, depending on age and an estimated cost of preventing one hospital admission of £43 000.

Ribavirin, an antiviral that inhibits a wide range of RNA and DNA viruses, is currently the only agent licensed in the UK (for administration by inhalation) for the treatment of severe bronchiolitis caused by RSV in infants, especially when they have other serious diseases.

11.30 Whooping cough

Answer C: The initial catarrhal phase is indistinguishable from common upper respiratory tract infections

Whooping cough is a respiratory tract infection characterised by paroxysmal coughing. *Bordetella pertussis* (a Gram-negative bacillus) is the cause of >90% of cases of whooping cough. Incubation period varies from 3 days to 12 days. The clinical disease often lasts 6 weeks, divided into three stages:

1. The catarrhal phase, in which the child is most infectious, symptoms are indistinguishable from those caused by viruses such as RSV, parainfluenza and adenovirus, and include nasal congestion, sneezing, rhinorrhoea and low-grade fever. Note that infectivity may continue for 3 weeks or more after the onset of the cough.
2. The paroxysmal phase, during which the patient experiences paroxysms of intense coughing lasting several minutes. In infants >6 months and toddlers the paroxysms are occasionally followed by the characteristic 'whoop', caused by inspired air being forced through a still partially closed airway. Infants <6 months do not display the classic whoop but are at risk from apnoeic episodes and exhaustion. Post-tussive vomiting is common.
3. The recovery stage, in which patients will experience a chronic cough that may last weeks.

Older children and adults often have a milder less typical form of illness. Preterm babies and infants with co-morbidity are most at risk of severe disease and complications.

Erythromycin may attenuate the disease if given early enough (during the catarrhal phase) but should be given once the cough has been established to shorten the period of infectivity and limit spread. Immunisation has greatly reduced the incidence of whooping cough but outbreaks still occur in a 2- to 5-year cycle and most cases fall between June and September. Neither vaccination nor acquisition of the disease provides lifelong immunity. Bronchopneumonia (sometimes due to secondary infection) may occur as a complication, but lower respiratory tract signs are not always present.

11.31 Community-acquired pneumonia

Answer D: Treatment with oral amoxicillin

The BTS published guidelines for the management of community-acquired pneumonia (CAP) in childhood in 2002. The most common bacterial cause of pneumonia is *Streptococcus pneumoniae*, although in younger children viruses are more commonly responsible and a significant proportion of cases of CAP (up to 40%) represent mixed infection.

According to the BTS guidelines, indications for hospital admission include: hypoxia (sats ≤92%), tachypnoea (>70 beats/min in infants and >50 beats/min in older children), grunting, apnoea, having difficulty breathing, dehydration, unable to tolerate oral medications or having insufficient family support.

Amoxicillin is recommended as first-line treatment for those children in whom pneumococcus is considered the most likely pathogen and who meet the criteria for management at home (with advice to the carers about identifying signs of deterioration). Macrolide antibiotics can be used in children aged >5 years due to the increased incidence of *Mycoplasma* sp. in this age group. Intravenous antibiotics are reserved for those who are unable to absorb oral antibiotics or who present with severe symptoms and signs. Any child who remains pyrexial or unwell 48 hours after admission for pneumonia requires re-evaluation for possible complications. Trials have not demonstrated that physiotherapy is beneficial in reducing the length of stay or improving chest radiograph findings in children with pneumonia in the consolidatory phase of the illness.

There is evidence to support the fact that a chest radiograph should not be performed routinely in children with mild uncomplicated lower respiratory tract infection and in whom for ambulatory care is appropriate; however, chest radiograph has a good yield (25%) in children aged <5 years with a pyrexia of unknown origin (PUO) and raised WBCs but no other source for infection. Repeat chest radiographs are recommended only in those children with lobar collapse or apparent round pneumonia on the original radiograph or in children whose symptoms fail to resolve. It is therefore important that children are reviewed if symptoms do not resolve with treatment.

11.32 Poorly controlled asthma

Answer B: Add monteleukast at a dose of 4 mg once daily

The BTS guidelines describe five steps in the management of childhood asthma. This child's treatment would be equivalent to step 3. He is still experiencing symptoms so his control is suboptimal and his management needs to be reviewed. In all children whose symptoms do not respond to appropriate anti-asthma treatment, review the diagnosis, inhaler technique and treatment compliance.

If you are confident of the diagnosis, compliance and inhaler technique, the management needs to be stepped up in a controlled manner as set out in the guidelines. He is already receiving a high dose of inhaled steroid, so a further increase in dose is not indicated. He is also on maximal long-acting β agonist (Note that a therapeutic trial of this therapy should be undertaken and if no benefit was demonstrated the drug should be stopped before starting further agents.)

At the age of 5 years a child's ability to use a dry powder device must be carefully assessed because it is possible that he is still too young to take this form of medication reliably. At all ages the use of a large volume spacer maximises the amount of drug deposited in the airways and is therefore the first choice of delivery mechanism for inhaled steroids.

The most appropriate addition to this child's therapy would be the introduction of monteleukast, a leukotriene receptor antagonist, as a 6-week therapeutic trial. It is licensed for use from the age of 6 months. Only about a third of people appear to benefit from the use of these agents and it would therefore be important to reassess the child's asthma control having commenced this treatment and discontinue it should no benefit be gained. Side effects include headache, sleep disorders and GI disturbance. If this therapeutic trial was to fail, an alternative would be a 6-week therapeutic trial of a modified-release oral theophylline, with consideration of referral to a paediatric respiratory physician for further advice.

EMQ Answers

11.33–11.35 Theme: Chronic cough

11.33

Answer J: Persistent isolated chronic cough

Cough is a common childhood symptom. Studies have shown that 5–10% of children aged 6–12 years have chronic cough without wheeze and the prevalence in younger children is likely to be higher. It may be the presenting symptom of respiratory illness, or more commonly an isolated symptom that can still be troublesome, and its effects should not be underestimated. Environmental pollutants especially tobacco smoke can play a significant role in the aetiology of chronic cough in children.

Non-specific isolated persistent cough is a diagnosis of exclusion. It is found in an otherwise well child with no associated wheezing or sputum production or alert signs of serious pathology (see below). The natural history of non-specific cough in childhood is good with most becoming symptom free in time.

Evidence suggests that the vast majority of these children do not have 'cough-variant asthma'. They do not have increased eosinophilic inflammation in their airways, they do not have a history suggestive of atopic disease and do not respond to anti-asthmatic therapy. It can, however, be difficult to be sure they do not have asthma, and so a limited trial of anti-asthmatic medication at reasonable doses, with a withdrawal of treatment and documentation of the outcome of the trial, may be justified to rule out a diagnosis of asthma.

Red flag alerts to underlying pathology: .

- Neonatal onset
- Cough with feeding
- Sudden onset cough (? foreign body aspiration – not always obvious from history!)
- Chronic wet cough ± phlegm production
- Associated with night sweats (TB)
- Continuous unremitting or worsening cough
- Signs of chronic lung disease.

11.34

Answer E: Protracted bacterial bronchitis

PBB is a paediatric condition clinically defined as (a) presence of isolated chronic (>8 weeks) wet cough, (b) resolution of cough with appropriate antibiotic treatment and (c) the absence of pointers suggestive of an alternative diagnosis.

Patients are typically <5 years, with a chronic wet cough, and some parents may report wheeze. Systemic effects are usually minimal or non-specific such as tiredness or lack of energy. These symptoms usually respond before the cough when appropriate treatment is commenced. Symptoms worsen during intercurrent viral infections and the combined history of viral exacerbations and persistent night-time cough often leads to the misdiagnosis of asthma. Asthma and PBB can coexist, further complicating the diagnosis. Common pathogens are those seen in the early stages of bronchiectasis *Haemophilus influenza, Stretococcus pneumoniae and Mycoplasma catarrhalis.*

On clinical assessment they have a persistent 'rattle' rather than wheeze, suggestive of airway secretion rather than bronchoconstriction. There is typically some delay in this diagnosis. Treatment is a prolonged course of antibiotics (10–14 days). The diagnosis is confirmed when the response to treatment is dramatic and the child becomes asymptomatic. The child may have received a shorter course of antibiotics (5–7 days) before the diagnosis, to which they may have partially responded or responded but relapsed within 2–3 days of the end of the course.

Chest radiograph may well be reported as normal but usually shows peribronchiolar changes. Hyperinflation is rare and should raise the concern of asthma alone or in association with PBB. Further investigations are reserved for children who do not respond to treatment or who have more than two episodes of PBB in a year, who should have a full evaluation for bronchiectasis, including assessment of immunoglobulins, functional antibody responses to immunisations, full blood count (FBC), sweat test, bronchoscopy and CT.

11.35

Answer B: Inhaled foreign body

A diagnosis of an inhaled foreign body in a child can be easily missed if not included in the differential diagnosis, particularly if a history of choking is not forthcoming or the episode of aspiration is unwitnessed. It is important to understand that a normal chest radiograph does not rule out the diagnosis. The presence of a radio-opaque foreign body may be obvious but the more usual small plastic objects or food particles may be radiolucent. Signs associated with intraluminal foreign bodies include obstructive emphysema, overinflation or collapse of the lung or lobe distal to the obstruction. Other complications include pneumonia, lung abscess, acute and chronic lung or lobar collapse, and permanent dilatation of the airways distal to the obstruction with subsequent chronic bronchiectasis. Foreign body aspiration should be considered in all children with persisting changes on chest radiograph or those who do not respond as expected to treatment.

When considering a diagnosis of foreign body aspiration, inspiratory and expiratory chest radiographs may be useful in showing the isolated, persistent changes of air trapping associated with a foreign body acting as a ball valve.

Laryngeal or tracheal foreign bodies can be acutely life threatening and should be treated clinically as per APLS (Advanced Paediatric Life Support) guidelines following the choking child algorithm. However, it is important to understand that even in asymptomatic children organic material such as nuts or beans may swell in the airway and in addition the inflammatory response to the foreign body may narrow the airway further, making it an emergency to diagnose and definitively treat all patients with recognised or suspected foreign body aspiration. Definitive management includes a rigid bronchoscopy and removal of the foreign body.

11.36–11.38 Theme: Cervical lymphadenopathy

11.36

Answer E: Cat-scratch disease

Cat-scratch disease is a common cause of chronic adenopathy in childhood. The causative bacterium in most cases is *Bartonella henselae*, a Gram-negative fastidious organism. Kittens are far more likely to transmit the disease than adult cats. Incubation is usually between 3 and 10 days. Most cases (>90%) have a recent history of bite or scratch from a cat or kitten. Classically (>90%) one or more red skin papules ≤0.5 cm in diameter occur at the sight of inoculation 1–4 weeks before the development of adenopathy. Lymphadenitis with tender red and warm node enlargement, with overlying skin induration, usually persists for 4–6 weeks but can last for up to a year. Many nodes will suppurate. Axillary nodes are the most common site, followed by cervical, submandibular and preauricular nodes. Single node involvement occurs in more than 50% and typical node size is 1–5 cm in diameter. Fever (often presenting as PUO lasting 1–2 weeks) and fatigue are also common associations. The signs and symptoms vary widely but regional lymphadenopathy is the most common. Infection can also affect the CNS (headache, encephalitis, seizure, myelitis, transient peripheral neuropathy and retinitis), eyes, liver, spleen, bone and lungs. Diagnosis can be difficult but serology for *Bartonella* sp. is usually positive. It is usually a self-limiting disease and has a benign course of 2–4 months; treatment is not usually indicated in most immunocompetent patients. It is, however, important to make the diagnosis because this allows a termination of the anxiety and investigations associated with investigating lymphadenopathy in children.

11.37

Answer B: Non-TB mycobacterial infection

Non-tuberculous mycobacteria (NTM; previously known as 'atypical mycobacteria') are a cause of lymphadenopathy that usually presents in young children (mean age 5.5 years) who are otherwise systemically well. The most commonly affected nodes are the cervical and submandibular. The average delay between diagnosis and the onset of symptoms is 7–10 weeks. In addition to lymphadenopathy the patient may experience mild tenderness (12%), fistula formation (20%) and changes in skin colour, often described as violaceous (80%), overlying the presenting lymph node. Ultrasonography and CT are not diagnostic and biopsy will often lead to fistula formation (70%) and so should be avoided. Intradermal skin testing can help to confirm the diagnosis and aid differentiation between TB and NTM. A positive skin test for NTM indicates the need to proceed to excision biopsy, the results of which are slow and often fail to culture NTM. Complete excision is the first-line treatment for this condition because it is most likely to lead to symptom resolution with minimal scarring and chance of fistula formation. The major risk of surgery is nerve damage. In contrast TB of the cervical lymph nodes responds well to medical treatment with anti-TB antibiotics.

11.38

Answer I: Group A haemolytic streptococcal lymphadenitis

One of the most common clinical presentations of infective lymphadenitis is an acute, one-sided, pyogenic adenitis. The involved node may be firm and tender, with erythema of the overlying skin. Most commonly this picture is secondary to group A β-haemolytic streptococci or staphylococcal organisms (especially *Staphylococcus aureus*). All acute episodes of acute cervical lymphadenopathy should be treated with a 2-week course of an antibiotic with good anti-staphylococcal and anti-streptococcal cover to treat and exclude a simple bacterial cause.

11.39–11.41 Theme: Diagnosis of asthma in children

11.39

Answer B: Trial of inhaled steroid MDI plus spacer at standard dose with defined reassessment and follow-up

11.40

Answer A: Trial of salbutamol MDI plus volumatic spacer device and planned review with GP

11.41

Answer J: Management of acute symptoms followed by discharge advice to avoid trigger factors and treat exacerbations with salbutamol MDI plus volumatic spacer with planned follow-up

Guidelines published by the BTS on the management of asthma in children state that the diagnosis is a clinical one, based on a characteristic set of episodically occurring symptoms in the absence of an alternative explanation. The criteria for making a diagnosis of asthma should always be clearly documented in the child's notes. With a thorough history and examination children should be grouped into one of three bands (high, intermediate and low probability) according to the likelihood of their symptoms being secondary to asthma and their ongoing management is guided according to these groupings.

Clinical features that suggest a diagnosis of asthma are listed below:

- Wheeze
- Cough
- Difficulty breathing
- Chest tightness.

The likelihood of the symptoms being due to asthma is further increased if they occur in a frequent/recurrent pattern, if they are worse at night or in the early morning, if they are triggered or exacerbated by exercise, animals, cold and/or damp air, or emotions, or occur apart from colds. The likelihood is further increased if the patient has a personal or family history of atopy/asthma, if symptoms or lung function respond to adequate therapy and if there is widespread wheeze heard on auscultation of the chest during an exacerbation.

Clinical features that lower the likelihood of a diagnosis of asthma include:

- Symptoms with colds with no interval symptoms
- Isolated cough in the absence of wheeze or difficulty breathing
- History of wet cough
- Repeatedly normal physical examination of the chest when symptomatic
- Normal PEFR or spirometry when symptomatic
- No response to a trial of adequate asthma treatment
- Clinical features suggestive of an alternative diagnosis.

It is essential at the initial consultation and whenever the child appears to be deteriorating, or not responding to current levels of treatment, to carefully consider the possibility of an alternative diagnosis.

Children with a high probability of asthma should start a defined trial of treatment and have their response observed and recorded. Further investigation should be reserved for those who show a poor response to the trial.

Children with a low probability of asthma should have further investigation with consideration of onward referral to a respiratory specialist paediatrician.

Children with intermediate probability of asthma who can reliably undergo spirometry, and show evidence of airway obstruction, should have their response to bronchodilators (reversibility) or response to a time-limited trial of inhaled steroids assessed and documented. If improvement is shown a diagnosis of asthma is likely and treatment should be continued with plans to minimise or trial a withdrawal of therapy once a period of good control has been established. If there is no significant reversibility or response to trial of treatment, an alternative diagnosis should be pursued.

Children with intermediate probability of asthma who can reliably undergo spirometry, but show no evidence of airway obstruction, should have their response to bronchodilators (reversibility) assessed and be considered for investigation of their atopic status and referral to a specialist respiratory paediatrician.

Children with intermediate probability of asthma who cannot reliably undergo spirometry should be offered a time-limited trial of treatment and their response documented. If improvement is shown a diagnosis of asthma is likely and treatment should be continued with plans to minimise or trial a withdrawal of therapy once a period of good control has been established. If there is no significant response to trial of treatment an alternative diagnosis should be pursued and referral to a specialist respiratory paediatrician considered.

11.42–11.44 Theme: Abnormalities of the airway

11.42

Answer F: Laryngomalacia

Laryngomalacia is the most common congenital anomaly of the upper airway and 60–70% of persistent stridor in infancy is due to this cause. The symptoms may present any time within the first 4–6 weeks of life. Inspiratory noises may be initially confused with nasal congestion or be higher pitched in nature. The noise often increases with crying, feeding, lying supine and intercurrent respiratory infections. The nature of the child's cry is not normally affected unless associated with reflux laryngitis. Gastro-oesophageal reflux is associated with this diagnosis. Although symptoms may seem to increase over the first 6 months as inspiratory air flow increases, resolution by 2 years is the norm. Most children do not need intervention and feed and thrive normally, and in these circumstances the diagnosis can be made clinically. Specific indications for investigation with flexible laryngoscopy include stridor at rest, late presentation (>4 weeks) and failure to thrive. Appearances suggesting laryngomalacia include an ω-shaped epiglottis that prolapses over the larynx during inspiration. Surgical intervention is needed in less than 1% of cases but is indicated in cases complicated by severe resistant failure to thrive, OSA and cor pulmonale.

11.43

Answer I: Vascular rings and slings

Vascular rings are rare congenital abnormalities that occur due to incomplete or abnormal regression of the branchial arches in the embryonic development of the aortic arch and great vessels. These abnormal arrangements surround the trachea and oesophagus partially or completely and produce symptoms from compression. The double aortic arch and right aortic arch account for about 85–95% of these anomalies.

Vascular rings and slings produce symptoms and signs consistent with tracheal and/or oesophageal compression and the vast majority present in infancy or childhood. Symptoms include biphasic stridor (unlike croup and 80% of laryngomalacia, which are uniphasic), which is unaffected by position, wheezing, cyanosis, apnoeas and a high-pitched 'brassy' cough. The child may present with a history of treatment-resistant asthma, recurrent pneumonia, and difficulty feeding or weight loss.

Investigation should be with a plain chest radiograph which may show the position of the aortic arch, compression of the trachea, and atelectasis or hyperinflation due to air trapping. Barium swallow studies are diagnostic in most cases. The treatment for symptomatic vascular rings is surgical.

11.44

Answer E: Bilateral choanal atresia

Choanal atresia is the lack of patency of the posterior nasal aperture; it is seen in 1 in 8000 births and is more common in girls. Choanal atresia is frequently associated with other congenital abnormalities, most commonly as part of the CHARGE association; however, unilateral lesions may be isolated abnormalities:

C	coloboma of the eye 70%
H	heart abnormalities 60–70%
A	choanal atresia 60–100%
R	retardation in growth and development:

intrauterine growth retardation 75%

failure to thrive 80%

learning disability (mental retardation) 70–80%

G genital hypoplasia 70% male, 30% female)

E ear malformations in 90–100%.

As neonates are obligate nasal breathers, bilateral choanal atresia leads to significant airway compromise, cyanosis and respiratory distress which is relieved by crying and requires emergency treatment. In contrast unilateral choanal atresia can often go undiagnosed for long periods. A few children can present with signs of respiratory distress at birth or develop OSA during infancy if the non-atretic side is also narrowed, others may present later with unilateral rhinorrhoea or congestion. Symptoms of OSA, failure to thrive or respiratory distress prompt early intervention.

Stabilisation in bilateral atresia requires an oropharyngeal airway; surgery is the definitive treatment but may be delayed in the presence of other significant abnormalities.

11.45–11.47 Theme: Respiratory diseases

11.45

Answer E: Pulmonary haemosiderosis

This is a rare disorder that typically has its onset before age 10 years. It is characterised by a triad of iron deficiency anaemia, haemoptysis (rare in children) and diffuse parenchymal infiltrates on chest radiograph secondary to repeated diffuse intra-alveolar bleeds. Most cases in childhood are idiopathic, but some are due to cows' milk protein hypersensitivity (Heiner syndrome) or secondary to systemic disease (cardiac, pneumonia and autoimmune disease, eg Goodpasture syndrome). BAL yields haemosiderin-laden macrophages secondary to diffuse pulmonary haemorrhage. The swallowing of this sputum results in positive faecal occult blood testing. Peripheral eosinophilia, chronic rhinitis, recurrent otitis media and failure to thrive are seen secondary to intolerance to cows' milk protein and symptoms improve on an elimination diet. In idiopathic cases the prognosis is more variable. Presentation can vary from insidious to fulminant course; chronic respiratory symptoms of cough, dyspnoea and tachypnoea are present in most cases; an acute haemorrhage, hypoxia and frank respiratory failure may occur later. Treatment is with iron replacement, steroids; additional immunosuppressive agents are occasionally required (eg azathioprine and cyclophosphamide, but the evidence base for this treatment is very limited). If left untreated, pulmonary fibrosis will develop and the condition can prove fatal with a mean survival post-diagnosis in idiopathic cases being as short as 5 years.

Note that α_1-anti-trypsin deficiency rarely presents with chest symptoms in infancy. Hepatosplenomegaly and jaundice may be presenting features in infancy but portal hypertension is rare in early childhood. GI bleeding is not a feature of α_1-anti-trypsin deficiency unless there is advanced liver disease leading to bleeding from oesophageal varices as a consequence of advanced portal hypertension.

11.46

Answer A: Bronchiolitis obliterans

Bronchiolitis obliterans is a rare pulmonary disorder that is characterised histologically by an inflammatory/fibrosing process that constricts and ultimately obliterates the small airways. In childhood cases of bronchiolitis obliterans, there is usually a preceding history of infection with adenovirus, measles, pertussis, influenza or *Mycoplasma* sp. It can also be related to connective tissue disease, malignancy and drugs, and can be part of graft-versus-host disease after bone marrow transplantation. Progressive symptoms of dyspnoea, cough, general malaise and weight loss are characteristic. Examination usually reveals the presence of inspiratory crepitations. Clubbing is unusual. Chest radiograph changes are variable and can range from normal appearances through to airspace consolidation with air bronchograms, to findings consistent with military TB. High-resolution CT provides a more sensitive assessment of disease pattern and severity. Pulmonary function tests are likely to reveal severe obstruction although a restrictive picture is sometimes seen.

Treatment with antibiotics is of no benefit. Some forms of bronchiolitis obliterans in adults respond well to corticosteroids, but this is seen less commonly in children. A trial of treatment with inhaled steroids is reasonable to rule out a diagnosis of asthma although sufficient dose must be given to ensure that lack of response is not due to inadequate dosage. Prognosis is variable but significant long-term morbidity is reported in 78–92% of cases.

11.47

Answer G: Lobar sequestration

This is a mass of non-functioning primitive pulmonary tissue, supplied by the systemic (not pulmonary) circulation and has no identifiable communication with the tracheobronchial tree. They are classified as either extrapulmonary (EPS) – which is completely enclosed in its own pleural sac and can be situated above, within or below the diaphragm – or intrapulmonary (IPS) which occurs within the visceral pleura of the normal lung. IPS accounts for 75% of sequestrations; 60% are in the left lower lobe and 38% are found in the right lower lobe, and 10% of these types of IPS are associated with other congenital abnormalities. IPS is the most common form and usually presents in late childhood or adolescence, but symptoms of recurrent pneumonia may start early in childhood; a chronic cough is common. Inadequate drainage leads to slow resolution of infections; enlargement of the cystic mass may cause compression of the normal lung tissue and compromise cardiorespiratory function.

EPS is commonly diagnosed in infancy with respiratory distress and chronic cough. It is four times more common in boys and can be associated with other abnormalities in 40–60% of patients, including diaphragmatic hernias, vertebral abnormalities and congenital heart defects; 95% are left sided.

Chest radiograph appearances vary depending on size, location and presence of infection. They may appear as a dense or cystic lesion, often in the lower lobes. Infection will increase the density and failure of resolution of an area of consolidation should lead to further investigations to confirm the diagnosis and provide anatomical and circulatory information, to facilitate treatment. In certain cases, embolisation of the feeding vessel can be curative. In other cases surgical resection is required. Some patients have large shunts through the sequestration and once it is removed there may be a striking improvement in cardiovascular status.

11. 48–11.50 Theme: Management of acute respiratory illness

11.48

Answer B: Nebulised adrenaline and supplementary oxygen

This child is unwell with evidence of upper airway obstruction and appears toxic. You are unable to obtain a clear history and given that the child has only recently arrived in the UK it is important to remember that she is unlikely to have been immunised against *Haemophilus influenza* type b. She is therefore at increased risk of epiglottitis. The immediate management must focus on maintaining a patent airway, which is obviously compromised. Therefore, nebulised adrenaline with oxygen should be given as a first-line treatment. Intravenous cefotaxime would also be required as part of the definitive management plan, but insertion of a cannula should be deferred in the short term until her airway is secured.

11.49

Answer E: Supplementary oxygen and nasogastric enteral feeds

This baby has a history and examination findings consistent with bronchiolitis, typically seen in the winter months. Although auscultation reveals wheeze, bronchodilators have not been proven to reduce admission rates or produce a clinically important improvement in oxygen saturations. Antibiotics are required only if secondary bacterial infection is suspected and there is no evidence of that in this case. Supportive treatment with supplementary oxygen, minimal handling and nasogastric feeds would be appropriate in the first instance.

11.50

Answer C: Oral azithromycin

This child has signs and symptoms suggestive of *Mycoplasma pneumoniae*, the second commonest cause of community-acquired pneumonia in the UK in children aged >5 years. Typically, in addition to the cough, you may elicit a history of malaise, headache, wheeze, arthralgia, myringitis, and abdominal pain, skin rash, nasal discharge and a sore throat. The treatment of choice is with a macrolide antibiotic such as erythromycin or azithromycin. His presentation is not of sufficient severity to request admission for intravenous antibiotics. If there is sufficient wheeze to require treatment with bronchodilators, a salbutamol inhaler and large volumatic spacer would be the most appropriate method of treatment, and it would be important to ensure that the child is instructed and tested on how to use the device before discharge.

Index

Entries are indexed by question number, not page number